Preoperative Medical Consultation

Guest Editors

LEE A. FLEISHER, MD
STANLEY H. ROSENBAUM, MD

MEDICAL CLINICS
OF NORTH AMERICA

www.medical.theclinics.com

September 2009 • Volume 93 • Number 5

SAUNDERS an imprint of ELSEVIER, Inc.

W.B. SAUNDERS COMPANY
A Division of Elsevier Inc.

1600 John F. Kennedy Boulevard ● Suite 1800 ● Philadelphia, Pennsylvania 19103-2899

http://www.theclinics.com

MEDICAL CLINICS OF NORTH AMERICA Volume 93, Number 5
September 2009 ISSN 0025-7125, ISBN-13: 978-1-4377-0501-0, ISBN-10: 1-4377-0501-4

Editor: Rachel Glover
Developmental Editor: Donald Mumford

Medical Clinics of North America (ISSN 0025-7125) is published bimonthly by Elsevier Inc., 360 Park Avenue South, New York, NY 10010-1710. Months of issue are January, March, May, July, September, and November. Periodicals postage paid at New York, NY, and additional mailing offices. Subscription prices are USD 187 per year for US individuals, USD 334 per year for US institutions, USD 96 per year for US students, USD 238 per year for Canadian individuals, USD 434 per year for Canadian institutions, USD 151 per year for Canadian students, USD 288 per year for international individuals, USD 434 per year for international institutions and USD 151 per year for international students. To receive student/resident rate, orders must be accompanied by name of affiliated institution, date of term, and the *signature* of program/residency coordinator on institution letterhead. Orders will be billed at individual rate until proof of status is received. Foreign air speed delivery is included in all *Clinics* subscription prices. All prices are subject to change without notice. **POSTMASTER:** Send address changes to *Medical Clinics of North America*, Elsevier Health Sciences Division, Subscription Customer Service, 3251 Riverport Lane, Maryland Heights, MO 63043. **Customer Service: Telephone: 1-800-654-2452** (U.S. and Canada); **1-314-447-8871** (outside U.S. and Canada). **Fax: 1-314-447-8029. E-mail: journalscustomerservice-usa@elsevier.com** (for print support); **journalsonlinesupport-usa@ elsevier.com** (for online support).

Reprints. For copies of 100 or more of articles in this publication, please contact the Commercial Reprints Department, Elsevier Inc., 360 Park Avenue South, New York, NY 10010-1710. Tel.: 212-633-3812; Fax: 212-462-1935; E-mail: reprints@elsevier.com.

Medical Clinics of North America is also published in Spanish by McGraw-Hill Interamericana Editores S. A., P.O. Box 5-237, 06500 Mexico, D.F., Mexico.

Medical Clinics of North America is covered in *MEDLINE/PubMed (Index Medicus), Current Contents, ASCA, Excerpta Medica, Science Citation Index, and ISI/BIOMED.*

Printed in the United States of America.

GOAL STATEMENT

The goal of *Medical Clinics of North America* is to keep practicing physicians up to date with current clinical practice by providing timely articles reviewing the state of the art in patient care.

ACCREDITATION

The *Medical Clinics of North America* is planned and implemented in accordance with the Essential Areas and Policies of the Accreditation Council for Continuing Medical Education (ACCME) through the joint sponsorship of the University of Virginia School of Medicine and Elsevier. The University of Virginia School of Medicine is accredited by the ACCME to provide continuing medical education for physicians.

The University of Virginia School of Medicine designates this educational activity for a maximum of 15 *AMA PRA Category 1 Credits*™ for each issue, 90 credits per year. Physicians should only claim credit commensurate with the extent of their participation in the activity.

The American Medical Association has determined that physicians not licensed in the US who participate in this CME activity are eligible for a maximum of 15 *AMA PRA Category 1 Credits*™ for each issue, 90 credits per year.

Credit can be earned by reading the text material, taking the CME examination online at http://www.theclinics. com/home/cme, and completing the evaluation. After taking the test, you will be required to review any and all incorrect answers. Following completion of the test and evaluation, your credit will be awarded and you may print your certificate.

FACULTY DISCLOSURE/CONFLICT OF INTEREST

The University of Virginia School of Medicine, as an ACCME accredited provider, endorses and strives to comply with the Accreditation Council for Continuing Medical Education (ACCME) Standards of Commercial Support, Commonwealth of Virginia statutes, University of Virginia policies and procedures, and associated federal and private regulations and guidelines on the need for disclosure and monitoring of proprietary and financial interests that may affect the scientific integrity and balance of content delivered in continuing medical education activities under our auspices.

The University of Virginia School of Medicine requires that all CME activities accredited through this institution be developed independently and be scientifically rigorous, balanced and objective in the presentation/discussion of its content, theories and practices.

All authors/editors participating in an accredited CME activity are expected to disclose to the readers relevant financial relationships with commercial entities occurring within the past 12 months (such as grants or research support, employee, consultant, stock holder, member of speakers bureau, etc.). The University of Virginia School of Medicine will employ appropriate mechanisms to resolve potential conflicts of interest to maintain the standards of fair and balanced education to the reader. Questions about specific strategies can be directed to the Office of Continuing Medical Education, University of Virginia School of Medicine, Charlottesville, Virginia.

The faculty and staff of the University of Virginia Office of Continuing Medical Education have no financial affiliations to disclose.

The authors/editors listed below have identified no professional or financial affiliations for themselves or their spouse/partner:
Jeffrey L. Carson, MD; Charles D. Collard, MD; Kimberly A. Davis, MD, FACS; Lee A. Fleisher, MD (Guest Editor); Rachel Glover (Acquisitions Editor); Dean R. Jones, MD, FRCPC; Vijay P. Khatri, MBChB, FACS; Benjamin A. Kohl, MD; H.T. Lee, MD, PhD; Phillip D. Levin, MB, BChir; Marek Mirski, MD, PhD; Diego J. Muilenburg, MD; Alexander Papangelou, MD; Manish S. Patel, MD; Stanley H. Rosenbaum, MD (Guest Editor); Adam Schiavi, MD, PhD; Kevin M. Schuster, MD; Amrik Singh, MD; Gerald W. Smetana, MD; Bobbie Jean Sweitzer, MD; Guido Torzilli, MD; Alec D. Weisberg, MD; Emily L. Weisberg, MD; Charles Weissman, MD; James M. Wilson, MD; and, Andrew Wolf, MD (Test Author).

The authors/editors listed below identified the following professional or financial affiliations for themselves or their spouse/partner:
Daniel J. Brotman, MD is an industry funded research/investigator for Siemens Diagnostics, a consultant for Quantia Communications, and serves on the Advisory Committee/Board for Cubist Pharmaceuticals and Otsuka Pharmaceuticals.
James B. Froehlich, MD, MPH serves on the Speakers Bureau for Merck/Schering-Plough, Pfizer, and Sanofi-Aventis, is a consultant for Pfizer and Sanofi-Aventis Blue, and is an industry funded research/investigator for Blue Cross/Blue Shield of Michigan.
Paul J. Grant, MD serves on the Advisory Committee/Board for Merck.
Amir K. Jaffer, MD is a consultant for Sanofi-Aventis and Astra Zeneca, and serves on the Speakers Bureau for Astra Zeneca.
Stanley Schwartz, MD serves on the Speakers Bureau and Advisory Committee/Board for Lilly, Takeda, and Amylin, serves on the Speakers Bureau for Sanofi-Aventis and Merck, and serves on the Advisory Committee/Board for Novo and CVT/Gilead.
David G. Silverman, MD is the owner of a pending patent for aspects of the scoring system cited in his article.

Disclosure of Discussion of Non-FDA Approved Uses for Pharmaceutical Products and/or Medical Devices.

The University of Virginia School of Medicine, as an ACCME provider, requires that all faculty presenters identify and disclose any off-label uses for pharmaceutical and medical device products. The University of Virginia School of Medicine recommends that each physician fully review all the available data on new products or procedures prior to clinical use.

TO ENROLL

To enroll in the Medical Clinics of North America Continuing Medical Education program, call customer service at 1-800-654-2452 or visit us online at http://www.theclinics.com/home/cme. The CME program is available to subscribers for an additional fee of USD 205.

THE CLINICS ARE NOW AVAILABLE ONLINE!

Access your subscription at:
www.theclinics.com

Contributors

GUEST EDITORS

LEE A. FLEISHER, MD
University of Pennsylvania Health System, University of Pennsylvania School of Medicine, Department of Anesthesiology and Critical Care Medicine, Philadelphia, Pennsylvania

STANLEY H. ROSENBAUM, MD
Professor of Anesthesiology, Internal Medicine and Surgery, and Vice-Chair, Department of Anesthesiology, Yale University School of Medicine, Yale-New Haven Hospital, New Haven, Connecticut

AUTHORS

DANIEL J. BROTMAN, MD
Associate Professor of Medicine; and Director, Hospitalist Program, Department of Medicine, Johns Hopkins University, Baltimore, Maryland

JEFFREY L. CARSON, MD
Richard C. Reynolds Professor of Medicine; and Chief, Division of General Internal Medicine, Department of Medicine, University of Medicine and Dentistry of New Jersey Robert Wood Johnson Medical School, New Brunswick, New Jersey

CHARLES D. COLLARD, MD
Professor and Vice Chair, Baylor College of Medicine Department of Anesthesiology; and Chief, Division of Cardiovascular Anesthesiology at the Texas Heart Institute, St. Luke's Episcopal Hospital, Houston, Texas

KIMBERLY A. DAVIS, MD, FACS
Associate Professor and Vice Chair of Clinical Affairs, Department of Surgery; and Chief, Section of Trauma, Surgical Critical Care, and Surgical Emergencies, Yale University, School of Medicine, New Haven, Connecticut

LEE A. FLEISHER, MD
University of Pennsylvania Health System, University of Pennsylvania School of Medicine, Department of Anesthesiology and Critical Care Medicine, Philadelphia, Pennsylvania

JAMES B. FROEHLICH, MD, MPH
Director, Vascular Medicine; and Associate Professor of Medicine, Department of Medicine, CVC Cardiovascular Medicine, University of Michigan Medical School, Ann Arbor, Michigan

PAUL J. GRANT, MD
Clinical Instructor, Division of General Medicine, Department of Internal Medicine, University of Michigan Medical School, Ann Arbor, Michigan

AMIR K. JAFFER, MD
Associate Professor of Medicine and Chief, Medicine Service, Division of Hospital Medicine, Department of Medicine, University of Miami Miller School of Medicine, Miami, Florida

DEAN R. JONES, MD, FRCPC
Assistant Professor, Department of Anesthesiology, Columbia University, New York, New York

VIJAY P. KHATRI, MBChB, FACS
Professor of Surgery, Department of Surgery; and Professor of Surgery, Division of Surgical Oncology, University of California, Davis School of Medicine, Sacramento, California

BENJAMIN A. KOHL, MD
Assistant Professor, Department of Anesthesiology and Critical Care, University of Pennsylvania School of Medicine, Philadelphia, Pennsylvania

H.T. LEE, MD, PhD
Associate Professor, Department of Anesthesiology, Anesthesiology Research Laboratories, Columbia University, New York, New York

PHILLIP D. LEVIN, MB, BChir
Senior Anesthesiologist and Lecturer in Anesthesiology, Department of Anesthesiology and Critical Care Medicine, Hadassah-Hebrew University Medical Center, Hebrew University-Hadassah School of Medicine, Kiryat Hadassah, Jerusalem, Israel

MAREK MIRSKI, MD, PhD
Vice Chair and Professor, Department of Anesthesiology and Critical Care Medicine, Neurology, Neurosurgery; Executive Director, Neurosciences Critical Care Division; and Chief, Division of Neuroanesthesiology, Johns Hopkins Medical Institutions, Baltimore, Maryland

DIEGO J. MUILENBURG, MD
Surgical Resident, Department of Surgery, University of California-Davis, Sacramento, California

ALEXANDER PAPANGELOU, MD
Assistant Professor, Division of Neuroanesthesia and Neurosciences Critical Care Medicine, Department of Anesthesiology and Critical Care Medicine, Johns Hopkins Medical Institutions, Baltimore, Maryland

MANISH S. PATEL, MD
Assistant Professor of Medicine, Department of Medicine, Division of General Internal Medicine, University of Medicine and Dentistry of New Jersey Robert Wood Johnson Medical School, New Brunswick, New Jersey

STANLEY H. ROSENBAUM, MD
Professor of Anesthesiology, Internal Medicine and Surgery; and Vice-Chair, Department of Anesthesiology, Yale University School of Medicine, Yale-New Haven Hospital, New Haven, Connecticut

ADAM SCHIAVI, MD, PhD
Assistant Professor, Division of Neuroanesthesia and Neurosciences Critical Care Medicine, Department of Anesthesiology and Critical Care Medicine, Johns Hopkins Medical Institutions, Baltimore, Maryland

KEVIN M. SCHUSTER, MD
Assistant Professor, Department of Surgery, Section of Trauma, Surgical Critical Care, and Surgical Emergencies, Yale University, School of Medicine, New Haven, Connecticut

STANLEY SCHWARTZ, MD
Clinical Associate Professor; and Director of Diabetes Disease Management, Department of Medicine, University of Pennsylvania Health System, Philadelphia Heart Institute, Philadelphia, Pennsylvania

DAVID G. SILVERMAN, MD
Medical Director of Pre-Admission Testing Center; and Professor, Department of Anesthesiology, Yale University School of Medicine, Yale-New Haven Hospital, New Haven, Connecticut

AMRIK SINGH, MD
Associate Professor, Department of Anesthesia and Pain Medicine, University of California Davis Medical Center, Sacramento, California

GERALD W. SMETANA, MD
Associate Professor of Medicine, Harvard Medical School; and Division of General Medicine and Primary Care, Beth Israel Deaconess Medical Center, Boston, Massachusetts

BOBBIE JEAN SWEITZER, MD
Associate Professor, Department of Anesthesia and Critical Care; Associate Professor of Medicine, University of Chicago; and Director, Anesthesia Perioperative Medicine Clinic, University of Chicago Medical Center, Chicago, Illinois

GUIDO TORZILLI, MD
Professor of Surgey, Third Department of Surgery, University of Milan, School of Medicine, IRCCS Istituto Clinico Humanitas, Rozzano, Milan, Italy

ALEC D. WEISBERG, MD
Fellow, Section of Cardiology, Department of Medicine, Baylor College of Medicine; and Texas Heart Institute, St. Luke's Episcopal Hospital, Houston, Texas

EMILY L. WEISBERG, MD
Resident, Department of Anesthesiology, Baylor College of Medicine, Houston, Texas

CHARLES WEISSMAN, MD
Chair and Professor of Anesthesiology, Department of Anesthesiology and Critical Care Medicine, Hadassah-Hebrew University Medical Center, Hebrew University-Hadassah School of Medicine, Kiryat Hadassah, Jerusalem, Israel

JAMES M. WILSON, MD
Associate Professor, Section of Cardiology, Department of Medicine, Baylor College of Medicine; and Robert Hall Chair of Cardiology, Texas Heart Institute, St. Luke's Episcopal Hospital, Houston, Texas

Contents

Assessment of the presurgical patient requires interdisciplinary cooperation over the continuum of documentation and optimization of existing disorders, determination of patient resilience and reserve, and planning for subsequent interventions and care. For many patients, evident or suspected morbidities or anticipated surgical disturbance warrant specialty consultation. There may be uncertainty as to the optimal processes for a given patient, a limitation attributable to myriad factors, not the least of which is that there is often a paucity of evidence that is directly relevant to a given patient in a given setting. The present article discusses these limitations and describes a framework for documentation, optimization, risk assessment, and planning, as well as a uniform grading of existing morbidities and anticipated perioperative disturbances for patients requiring integrated assessment and consultation.

Cardiac surgery is associated with significant morbidity, mortality, and socioeconomic costs. Preoperative assessment assists the clinician in identifying potential complications and facilitates discussion of these risks with the patient. Careful patient selection and preparation during preoperative evaluation may minimize morbidity, mortality, and resource use. This article outlines a system-based approach to preoperative evaluation and preparation of the patient undergoing cardiac surgery.

Clinicians are increasingly asked what they can do to evaluate and lower the risk of perioperative cardiac complications. Approximately 4 decades ago, there were few tools to guide the evaluation of perioperative risk. The American Society of Anesthesiology Classification System (ASA class) gave only a vague idea of the risk patients faced during surgery, but the modern era of clinical risk assessment for perioperative complications has seen the introduction of tools that allow clinicians to estimate risk, and also the addition of stress testing for assessing perioperative risk. None of these tests, however, were designed to identify perioperative cardiac risk. This article reviews the literature on perioperative risk assessment, risk reduction, and testing modalities in patients with cardiac disease, along with the role of perioperative angioplasty and the current American College of Cardiology/American Heart Association guidelines.

Bobbie Jean Sweitzer and Gerald W. Smetana

Preoperative pulmonary evaluation and optimization improves postoperative patient outcomes. Clinicians frequently evaluate patients with pulmonary disease before surgery who are at increased risk for pulmonary and nonpulmonary perioperative complications. Postoperative pulmonary complications are as common and costly as cardiac complications. In this article, the evaluation of patients with the most common conditions encountered in the preoperative setting, including unexplained dyspnea, asthma, chronic obstructive pulmonary disease, obstructive sleep apnea, and cigarette use, are discussed. Risk stratification for postoperative pulmonary complications and strategies to reduce them for high-risk patients are also discussed. From the available literature, high-risk patients and those patients for whom a multidisciplinary collaboration will be most helpful can be accurately identified.

Benjamin A. Kohl and Stanley Schwartz

Patients with preoperative endocrinopathies represent a particular challenge not only to anesthesiologists but also to surgeons and perioperative clinicians. The "endocrine axis" is complex and has multiple feedback loops, some of which are endocrine and paracrine related, and others that are strongly influenced by the surgical stress response. Familiarity with several of the common endocrinopathies facilitates management in the perioperative period. This article focuses on 4 of the most common endocrinopathies: diabetes mellitus, hyperthyroidism, hypothyroidism, and adrenal insufficiency. Perioperative challenges in patients presenting with pheochromocytoma are also discussed.

Phillip D. Levin and Charles Weissman

Contemporary life, with its sedentary lifestyles, fast foods, processed foodstuff, and desk-bound service employment, is beset by an epidemic of overweight and obese individuals. The World Health Organization reported that worldwide a billion adults are overweight and at least 30% of them are obese. Moreover, increasing numbers of children are obese. In the United States, 2 National Health and Nutrition Examination Surveys of adults aged 20 to 74 years showed that the prevalence of obesity increased from 15% in the 1976 to 1980 survey to 34% in the 2003 to 2004 survey. Obesity and the metabolic syndrome are unfortunately becoming increasingly common perioperative issues. The ultimate aim of caring for such patients is to find ways to minimize the untoward effects of surgery in patients who are obese or have metabolic syndrome.

Liver dysfunction is a prominent entity in Western medicine that has historically affected patients suffering from chronic viral or alcoholic hepatitis. The incidence of these conditions has not changed dramatically in recent years but the overall number of patients with liver dysfunction has increased considerably with the emergence of the obesity epidemic. Nonalcoholic fatty liver disease (NAFLD) has become increasingly recognized as the most common cause of chronic liver disease in the United States. Although the rate of progression of NAFLD to overt cirrhosis is low, the high prevalence of this condition, combined with the moderate degree of liver dysfunction it engenders, has resulted in a significant increase in the number of patients with liver disease that can be encountered by a surgical practice. Any degree of clinically evident liver disease in a prospective surgical patient should raise concern for the entire surgical team. This particularly applies to intraabdominal surgery whereby the presence of hepatomegaly, portal hypertension, variceal bleeding, and ascites can turn even the most routine operation into a morbid and life-threatening procedure. Nonabdominal surgery avoids some of the technical challenges presented by liver disease but the anesthetic management of a cirrhotic patient still makes any operation potentially more dangerous. In this article, approaches to minimize the risk when surgery becomes necessary in the presence of liver disease are discussed.

Preoperative evaluation of patients with renal dysfunction often requires the collaborative efforts of the primary care physician, nephrologist, surgeon, and anesthesiologist. Renal dysfunction is typically a spectrum of disease with multisystem effects. Optimization of preexisting medical issues is the key as is a thorough understanding of the potential perioperative risks for further renal injury. Surgical or anesthetic techniques may require alteration for the patient with significant renal dysfunction. Identification of those at risk for renal injury may allow for preventative therapies in the perioperative period. This article focuses on defining the population at risk, a framework for preoperative evaluation, and developments in the area of perioperative renal protection.

Anemia is commonly encountered in the preoperative patient. Determination of the cause of the anemia can affect perioperative surgical and medical management and outcome. Red blood cell transfusions are often administered during the perioperative time period in patients with preoperative anemia, although evidence to support the optimal transfusion threshold is limited. The authors review the evaluation of anemia and evidence regarding perioperative blood transfusions. Recommendations on the treatment of anemia, including perioperative blood transfusions, are outlined.

Preface

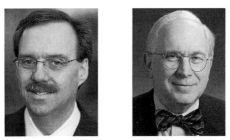

Lee A. Fleisher, MD   Stanley H. Rosenbaum, MD
Guest Editors

The knowledge of mountain climbers and the variety of equipment that they use have greatly increased in the past few decades, as climbing gear, communication devices, and navigation tools have all improved. Yet we still read in the media of mountaineering accidents. Clearly, as mountain climbing has become technically easier, more and more people have been climbing up steeper and more difficult mountains. Similarly, in modern surgical care, we have seen knowledge and technology get better as we go yet more aggressively up the "steepest mountains." It is our hope in this issue to address the many aspects of the medical care and preparation of patients, so that when they face surgery, the groundwork will be ideal and the approach (and descent), the least arduous.

Perioperative patient care involves, in essence, the arrival of a medical patient, the preoperative preparation by the medical, anesthesia, and surgical teams, the care during surgery by the anesthesiologist and surgeon, and then the full input of all the teams after surgery. All this then leads back to what is likely to be the long-term care by the medical team alone. The process often entails a detailed assessment of multiple medical and surgical diagnoses, the optimization of ongoing disease processes, a determination of the risk and even reasonableness of the planned surgery, and then the planning and performance of the intraoperative and postsurgical procedures and therapies.

We have addressed many of the aspects of the preoperative care of patients in invited articles, all of which include authors from multiple specialties, including internists or medical specialists, anesthesiologists, and surgeons. In the perioperative period, the input and perspectives of all 3 members of the perioperative team are essential in ensuring optimal safety. We are fortunate to have an outstanding group of authors from a diverse group of institutions, who provided unique insights. We

Med Clin N Am 93 (2009) xiii–xiv
doi:10.1016/j.mcna.2009.06.001
0025-7125/09/$ – see front matter   **medical.theclinics.com**

hope that our readers will find the many specialized discussions helpful, and that this will make the mountain of problems faced by our patients heading into surgery more readily conquered.

Lee A. Fleisher, MD
University of Pennsylvania Health System
University of Pennsylvania School of Medicine
Department of Anesthesiology and Critical Care Medicine
3400 Spruce Street, 6 Dulles
Philadelphia, PA 19104, USA

Stanley H. Rosenbaum, MD
Yale University School of Medicine
New Haven, CT 06510, USA

E-mail address:
Lee.fleisher@uphs.upenn.edu (L.A. Fleisher)

Integrated Assessment and Consultation for the Preoperative Patient

David G. Silverman, MD[a,*], Stanley H. Rosenbaum, MD[b]

KEYWORDS

- Preoperative consultation • Preoperative laboratory testing
- Preoperative guidelines • Preoperative comorbidities
- Preoperative physical status

The goal of perioperative medicine is to enable a patient to undergo a required or desired surgical intervention with minimal exacerbation of existing disorders, avoidance of new morbidities, and subsequent prompt recovery from the surgical procedure. Preoperative accrual of information to establish a risk profile and the associated planning are vital foundations of this continuum, with varying degrees of input from the surgeon, anesthesiologist, primary care provider, and medical specialists during the different phases. A specialist may be consulted to "provide a clinical risk profile" and make "recommendations concerning diagnosis and medical management."[1]

For uncomplicated cases, the preoperative assessment by the surgeon and assessment by the anesthesiologist on the day of surgery are typically sufficient as long as regulatory requirements for general and surgically focused history and physical examinations are met. However, for many patients, more extensive evaluation is required. Regardless, there is often reliance on the old-style surgical tradition of having a primary care physician or medical specialist provide preoperative clearance. This procedure could simply entail transfer of an updated history and physical examination on what the Center for Medicare and Medicaid Services (CMS) refers to as an established patient, with the annotation "cleared for surgery." In many cases, one-time transfer of information to the patient's acute care providers (surgeon, anesthesiologist, and perhaps a hospitalist) constitutes the foundation of preoperative assessment; and

Dr. David Silverman has a pending patent for aspects of the scoring system cited in this article.

[a] Department of Anesthesiology, Yale University School of Medicine, Yale-New Haven Hospital, TMP-3, 333 Cedar Street, New Haven, CT 06510, USA

[b] Department of Anesthesiology, Yale University School of Medicine, Yale-New Haven Hospital, 789 Howard Avenue, PO Box 208051, New haven, CT 06520, USA

* Corresponding author.

E-mail address: david.silverman@yale.edu (D.G. Silverman).

there is little expectation that additional testing, specialty consultation or preparative intervention is required. Schein and colleagues[2] randomized patients scheduled for cataract surgery into preoperative testing and no preoperative testing groups; the latter received no additional testing beyond the routine care delivered by their primary care provider unless the history and physical examination revealed that a test was indicated even if surgery had not been planned. They concluded that, for a minimally invasive procedure such as cataract surgery, additional routine testing had no effect aside from markedly increasing costs.[2] The process is more complex for the patient who has not received regular medical care; if the surgeon or anesthesiologist does not assume responsibility for the general history, physical status, and adherence to mandates by oversight agencies, then referral to a primary care provider may be indicated not only for the acute challenge but also for the patient's overall health.

In other settings, evident suspected morbidities or the anticipated physiologic disruption by surgery warrant additional input, including specialty consultation and integrated expertise to determine what information is needed and how best to apply the findings. However, there is often uncertainty as to the optimal processes in a given patient, with the potential for inadequate workups and inadequate communication, and, hence, suboptimal care. Who should obtain, interpret, and act on needed information? How and when should it be obtained? Is it safe to proceed with surgery? Accompanying questions include: when should the patient's primary care physician be consulted for expanded preoperative assessment? When is consultation with a medical specialist indicated? And, under what circumstances should the patient see an anesthesiologist before the day of surgery? The logistical problems were illustrated by a survey of physicians in Veterans Administration hospitals: although cardiologists were more comfortable starting with β-blockers than were anesthesiologists or surgeons, they felt that β-blockers were best started in a preoperative clinic, which is usually run by anesthesiologists.[3]

CMS policies impose some order to the process by establishing guidelines for billing; but they do not guide patient care. According to the online CMS Medicare Claims Processing Manual, "a consultation service is distinguished from other evaluation and management visits because it is provided by a physician or qualified nonphysician practitioner (NPP) whose opinion or advice regarding evaluation and/ or management of a specific problem is requested by another physician or other appropriate source ... because that individual has expertise in a specific medical area beyond the requesting professional's knowledge." In order for the visit to be billed as a consultation, "A request for a consultation from an appropriate source and the need for consultation shall be documented by the consultant in the patient's medical record and included in the requesting physician or qualified NPP's plan of care [written report] in the patient's medical record." The CMS manual adds that "A physician or qualified NPP consultant may initiate diagnostic services and treatment at the initial consultation service or subsequent visit. Ongoing management, following the initial consultation service by the consultant physician, shall not be reported with consultation service codes." Specifically with respect to preoperative consultations, CMS states "Preoperative consultations are payable for new or established patients [already under the requested consultant's care] performed by any physician or qualified NPP at the request of a surgeon, as long as all of the requirements for performing and reporting the consultation codes are met and the service is medically necessary and not routine screening."[4] Hence, the importance of providing detailed documentation.

The need for specialty consultation, as well as the potential for lack of consensus even after such consultation is obtained, is attributable to several factors, not the least of which is that there is a paucity of evidence-based guidelines that are directly relevant to a given patient in a given setting. Despite having statistical power for predicting outcomes in groups of patients and providing justification for expanded evaluation,[5–8] validated risk indices do not define how best to assess and treat on a per patient basis. The indices rely on fixed variables that do not necessarily capture the nature, severity, and acuity of the specific morbidities in the individual patient. To further complicate matters, different indices do not necessarily agree as to which variables should be taken into account; and those that rely on administrative databases (eg, International Classification of Diseases [ICD] codes) may not have reliably captured critical variables.[9,10]

The need to use caution when applying indices to individual patients has been expressed by leading authorities. In their review of risk factors for pulmonary complications, Smetana and colleagues[11] noted that prescreening methods and variable selection algorithms of the different studies often limited reporting to risk factors that were determined as statistically significant in a given sample. Such limitations may have contributed to their identifying only one eligible study that evaluated the value of self-reported exercise capacity or complication risk among patients with HIV infection.[11]

In their recommendations for predicting cardiac complications, Detsky and colleagues[8] stated that the limitations of their index, as well as of the Goldman index[7] they were seeking to modify, were attributable, at least in part, to failure to capture all relevant variables in many of their patients. They cited the potential for "omission of variables that reflect the severity of coronary artery disease such as angina pectoris" and "selection of limited variables to identify a problem – eg, a third heart sound or jugular venous distention to reflect LV dysfunction." They noted that reliance of dichotomous variables was further complicated by poor agreement among observers: Kappa statistics were only 0.42, 0.50, and 0.34 for the finding of an S3, jugular venous distension or important aortic stenosis (in the absence of echocardiography). They also pointed out that calculated risk estimates "should not be applied directly in the face of clinical information that is not adequately considered by the index, but which clearly changes the patient's risk (eg, myocardial infarction with ventricular fibrillation two days before planned surgery)" and that the ideal index should include the extent to which the risk factors are reversible, "indicating that the patient may benefit from delay of surgery with some therapeutic adjustments."[8]

Lee and colleagues, in their introduction of the Revised Cardiac Risk Index, also noted the challenges encountered by investigators seeking to derive and validate risk indices.[6] They stated that "The form and content of the Revised Cardiac Risk Index reflect the goal of this investigation: to derive a simple index that might influence and be readily incorporated into routine practice (eg, on forms for preoperative evaluations). We therefore emphasized in the analyses dichotomous variables that were either present or absent and used a scoring system that assigned one point to each variable. A more complex index might have achieved greater accuracy but at the expense of ease of use."[6]

The aforementioned factors have led to the potential for differing recommendations among diagnostic and treatment algorithms. Functional capacity, an essential factor in the American College of Cardiology (ACC)/American Heart Association (AHA) Guidelines,[1,12] which are based largely on the Revised Cardiac Risk Index of Lee and colleagues,[6] was not considered to be significant in the risk index published by Detsky and colleagues.[8] Whereas the 2002 update of the ACC/AHA Guidelines included advanced age, an abnormal ECG, rhythm other than sinus, and uncontrolled hypertension among its potentially significant factors,[1] these were not included in their 2007 algorithm revision;[12] and cerebrovascular disease was promoted from minor risk factor in 2002 to one of only five clinical risk factors in 2007. Citing the potential for inconsistencies, Lee and colleagues commented that their finding that several previously identified risk factors did not correlate with complications in their study "may reflect patient selection and increased attention to these issues (at their institution)." They emphasized that "the absence of these factors from the Revised Cardiac Risk Index should not be taken as evidence that they are not worrisome prognostic factors."[6]

Perhaps most disturbing is the realization that the evidence on which guidelines, advisories, and mandates are based and on which case-by-case decisions are made may be flawed. Hence, in addition to the lack of evidence-based regimens that specifically address the vast majority of interacting stresses and morbidities, there is often a lack of confidence in the reports that led to the proposed guidelines. Ioannidis reported that 32% of the initial reports of therapeutic efficacy in major impact journals were contraindicated or found to have effects that were stronger than those of subsequent studies.[13] In their recent cohort of high-quality systematic reviews directly relevant to clinical practice, Shojania and colleagues[14] found that the median survival of those reviews was 5.5 years and that signals for updating occurred within 2 years for 23% of reviews, within 1 year for 15%, and before publication for 7%. In addition to new evidence with respect to efficacy, there is the potential for new evidence with respect to adverse effects; the latter may have been missed (perhaps not sufficiently looked for) in the original landmark reports or been overshadowed by the findings pertaining to the primary objective. This potential for what may be referred to as *evidence-biased* medicine (albeit more likely innocent than deliberate), has impacted on guidelines and the willingness of clinicians to adhere to them in many settings. Furthermore, Sniderman and Furberg recently suggested that the guideline process itself needs reform. They argue that the need for judgments to fill in the gaps in the evidence, the potential for diverse opinions (which are not reflected in the published guidelines), the potential for conflict of interest and the lack of peer review should make us question whether guidelines deserve their anchoring authority.[15]

Even without several of the aforementioned limitations, the concerns expressed by Tinetti and colleagues[16] and McAlister and colleagues[17] about the inappropriate extension of guidelines derived from evidence-based medicine to settings in which the evidence does not apply may be disturbingly relevant to the patient scheduled for surgery. Not only is there a wide range of potential morbidities and multiple potential ways to treat them, there is also a wide range of interacting surgically induced disturbances and multiple potential ways to ameliorate them. Misperceptions, miscommunications, and adherence to specialty dogma or one's favorite indices, advisories, or guidelines may cause failure to focus on conditions affecting the given patient undergoing the given surgery, failure to avert potential conflicts between long-term therapies and perioperative requirements, and failure to identify and address operating room (OR)–specific risks and requirements. Hence, unless you are the physician performing the plan (and, perhaps, even if you are the physician performing the plan), it is unwise to dictate future interventions and therapies in the context of such a complex of interacting and potentially changing variables. Advice as to when not to follow a given guideline may be as valuable as advice as to when to do so.

Perioperative β-blocker therapy is a case in point. According to Akhtar and colleagues,[18] "concern over the side effects and possible drug interaction" may have been responsible for their finding that, even after published ACC/AHA recommendations for β-blocker use, only 48% of patients at their tertiary care center were receiving β-blockers at the time of their preanesthetic assessment and that only 22% of these reached the recommended lowering of heart rate to 60 beats/min.[18]

Citing Tinetti and colleagues,[16] they added that "Although one of the valid aims of developing clinical guidelines is to reduce practice variation, one should be mindful of the potential pitfalls of disease-specific guidelines when applied to patients with multiple medical problems. ... Because 20% of Medicare beneficiaries have 5 or more chronic conditions[19] and 50% are receiving five or more medications,[20] the potential for adverse drugs interactions is significant." More recent evidence as to the higher incidence of strokes and other noncardiac complications suggests that such concerns by clinicians (consultants as well as surgeons, anesthesiologists, and primary care providers) may have been justified.[21,22]

As discussed above, there clearly is the potential for a lack of confidence in established indices and guidelines, and in those who cite them. The art and science of successful decision making and consultant recommendation entails not only the application of indices, advisories, and guidelines but also documented determinations as to when to modify them or even abandon them. The shortcomings may strain relationships among the different specialties and predispose to discrepancies that may provide harmful medicolegal fodder. A recent survey noted that only 17% of anesthesiologists felt obligated to follow a cardiologist's suggestions; "recommendations regarding intraoperative monitoring or medications were largely ignored."[23] Conversely, compliance with the anesthesiologist's recommendations may also be low. It was reported that 45% of the recommendations by anesthesiologists at a major medical center for preoperative assessments or interventions were ignored.[24] Whether it is due to an imprecise question to the consultant, an inadequate answer, an insufficient response to recommendations, or simply a lack of reliable and applicable evidence, failure to integrate expertise may constitute the most egregious failure of the preoperative process.

This article relates the structure that the authors deem critical to appropriate assessment and planning in a given patient and a method to standardize its accrual and integration. A fluid four-phase process for generating and applying a preoperative risk profile (with the acronym DORP for *documentation, optimization, risk assessment,* and *planning*) is described; then a means for consistently scoring the components of this profile[25] (that facilitates tabulating them in an integrated current disorders and anticipated disturbances matrix) is proposed. This matrix, in turn, may be used to document the basis for extended testing, consultation, and therapeutic interventions. Detailed descriptions of the consultative assessments and recommendations by different medical specialists are provided in the disorder-focused articles elsewhere in this issue.

PHASES OF PREOPERATIVE ASSESSMENT
Documentation and Optimization

Essential components of long-term care, *documentation* of existing conditions and their *optimization* constitute the first two phases of preoperative assessment.

Documentation is initiated by identification of the need for surgery, with the assessment of the surgical condition's current impact, determination of the urgency for surgical intervention, and anticipation of the consequences if the planned procedure is postponed or canceled. The phase then focuses on accumulating and updating information about evident comorbidities and searching for likely disorders. This simply may mean gathering the information that has already been obtained on an established patient by his/her general internist and specialist(s); or it may include updating such information as one might do at a regularly scheduled visit of an established patient or during a visit for a new problem by such a patient. Alternatively, it may require more extensive evaluation of what may be called a re-established patient (returning after not being seen for ≥ 5 years) or of a new patient. Consistent with evaluation and re-evaluation in nonsurgical settings, findings during *documentation* may identify the need for additional testing, consultation, or optimization, regardless of the upcoming surgery.

Until recently, it was not uncommon to consider an extensive unstructured battery of tests (regardless of underlying disease or planned surgery) as a foundation of preoperative testing. However, the recent literature is replete with reports documenting that extensive routine testing is not justifiable either medically or financially.[2,26–30] An excessively aggressive search for preoperative diagnoses is time consuming and costly. It may also produce problems if false positive results mislead the team into fruitless, risky, and unwarranted additional assessments. The more tests that are ordered, the greater the likelihood of an abnormal result (outside the range that encompasses 95% of normal patients). Assuming that results of tests are independent of each other, "for 20 tests, the chance that all will be normal is only 36%."[26]

Hence, many hospitals have replaced unbridled testing with more restrictive guidelines whereby basic testing is based on age-based prevalence of disorders in essentially healthy patients. Minimum testing for a patient scheduled for surgery under the care of an anesthesiologist may include an electrocardiogram for all patients greater than 50 years of age and complete blood count (CBC), electrolytes, blood urea nitrogen (BUN), creatinine, and glucose levels for all patients more than 70 years. Such testing typically would be consistent with testing during long-term management by a patient's primary care physician and thus compatible with the aforementioned recommendation by Schein and colleagues[2] to eliminate routine ordering of tests before minimally invasive surgery. However, if recent measurements are not available, then obtaining them before surgery not only can discover disorders with high prevalence but also establish baseline values so that an abnormality will not be either inappropriately dismissed as being old or falsely categorized as being new (ie, as being attributable to surgery). The age limitations may be modified by risk factors, even in the absence of evident disease. For example, the age requirement for an electrocardiogram may be lowered or completely outweighed by risk factors such as smoking or a history of cocaine use.

Focused testing based on suspected or evident morbidities is less well defined. For patients currently under medical care, it is likely that documented conditions have been assessed with relevant testing. Otherwise, simply identifying a disorder does not dictate testing: disorders may be multifaceted, with a wide range of severity and acuity; and there often are multiple means of assessing the extent of disease and dysfunction. According to the American Society of Anesthesiologists (ASA) Advisory on Preoperative Assessment, "there is insufficient evidence to identify explicit decision parameters or rules for ordering preoperative tests on the basis of specific patient factors."[31] Hence, the needs for evaluations typically are determined on an ad hoc basis as the patient's risk profile is established. Focused testing also may include guidelines for testing based on the anticipated surgically induced disturbance. These indications for testing are addressed with respect to a subsequent phase of the preoperative process (see later discussion).

Optimization involves the necessary treatment of conditions identified during *documentation*. Although the assessment and treatment of these conditions may be accelerated by the upcoming surgery, for the most part these efforts should be directed at improvements that the patient's primary care physician or specialist(s) anticipate would be beneficial during daily life, regardless of impending surgery. Examples include: bronchospasm that may benefit from bronchodilator therapy (eg, daily inhalers); hyperglycemia that merits treatment of diabetes; hypertension that requires new or improved control; or an ACC/AHA-defined active cardiac condition (unstable coronary syndromes, decompensated congestive heart failure [CHF], significant arrhythmias, or severe valvular disease) that requires cardioprotection or revascularization.

As for testing and treatments, the indications for consultation during *documentation* and *optimization* generally parallel those for consultation in the absence of surgery. Clearly, consultation before surgery should take into account the anticipated intra- and postoperative impacts, the integrated impacts of existing conditions, and anticipated disturbances (see later discussion).

Creation of an Integrated Clinical Risk Profile: Risk Assessment

The phase of *risk assessment* combines information obtained by *documentation* and *changes due to optimization* with the anticipated physiologic disturbance of the planned surgery (and accompanying anesthetic) and thereby generate an integrated clinical risk profile (CRP) that anticipates the adequacy of resilience and reserve; that is, it is the transition from simply what *is* already wrong to what *could go* wrong. A multidimensional approach is vital, in that suitability for daily activities may not necessarily ensure readiness for surgery. *Resilience* reflects on the ability of the patient (overall as well as his/her individual bodily systems) to withstand the insults of the planned anesthesia and surgery; for example, is it likely that the stress will exceed the patient's cardiac ischemic threshold? Is liver function compromised to a degree that significantly increases its likelihood of failure? *Reserve* reflects the patient's ability to meet the anticipated increase in functional demands; for example, will the patient be able to maintain a minute ventilation sufficient to meet the needs imposed by the surgically induced hypermetabolic state? Will his/her platelet function be sufficient for the anticipated invasiveness of the planned surgery?

In addition to the laboratory values obtained during *documentation* based on disease prevalence, risk factors, and known or suspected disorders, the laboratory profile is completed during *risk assessment* by taking the nature and severity of the planned surgery into account. On the simplest level, an institution (or oversight agency) can establish uniform guidelines for such testing based on severity-specific tests (eg, platelet count before major surgery) and procedure-specific tests (eg, urine culture before prosthetic joint insertion) to uncover disorders that, if present, might complicate the planned surgery. As for testing based on prevalence, these would be indicated regardless of whether there was clinical evidence of an abnormality. Additional testing may be based on either the need to evaluate an uncertain condition or the combined impact of the anticipated disturbances of planned surgery with the patient's presurgical morbidities; for example, obtaining liver function tests before major abdominal surgery in a patient with prior liver injury (even if the surgery alone or the history alone would not have prompted such testing).

After the integrated CRP is established, the threats to resilience and reserve as a result of proceeding with surgery can be weighed against the risk(s) of not proceeding with surgery. The need for consultation largely is attributable to uncertainty as to the degree to which a given patient's resilience and reserve will be maintained; that is, to address the integrated impact of the patient's existing conditions and the anticipated surgical disturbance on an overall as well as a system-specific (eg, cardiac, respiratory) level.

There seems to be increasing appreciation of the need for such multifactorial assessment of existing morbidities and anticipated surgical impact. In its risk indices for pulmonary complications, the American College of Physicians takes into account organ (system) dysfunction, functional capacity, and site of surgery (eg, upper abdominal); pulmonary factors alone do not adequately predict the likelihood of postoperative pulmonary complications.[32,33] In their proposed modifications of the Goldman index,[7] Detsky and colleagues[8] separated groups of patients based on whether they were undergoing minor or major surgery. The importance of the integrated CRP is also exemplified by the 2007 update of the ACC/AHA Guidelines,[12] which states that the five clinical risk factors identified by Lee and colleagues (eg, ischemic heart disease, compensated or prior heart failure, diabetes mellitus, renal insufficiency, and cerebrovascular disease)[6] warrant cardiac consultation and testing (or special perioperative intervention such as heart rate control with β-blockers) only if accompanied by decreased exercise tolerance and only in anticipation of intermediate-risk or high-risk surgery.

Integrated assessments of existing morbidities and anticipated disturbance are also included in the ASA Practice Advisory for Preanesthesia Evaluation,[31] which recommends that patients be seen by a member of the anesthesia team before the day of surgery not only if they have severe disease (as indicated by a high ASA physical status score) but also if, despite a low severity of disease, they are undergoing a highly invasive procedure.[31] In a recent ASA survey, 57% of the 1857 respondents reported that delays occur in at least 1 in 10 patients not seen for preanesthesia evaluation before the day of surgery (versus 23% of respondents for patients who had a preanesthetic evaluation visit).[34] Review of the health care databases in Ontario, Canada, indicated that assessment by an anesthesiologist before the day of surgery (for patients >40 years old undergoing intermediate- or high-risk surgery) reduced mean hospital stay by 0.35 days, with the greatest impact in patients with significant comorbidities undergoing major surgery.[35] Overall, preanesthesia evaluation clinics and other forms of preanesthesia evaluation have been shown to reduce hospital costs and duration of hospital stay[36–38] as well as day of surgery cancellations.[38–40] The justification for consultation (as opposed to a less complex preoperative assessment) by an anesthesiologist is less well defined. It may be viewed as falling into three major categories: decisions deferred to the anesthesiologist with respect to management of a high-risk patient (eg, is the patient a suitable candidate for the planned surgery? Is special planning required to reduce risk or facilitate management?), pain management, and conditions which, although not necessarily of major impact during daily life, may pose a disproportionate risk during the perioperative period unless assessed and planned for appropriately (discussed later).

Integrated clinical risk profile matrix

In recent years, members of the authors' preoperative assessment team have described a means for uniform grading of existing patient morbidities as well as anticipated perioperative disturbances,[25,41] thereby facilitating generation of an integrated existing morbidity and anticipated disturbance matrix that tabulates a patient's risk profile. Its foundation is the application of the overall 1 to 5 ASA physical status score on a system-by-system basis or, when added specificity is deemed indicated on a subsystem or disorder basis (**Table 1**). Such scoring can be readily accomplished with minimal additional effort at the time of clinical assessment. Initial studies have suggested high correlations between preoperative system-specific scores and hospital costs and length of stay,[42,43] as well as diagnosis-related group (DRG) weighting and ICD coding.[44,45] Comparable scoring can also be applied to other components of the integrated CRP, most notably anticipated surgical disturbance (**Table 2**). The ability to rate patient morbidity and surgical risk on common scales provides an otherwise unavailable means for quantifying their (potential) cumulative impact on overall and system-specific levels; for example, a patient with grade

	ASA Status 2 Features	ASA Status 3 Features	ASA Status 4 Features	ASA 5 Features
Table 1				
Sample application of system-specific scoring to the selected features of the ischemic heart disease subsystem of the cardiac system				
Cardiac system				
Ischemic heart disease subsystem	History of chest pain and transient ST segment changes after cocaine (not current)	Stable exertional angina, occasional resting angina, occasional use of sublingual nitroglycerin. Cardiac-related dyspnea at 2–4 METS. Old myocardial infarction. Long-standing, stable wall motion abnormalities. EF 25%–50%. ICD in place for history of ventricular fibrillation. Compensated CHF, stable on cardiac medication	Severe left ventricular compromise. Unstable angina. Acute infarction. Cardiac-related SOB or angina at <2 METS. Prone to ventricular fibrillation. EF <25%. Extensive wall motion abnormalities and ischemia on catheterization. Symptomatic L main occlusion. Multiple vessel disease with decreased EF	Acute, severe heart failure requiring aggressive life-saving treatment

As for the overall ASA score, system-specific scores are based on a 1 to 5 scale: 1, healthy; 2, 3, and 4, mild, moderate, and severe systemic disorders/dysfunction, respectively; 5, acutely life-threatening condtion.[25] Suggested default scores for selected features are included in the table. Clinical significance, and hence the score, may be influenced by acuity as well as the nature of the condition (eg, current versus acute ischemia, transient versus lasting injury).

Abbreviations: EF, ejection fraction; METS, metabolic equivalents; SOB, shortness of breath.

3 cardiac disease could receive a cumulative cardiac score of 4, 5, 6, 7, or 8, depending on the anticipated impact of surgery. This means a standardized assessment may be applied to justify, but not necessarily drive, laboratory testing, consultation, and interventions on a per patient basis and to provide a framework for tabulation of a series of patients (within and among institutions) for the design of testing guidelines, quality assurance, billing, and research.

Planning

For some patients, the final phase of the preoperative process, *planning*, is straightforward, with standard instructions for diet, nothing by mouth (NPO) status, dentures, contact lenses, and plans for surgery-specific needs (eg, bowel preparation and preoperative antibiotics). However, in many settings, *planning* may include customized preparation based on the patient's integrated CRP, with input from the surgeon, anesthesiologist, primary care provider, and consultant(s). A brief overview of the issues is provided here; specialty-related details are provided in the other articles.

Table 2
Scored classification of anticipated surgical disturbances

Category	Description	Examples
1	Minimally invasive	Breast biopsy; removal of minor skin or subcutaneous lesions; myringotomy tubes; cystoscopy; colonscopy; herniorrhaphy (simple); vasectomy; circumcision
2	+ Likely intraoperative airway/respiratory requirements (eg, laryngeal mask airway or endotracheal intubation) or potential for procedure to become moderately invasive	Diagnostic laparoscopy; laparoscopic cholecystectomy; laparoscopic lysis of adhesions; laparoscopic or complex hernia; umbilical hernia; tubal ligation; arthroscopy; tonsils; rhinoplasty; percutaneous lung biopsy; extensive superficial procedures
3	Moderately invasive	Thyroidectomy (total); hysterectomy; myomectomy; cystectomy; open cholecystectomy; laminectomy; hip and knee replacement; simple nephrectomy; major laparoscopic procedures; partial colectomy
4	+ Likely intraoperative cardiac, respiratory, or fluid/electrolyte disturbances	Major orthopedic-spinal reconstruction; major gastrointestinal reconstruction; radical genitourinary surgery; nonaortic vascular surgery; video-assisted thoracoscopy
5	Highly invasive	Major cardiothoracic procedure; major intracranial procedure; major aortic surgery

The scores are in accordance with the recently proposed uniform 1 to 5 scoring of conditions and challenges.[25]

In addition to the aforementioned *optimization* of disease states for the long-term as well as acute setting, preoperative interventions tailored to the patient's conditions may include new or augmented therapy. In accordance with the ACC/AHA Guidelines for integrated assessment described above,[12,46] the risk of ischemic heart injury may prompt increased cardioprotection with β-blockers or more aggressive intervention (angioplasty, stenting, coronary bypass grafting). The stress of upcoming surgery often exacerbates hypertension, prompting the need for new or increased antihypertensive therapy or the amelioration of white coat hypertension with an anxiolytic on the morning of surgery. In selected patients, even if it is currently quiescent, a history of severely reactive airway disease may prompt initiation of preoperative steroids before intraoperative airway stimulation; likewise a history of chronic bronchitis may prompt a course of antibiotics before a surgical procedure that will compromise pulmonary function. *Planning* for the patient at high risk of pulmonary complications may also entail perioperative lung expansion techniques (eg, incentive spirometry), increased use of inhaled bronchodilators, drainage of ascitic or pleural fluid, and discontinuation of smoking. *Planning* also should include aspiration prophylaxis as deemed indicated (eg, gastroesophageal reflux, hyperacidity, decreased gastric emptying, recent food ingestion). One should remember that, although it is common to continue H2-blockers and proton pump antagonists to decrease the risk of acid aspiration, particulate antacids (eg, Tums, Mylanta) are withheld on the morning of surgery in light of their deleterious effects if aspirated.

Several daily medications may be contraindicated to varying degrees perioperatively. The need to bridge acute care to long-term care discordance is particularly important with antithrombotic and anticoagulant medications,[47] often requiring the surgeon and prescriber to decide on a case-by-case basis. Can the surgeon operate effectively in their presence? Can the patient tolerate them being discontinued? The anesthesiologist is particularly concerned if a major regional anesthetic is planned.[48] The patient with a recent coronary stent or who may need a stent placed preoperatively may be especially challenging. The decision as to how to proceed requires a knowledge of the given stent's tendency for stent thrombosis, site of and time since stent placement, and exacerbating comorbidities. This is but one example of the literature changing almost on a daily basis, causing recommendations and guidelines to rapidly become outdated.[14]

The anesthesiologist can typically make decisions about most other medications without the need for extensive consultation; however, it may not be practical to establish standing orders. Except for angiotensin converting enzyme inhibitors (ACEIs), angiotensin receptor blocking (ARB) drugs, and diuretics, cardiac medications are commonly continued through the morning of surgery. Although anesthesiologists prefer to withhold ACEIs and ARBs before general, spinal, and epidural anesthesia because of their potential to contribute to recalcitrant intraoperative hypotension,[49] this may be outweighed by concerns about poorly controlled hypertension, fear of rupture of a fragile aneurysm, or the need to maintain a reduced afterload. Diuretics may be continued in the presence of congestive failure or electrolyte disturbances. Tricyclics and monoamine oxidase inhibitors are often discontinued preoperatively, except if continued use is deemed necessary for treatment of existing disease. Decisions about insulin management take into account the nature of insulin dependence (eg, whether the patient is prone to ketosis), concomitant conditions and medications, the stability of current management, typical morning glucose levels, and susceptibility to hypoglycemia.

For many of the issues of particular concern to the anesthesiologist, although it is optimal to be forewarned, extensive advanced planning is not required as long as vigilance is maintained on the day of surgery. For example, the need to avoid succinylcholine because of a potential for rhabdomyolysis and hyperkalemia in the presence of a denervating disorder, muscular disorder, or major trauma usually can be addressed on the day of surgery. Likewise, barbiturates can be avoided in the setting of porphyria and inhalational anesthetics can be avoided in a patient with a history of what has been referred to as halothane hepatitis. Clearly, advanced notification would be helpful; and if a patient is not seen by an anesthesiologist before the day of surgery, it may be incumbent on other care givers to be certain that the necessary information (eg, documentation of the disorders and information about prior anesthetic experiences) is available by the day of surgery.

For some intraoperative conditions, advanced planning or action is indicated. These include airway anatomy predisposing to difficult bag and mask ventilation or difficult endotracheal intubation; increased likelihood of malignant hyperthermia, wherein one needs to avoid succinylcholine as well as any traces of inhalational anesthetics and possibly ensure the ready availability of sodium dantrolene; and latex allergy so that all latex-containing supplies can be eliminated. Special adaptations may also be indicated for the pregnant patient or breast-feeding mother. Especially with respect to the former, input from the patient's obstetrician or involvement of a high-risk fetal team may be required. Cardiac rate management devices may also prompt consultation in the perioperative period; intracardiac defibrillators often need to be deactivated before, and reactivated after, surgery; the need for, and practicality of, an external pacer also needs to be assessed.

Recommendations as to what should or should not be done intraoperatively should be made in concert with other team members. Although the warning "avoid general endotracheal anesthesia" may reduce potential exacerbation of bronchospasm, it consistently safeguards the patient only if it is accompanied by "avoid surgery." Many procedures are either impossible or impractical to perform without general anesthesia (due to pain, need for heavy sedation, loss of airway, and cardiovascular or pulmonary changes that prompt emergency conversion to general endotracheal anesthesia).

Planning also entails preparation for the transitions from intraoperative to acute postoperative and, if need be, longer-term rehabilitative care. With respect to intraoperative care, the combined administration of an epidural and general anesthetic may improve pain management and reduce postoperative morbidity, especially in patients with severe respiratory compromise.[1,50] Critical care consultation and preoperative intervention may be valuable economically as well as physiologically for the care of selected high-risk patients. The impact of addiction and the potential for withdrawal may have the greatest impact postoperatively and thus should be anticipated and planned for accordingly.

SUMMARY

The assessment of the presurgical patient is a complex process that requires integration of multiple areas of expertise. The classic, indeed obsolete, concept of clearing a patient for surgery is replaced instead with an integrated approach that must focus on assessment and optimization of resilience and reserve in anticipation of increased demand, avoidance of therapeutic conflicts, and identification of potential OR-specific risks.

Although 4 separate phases of preoperative assessment and planning are listed in this article, they clearly overlap. Communication among specialties is critical to prevent misperceptions leading to failures in the bidirectional transition between long-term and acute perioperative care. Although evidence-based advisories and guidelines are extremely valuable for preoperative assessment and planning, they are not replacements for diligent and integrated clinical care by primary care providers, specialists, and consultants involved with the care of a given patient.

Each member of the team must be open to the potential for integrated *risk assessment* and *planning* to lead to roads not taken as well as taken, ranging from uninterrupted procession to surgery to additional assessment or optimization that may cause surgical postponement, and even to the cancellation of the surgical procedure. Although it might be viewed as an inefficiency of the system for surgery to be postponed after scheduling, this may be seen instead as a significant advantage of preoperative evaluation. The cost savings resulting from having surgery rescheduled before the actual planned date, rather than cancellation on the day of surgery, is considerable, and may even be sufficient to justify the entire cost of the preoperative system. Moreover, it may avert a bad outcome.

REFERENCES

1. Eagle KA, Berger PB, Calkins H, et al. ACC/AHA Guideline update for perioperative cardiovascular evaluation for noncardiac surgery—executive summary: a report of the American College of Cardiology/American Heart Association

Task Force on Practice Guidelines (committee to update the 1996 guidelines on perioperative cardiovascular evaluation for noncardiac surgery). J Am Coll Cardiol 2002;39(3):542–53.

2. Schein OD, Katz J, Bass EB, et al. The value of routine preoperative medical testing before cataract surgery. Study of Medical Testing for Cataract Surgery. N Engl J Med 2000;342(3):168–75.

3. London MJ, Itani KM, Perrino AC Jr, et al. Perioperative beta-blockade: a survey of physician attitudes in the department of Veterans Affairs. J Cardiothorac Vasc Anesth 2004;18(1):14–24.

4. Centers for Medicare & Medicaid Services. Medicare claims processing manual. Chapter 12, section 30.6.10 – Consultation services, Rev. 788, Issued 12/5/05. Available at: http://www.cms.hhs.gov/manuals/downloads/clm104c12.pdf. Accessed January 15, 2009.

5. Eagle KA, Rihal CS, Mickel MC, et al. Cardiac risk of noncardiac surgery: influence of coronary disease and type of surgery in 3368 operations. CASS Investigators and University of Michigan Heart Care Program. Coronary Artery Surgery Study. Circulation 1997;96(6):1882–7.

6. Lee TH, Marcantonio ER, Mangione CM, et al. Derivation and prospective validation of a simple index for prediction of cardiac risk of major noncardiac surgery. Circulation 1999;100(10):1043–9.

7. Goldman L, Caldera DL, Nussbaum SR, et al. Multifactorial index of cardiac risk in noncardiac surgical procedures. N Engl J Med 1977;297(16):845–50.

8. Detsky AS, Abrams HB, McLaughlin JR, et al. Predicting cardiac complications in patients undergoing non-cardiac surgery. J Gen Intern Med 1986; 1(4):211–9.

9. Romano PS, Schembri ME, Rainwater JA. Can administrative data be used to ascertain clinically significant postoperative complications? Am J Med Qual 2002;17(4):145–54.

10. Best WR, Khuri SF, Phelan M, et al. Identifying patient preoperative risk factors and postoperative adverse events in administrative databases: results from the Department of Veterans Affairs National Surgical Quality Improvement Program. J Am Coll Surg 2002;194(3):257–66.

11. Smetana GW, Lawrence VA, Cornell JE. Preoperative pulmonary risk stratification for noncardiothoracic surgery: systematic review for the American College of Physicians. Ann Intern Med 2006;144(8):581–95.

12. Fleisher LA, Beckman JA, Brown KA, et al. ACC/AHA 2007 guidelines on perioperative cardiovascular evaluation and care for noncardiac surgery: a report of the American College of Cardiology/American Heart Association Task Force on Practice Guidelines. Circulation 2007;116(17):e418–99.

13. Ioannidis JPA. Contradicted and initially stronger effects in highly cited clinical research. JAMA 2005;294:218–28.

14. Shojania KG, Sampson M, Ansari MT, et al. How quickly do systematic reviews go out of date? A survival analysis. Ann Intern Med 2007;147(4):224–33.

15. Sniderman AD, Furberg CD. Why guideline-making requires reform. JAMA 2009; 301(4):429–31.

16. Tinetti ME, Bogardus ST Jr, Agostini JV. Potential pitfalls of disease-specific guidelines for patients with multiple conditions. N Engl J Med 2004;351(27):2870–4.

17. McAlister FA, van Diepen S, Padwal RS, et al. How evidence-based are the recommendations in evidence-based guidelines? PLoS Med 2007;4(8):e250.

18. Akhtar S, Assaad S, Amin M, et al. Preoperative beta-blocker use: impact of national guidelines on clinical practice. J Clin Anesth 2008;20(2):122–8.

19. Berenson RA, Horvath J. Confronting the barriers to chronic care management in medicare. Health Aff. Suppl Web Exclusives:W3-37-53, 2003 Jan–June. Available at: http://search.ebscohost.com/login.aspx?direct=true&db=aph&jid=HAF&site=ehost-live. Accessed August 1, 2003.

20. Kaufman DW, Kelly JP, Rosenberg L, et al. Recent patterns of medication use in the ambulatory adult population of the United States: the Slone survey. JAMA 2002;287(3):337–44.

21. POISE Study Group, Devereaux PJ, Yang H, et al. Effects of extended-release metoprolol succinate in patients undergoing non-cardiac surgery (POISE trial): a randomised controlled trial. Lancet 2008;371(9627):1839–47.

22. Bangalore S, Wetterslev J, Pranesh S, et al. Perioperative beta blockers in patients having non-cardiac surgery: a meta-analysis. Lancet 2008;372(9654):1962–76.

23. Katz RI, Barnhart JM, Ho G, et al. A survey on the intended purposes and perceived utility of preoperative cardiology consultations. Anesth Analg 1998; 87(4):830–6.

24. Prause G, Ratzenhofer-Komenda B, Smolle-Juettner F, et al. Operations on patients deemed "unfit for operation and anaesthesia": what are the consequences? Acta Anaesthesiol Scand 1998;42(3):316–22.

25. Holt NF, Silverman DG. Modeling perioperative risk – can numbers speak louder than words? Anesthesiol Clin North America 2006;24:427–59.

26. Roizen MF. More preoperative assessment by physicians and less by laboratory tests. N Engl J Med 2000;342(3):204–5.

27. Fischer SP. Cost-effective preoperative evaluation and testing. Chest 1999; 115(Suppl 5):96S–100S.

28. Smetana GW, Macpherson DS. The case against routine preoperative laboratory testing. Med Clin North Am 2003;87(1):7–40.

29. Pasternak LR. Preoperative laboratory testing: general issues and considerations. Anesthesiol Clin North America 2004;22(1):13–25.

30. Pauker SG, Kopelman RI. Interpreting hoofbeats: can Bayes help clear the haze? N Engl J Med 1992;327(14):1009–13.

31. Pasternak LR, Arens JF, Caplan RA, et al. Practice advisory for preanesthesia evaluation: a report by the American Society of Anesthesiologists Task Force on Preanesthesia Evaluation. Anesthesiology 2000;96:485–96.

32. Epstein SK, Faling LJ, Daly BD, et al. Predicting complications after pulmonary resection. Preoperative exercise testing vs a multifactorial cardiopulmonary risk index. Chest 1993;104(3):694–700.

33. Smetana GW. Preoperative pulmonary evaluation. N Engl J Med 1999;340(12): 937–44.

34. Holt NF, Silverman DG, Prasad R, et al. Preanesthesia clinics, information management, and operating room delays: results of a survey of practicing anesthesiologists. Anesth Analg 2007;104(3):615–8.

35. Wijeysundera DN, Austin PC, Beattie WS, et al. A population-based study of anesthesia consultation before major non-cardiac surgery. Arch Internal Med 2009;169(6):595–602.

36. Pollard JB, Zboray AL, Mazze RI. Economic benefits attributed to opening a preoperative evaluation clinic for outpatients. Anesth Analg 1996;83(2):407–10.

37. van Klei WA, Moons KG, Rutten CL, et al. The effect of outpatient preoperative evaluation of hospital inpatients on cancellation of surgery and length of hospital stay. Anesth Analg 2002;94(3):644–9.

38. Ferschl MB, Tung A, Sweitzer B, et al. Preoperative clinic visits reduce operating room cancellations and delays. Anesthesiology 2005;103(4):855–9.

39. Cantlay KL, Baker S, Parry A, et al. The impact of a consultant anaesthetist led pre-operative assessment clinic on patients undergoing major vascular surgery. Anaesthesia 2006;61(3):234–9.

40. Fu ES, Scharf JE, Glodek J. Preoperative testing: a comparison between Health-Quiz recommendations and routine ordering. Am J Anesthesiol 1997;24:237–40.

41. Rosenbaum SH, Silverman DG. The value of preoperative assessment. In: Newman MF, Fleisher LA, Fink MP, editors. Perioperative medicine: managing for outcome. Philadelphia: Saunders Elsevier; 2008. p. 37–43.

42. Holt NF, Mukherjee A, Schonberger RB, et al. ASA physical status and surgical complexity on length of stay and hospital charges. Anesthesiology 2006;105: A195 [abstract].

43. Nath B, Silverman DGS, Mukherjee A, et al. Relationship of system-specific disorders in the pre-anesthesia evaluation to hospital length of stay. Anesth Analg 2008;106(Suppl 3):S70 [abstract].

44. Nath B, Holt NF, Mukherjee A, et al. Are post-discharge coders failing to capture disorders identified by system-specific scoring of the pre-anesthetic note? Anesth Analg 2008;106(Suppl 3):75 [abstract].

45. Jakab EJ, Romberg F, Nath B, et al. System-specific ASA score: does it bridge the gap between clinical assessment and ICD-9 coding? Anesthesiology 2008; 109:A144 [abstract].

46. Fleisher LA, Beckman JA, Brown KA, et al. ACC/AHA 2006 guideline update on perioperative cardiovascular evaluation for noncardiac surgery: focused update on perioperative beta-blocker therapy. A report of the American College of Cardiology/American Heart Association Task Force on Practice Guidelines (writing committee to update the 2002 guidelines on perioperative cardiovascular evaluation for noncardiac surgery). J Am Coll Cardiol 2006;47:2343–55.

47. Bonow RO, Carabello B, de Leon AC Jr, et al. ACC/AHA guidelines for the management of patients with valvular heart disease. A report of the American College of Cardiology/American Heart Association Task Force on practice guidelines (committee on management of patients with valvular heart disease). J Am Coll Cardiol 1998;32(5):1486–588.

48. Horlocker TT, Wedel DJ, Benzon H, et al. Regional anesthesia in the anticoagulated patient: defining the risks (the second ASRA Consensus Conference on Neuraxial Anesthesia and Anticoagulation). Reg Anesth Pain Med 2003;28(3): 172–97.

49. Bertrand M, Godet G, Meersschaert K, et al. Should the angiotensin II antagonists be discontinued before surgery? Anesth Analg 2001;92(1):26–30.

50. Rodgers A, Walker N, Schug S, et al. Reduction of postoperative mortality and morbidity with epidural or spinal anaesthesia: results from overview of randomised trials. BMJ 2000;321(7275):1493–7.

Preoperative Evaluation and Preparation of the Patient for Cardiac Surgery

Alec D. Weisberg, MD[a,b], Emily L. Weisberg, MD[c],
James M. Wilson, MD[a,b], Charles D. Collard, MD[c,d],*

KEYWORDS

- Cardiac surgery • Preoperative evaluation
- Risk stratification • Atrial fibrillation • Renal dysfunction
- Stroke • Statins • β-Blockers

Coronary artery bypass graft (CABG) and valve surgery are among the most common operations performed worldwide. The incidence of cardiac complications after CABG is at least 10% and costs $2 billion annually.[1] These figures are anticipated to increase as older patients with more comorbidities are referred for cardiac surgery. Objective risk stratification provides the physician and patient with valuable information for assessing the risk/benefit ratio before proceeding with cardiac surgery. Careful patient selection and preparation during preoperative evaluation may minimize morbidity and mortality.

MORTALITY RISK STRATIFICATION

The mortality rate associated with cardiac surgery varies widely and is influenced by multiple preoperative risk factors. Jones and colleagues[2] defined 7 "core" variables that were unequivocally associated with operative mortality, and 13 "level 1" variables

[a] Section of Cardiology, Department of Medicine, Baylor College of Medicine, One Baylor Plaza, Houston, TX 77030, USA
[b] Texas Heart Institute, St. Luke's Episcopal Hospital, Houston, TX, USA
[c] Department of Anesthesiology, Baylor College of Medicine, 1709 Dryden Road, Suite 1700, Houston, TX 77030, USA
[d] Division of Cardiovascular Anesthesiology, Texas Heart Institute, St. Luke's Episcopal Hospital, 6720 Bertner Avenue, Room 0520, Houston, TX 77030, USA
* Corresponding author. Division of Anesthesiology, Texas Heart Institute, St. Luke's Episcopal Hospital, 6720 Bertner Avenue, Room 0520, Houston, TX 77030.
E-mail address: ccollard@bcm.tmc.edu (C.D. Collard).

Med Clin N Am 93 (2009) 979–994
doi:10.1016/j.mcna.2009.05.001
0025-7125/09/$ – see front matter © 2009 Elsevier Inc. All rights reserved.

medical.theclinics.com

Table 1
Predictors of post-CABG mortality

"Core" Variables	"Level 1" Variables
Age	Height
Sex	Weight
Urgency of operation	PCI during current admission
Prior heart surgery	Date of most recent MI
LVEF	History of angina
Percent stenosis of LM coronary artery	Ventricular arrhythmia
Number of major coronary arteries with >70% stenosis	CHF
—	Mitral regurgitation
—	DM
—	CVD
—	PVD
—	COPD
—	Creatinine level

Abbreviations: CHF, congestive heart failure; COPD, chronic obstructive pulmonary disease; Core, variables unequivocally related to operative mortality; CVD, cerebrovascular disease; DM, diabetes mellitus; Level 1, variables with a likely relation to short-term mortality; LM, left main; LVEF, left ventricular ejection fraction; MI, myocardial infarction; PCI, percutaneous coronary intervention; PVD, peripheral vascular disease.

Data from Jones RH, Hannan EL, Hammermeister KE, et al. Identification of preoperative variables needed for risk adjustment of short-term mortality after coronary artery bypass graft surgery. The Working Group Panel on the Cooperative CABG Database Project. J Am Coll Cardiol 1996;28:1480.

that were likely to be related to mortality (**Table 1**). The core variables contained 45% to 83% of the predictive information, whereas the level 1 variables had only modest predictive power.[2] Risk scoring systems that incorporate the influence of multiple risk factors have been developed to estimate perioperative mortality. Although the American College of Cardiology (ACC) and the American Heart Association (AHA) believe that the use of statistical risk models to obtain objective estimates of CABG operative mortality is reasonable,[3] their use must be complementary to clinical judgment, as their performance is limited by their application to different procedures and populations than their original design and validation.

SYSTEM-BASED PREOPERATIVE EVALUATION

If the mortality risk associated with cardiac surgery is not prohibitive, the next phase of preoperative evaluation estimates the risk of other complications and identifies conditions that will delay surgery or need to be addressed before or concomitant with operative intervention. A thorough system-based approach is the preferred strategy for preoperative evaluation.

Cardiovascular

Preoperative evaluation should include a careful physical examination with particular attention to the cardiac and vascular systems. Severe aortic regurgitation (AR) and peripheral vascular disease (PVD) involving the access site femoral or iliac vessels or aneurysmal disease of the aorta are contraindications to perioperative intraaortic balloon pump (IABP) placement. Furthermore, in patients with AR, the regurgitant volume may increase during cardiopulmonary bypass (CPB) resulting in acute left ventricular (LV) distension. Varicose veins or a history of vein stripping or ligation in the lower extremities may preclude use of saphenous vein grafts as bypass conduits and prompt evaluation for alternative conduits. A carotid bruit or significant PVD may signify the presence of cerebrovascular disease (CVD) and requires further evaluation by carotid Doppler to assess the need and timing for carotid revascularization.[4]

Atrial fibrillation
The incidence of atrial fibrillation (AF) after CABG, valve surgery, and combined CABG and valve surgery is approximately 30%, 40%, and 50%, respectively.[5] Postoperative AF is associated with increased in-hospital and long-term mortality, renal failure (RF), stroke, congestive heart failure (CHF), hospital length of stay (HLOS), intensive care unit (ICU) readmission, and cost of hospitalization.[6,7] Age is one of the most reliable preoperative predictors of postoperative AF with a reported 75% increase in the odds of developing AF for every 10-year increase in age.[6] Other established predictors for the development of postoperative AF include history of AF, male gender, decreased LV ejection fraction (LVEF), left atrial enlargement, valvular heart surgery, chronic obstructive pulmonary disease (COPD), diabetes mellitus (DM), chronic renal failure (RF), rheumatic heart disease, LV hypertrophy, and withdrawal from β-blocker and angiotensin 1 converting enzyme inhibitor (ACEI) therapy.[6,8] Preoperative β-blocker, sotalol, and amiodarone therapy may be used to lower the incidence of postoperative AF. Although digoxin and calcium channel antagonists may be useful for ventricular rate control, they have not been demonstrated to reduce the postoperative incidence of AF.[3,9]

Left ventricular dysfunction
Surgical revascularization in patients with advanced myocardial dysfunction and coronary artery disease (CAD) is superior to medical therapy.[10] LV dysfunction and CHF are associated with higher mortality during CABG.[11] Topkara and colleagues[11] analyzed more than 55,000 patients undergoing CABG from the New York State (NYS) database and found that patients with advanced LV dysfunction had more comorbid conditions, including previous myocardial infarction (MI), RF, and CHF. Patients with LVEF less than 20% undergoing CABG had nearly four times the in-hospital mortality rate, lower rate of discharge to home, and higher incidence of postoperative respiratory failure, RF, and sepsis than patients with an LVEF greater than 40%. Independent predictors of in-hospital mortality in the low LVEF group were hepatic failure, RF, previous MI, reoperation, emergent procedures, female gender, CHF, and age. In high-risk patients, preoperative placement of an IABP reduces the use of inotropic and vasopressor medications, CPB time, in-hospital mortality, and shortens ICU stay.[12]

   Although LV dysfunction is often due to MI with associated necrosis and scar formation, it may also be due to hibernating or stunned myocardium, potentially reversible processes with revascularization.[13] A perioperative reduction in the contractile efficiency of previously functioning myocardial segments may be seen in the immediate postoperative period. Preoperative cardiac evaluation in patients with severely reduced LV function should focus on identifying patients with dysfunctional but viable myocardium by either [99mTc]MIBI, ^{201}Tl, [18F]fluorodeoxyglucose (FDG) positron emission tomography (PET), dobutamine echocardiography, dobutamine magnetic resonance imaging (MRI), or delayed-enhancement cardiac MRI. The sensitivity of these various imaging modalities ranges from 80% to 90% with specificity of 54% to 92%.[14,15] In a patient with marginal preoperative hemodynamic function who can expect little or no improvement in the immediate postoperative period, the likelihood of complication or death is high and possibly prohibitive for cardiac surgery.

Recent myocardial infarction

The timing and location of a recent MI should be included in the preoperative evaluation. Mortality associated with CABG is increased for the first 3 to 7 days following MI, and if clinically appropriate, a delay in surgery beyond this time period should be considered.[3,16] Following anterior MI, the detection of an LV thrombus by preoperative transthoracic echocardiogram may alter the timing and approach of CABG.[3] Inferior MI that significantly impairs right ventricular (RV) function is associated with hemodynamic consequences that can be exacerbated during CPB, and it is reasonable to delay CABG for 4 weeks to allow RV recovery.[3]

Hematologic

Preoperative anemia is associated with increased morbidity and mortality during cardiac surgery.[17] Kulier and colleagues[17] found that preoperative anemia was an independent predictor of noncardiac complications. In patients with preoperative anemia and a European System for Cardiac Operative Risk Evaluation (EuroSCORE) of 4 or more, there were increased cardiac complications but these were likely attributable to other concomitant risk factors. Independent predictors of preoperative anemia are a history of anemia, RF, female gender, advanced age, DM, unstable angina, and history of CABG. As blood transfusions in patients undergoing cardiac surgery have been associated with increased morbidity and mortality,[18] perioperative transfusion strategies that incorporate the degree of anemia and other comorbidities need to be developed for individual patients.

Heparin-induced thrombocytopenia

Heparin-induced thrombocytopenia (HIT) is an immune-mediated complication of heparin therapy associated with arterial and venous thrombosis. There is typically a 50% or greater decrease in platelet count from baseline in association with thrombotic events.[19] In most cases, immunoassays can detect antibodies against complexes of platelet factor 4 (PF4) and heparin. Everett and colleagues[20] found that in patients undergoing cardiac surgery, the preoperative and postoperative incidence of antibodies to PF4/heparin was 4.3% and 22.4%, respectively, but thrombotic events occurred only in 6.3% of patients with a positive antibody. Diagnostic specificity for HIT can be increased by use of platelet activation assays such as the serotonin release assay.[19] Post-CABG, patients with HIT have a higher incidence of saphenous vein graft occlusion than patients without HIT, but no significant difference in left internal mammary artery graft occlusion.[21]

Management of patients undergoing cardiac surgery with antibodies to PF4/heparin and HIT is evolving. During CPB, unfractionated heparin (UFH) is the preferred agent due to familiarity with its use, reversibility with protamine, and ease of intraoperative monitoring. In this syndrome, a typical anamnestic immune response is often not formed, and rechallenge with heparin is a reasonable strategy for patients with HIT who need to undergo CPB.[19] Warkentin and colleagues[19] outline management guidelines for HIT patients undergoing cardiac surgery. An immunoassay for PF4/heparin antibodies should be performed and if positive, a platelet activation assay should be completed (if available). Patients who are PF4/heparin antibody negative or antibody positive by immunoassay, but antibody negative by platelet activation assay, may proceed with cardiac surgery using UFH during CPB. Preoperative and postoperative anticoagulation should be performed with a nonheparin anticoagulant. In patients with a history of HIT whose platelet counts have recovered but are heparin/PF4 antibody positive, surgery should be delayed if possible until a platelet activation assay is negative, and then surgery can be performed using UFH during CPB. If delaying surgery is not an option, use of a nonheparin anticoagulant is recommended over UFH during CPB. In patients with HIT who remain thrombocytopenic and are heparin/PF4 antibody positive, the preferred strategy is to delay surgery until the platelets have normalized and the heparin/PF4 antibodies are negative or weakly positive. However, if delaying surgery is not feasible, alternative anticoagulation regimes during CPB should be considered.

Hypercoagulable disorders

Balancing the risk of thrombosis with excessive perioperative bleeding is difficult in patients with a hypercoagulable disorder. In hospitalized patients with a hypercoagulable disorder who are not on chronic anticoagulation, preoperative administration of subcutaneous UFH and low molecular weight heparin (LMWH) are important to lower the risk of developing a deep venous thrombosis while mobility is limited.[22] For chronically anticoagulated patients, warfarin therapy should be held at least 5 days before cardiac surgery,[23] and therapeutic anticoagulation may be bridged with UFH or LMWH. In patients with antiphospholipid antibody syndrome, perioperative anticoagulation monitoring can be difficult due to abnormal prolongation in clotting times and consultation with a hematologist and clinical pathologist is often required to design the best management strategy.[4,24]

Renal

Preoperative renal dysfunction is common in patients undergoing cardiac surgery and is an important risk factor for increased morbidity and mortality.[25-27] Cooper and colleagues[25] found that in patients undergoing CABG, the preoperative incidence of mild, moderate, and severe renal dysfunction and dialysis dependence was 51%, 24%, 2%, and 1.5%, respectively, and operative mortality increased with declining renal function. Preoperative estimated creatinine clearance is a better predictor of postoperative adverse events than plasma creatinine level.[27] Although renal dysfunction after cardiac surgery is an independent risk factor for mortality, improved preoperative renal function reduces this effect on mortality.[26]

In a large multicenter study of patients undergoing cardiac surgery, Mangano and colleagues found that the incidence of postoperative renal dysfunction not requiring dialysis was 7.7% and requiring dialysis, 1.4%. Mortality in patients without renal dysfunction was 0.9% but increased to 19% in patients with renal dysfunction and 63% in patients requiring dialysis. Postoperative RF is associated with increased ICU and HLOS, higher mortality, and greater likelihood for discharge to an extended care facility. Although multiple factors are associated with increased risk of postoperative renal dysfunction following cardiac surgery, advanced age, CHF, prior CABG, DM, and preexisting renal disease are factors that identify a high-risk population for renal dysfunction after CABG.[28] Cardiac catheterization performed on the day of cardiac surgery and higher doses of contrast medium are independently associated with higher risk for postoperative RF.[29] Preoperative serum creatinine, age, race, type of surgery, DM, shock, NYHA class, lung disease, recent MI, and prior cardiovascular surgery are associated with increased risk for postoperative dialysis and have been incorporated into a bedside risk algorithm for estimating a patient's probability for dialysis after cardiac surgery.[30]

Perioperative management in patients at high risk for RF and dialysis focuses on minimizing exposure to nephrotoxic drugs and contrast media and maintaining renal perfusion. If possible, cardiac surgery immediately after cardiac catheterization should be avoided. Although N-acetylcysteine has been shown to attenuate contrast-induced declines in renal function, there is no convincing evidence that perioperative administration of N-acetylcysteine is protective in cardiac surgery.[31] Future studies will help clarify whether off-pump CABG, which eliminates the need for CPB, is associated with lower risk for postoperative renal dysfunction.

Endocrine

DM is present in approximately 25% of patients presenting for CABG or percutaneous coronary intervention and is associated with worse outcomes after cardiac surgery.[2,3,28,32] Patients with DM without RF or PVD who undergo CABG have similar long-term survival to patients without DM.[33] Preoperative screening for DM is an important aspect of preparing a patient for cardiac surgery. Lauruschkat and colleagues[34] found the incidence of undiagnosed DM in patients undergoing CABG to be 5.2%, and noted that these patients had higher perioperative mortality, required reintubation more frequently, and remained intubated longer than patients without DM and with known DM.

In patients undergoing cardiac surgery, strict perioperative glucose control using perioperative insulin infusions can significantly lower operative mortality and the incidence of mediastinitis.[35,36] There is growing evidence that insulin exerts antiinflammatory effects, beyond its metabolic activities, which may partially explain its cardioprotective properties.[37] Future studies will clarify the role of preoperative glucose control and the optimal perioperative management scheme.

Pulmonary

COPD is the most common cause of preoperative pulmonary dysfunction. Cohen and colleagues[38] noted that patients with clinically significant COPD undergoing CABG had higher rates of pre- and postoperative atrial and ventricular arrhythmias, reintubation, and longer ICU stay and HLOS than matched controls. Although Fuster and colleagues[39] showed that a preoperative FEV1 of 60% of predicted or higher is associated with increased mortality during CABG, Spivack and colleagues[40] did not find a clear role for pulmonary function testing in preoperative evaluation for cardiac surgery. Home oxygen therapy or hypercapnia are clinical parameters that identify a population at higher risk for postoperative respiratory failure.[3,38] Clinical assessment of lung function and severity of COPD is a critical component of preoperative assessment.

The incidence of respiratory failure in patients undergoing cardiac surgery varies widely depending on the definition. Filsoufi and colleagues[41] defined respiratory failure as intubation time of 72 hours or longer and found that the incidence of respiratory failure in the NYS database was 9.1%, with the highest incidence in combined CABG and valve procedures (14.8%). Independent predictors of postoperative respiratory failure were age more than 70 years, female gender, LVEF 30% or less, combined CABG/valve surgery, CHF, DM, PVD, COPD, RF, active endocarditis, reoperation, hemodynamic instability, and IABP insertion. Postoperative respiratory failure was associated with significantly increased morbidity, mortality, and HLOS. To optimize respiratory function before surgery, existing pulmonary conditions or exacerbations should be treated, including smoking cessation, antibiotic therapy for existing pneumonia or bronchitis, diuresis for pulmonary edema, and bronchodilator and steroid treatment of COPD exacerbation.[3] In high-risk patients undergoing CABG, inspiratory muscle training is associated with a reduction in postoperative pulmonary complications.[42]

Neurologic

The incidence of neurologic complications following cardiac surgery, including global encephalopathy, focal neurologic syndromes, and decline in intellectual function and memory, ranges widely from 1% to 80%.[43,44] These complications have largely been attributed to the adverse effects of CPB, which can lead to embolism, hemorrhage, hypoxia, cerebral edema, and metabolic derangements. Advanced age, prior neurologic disease, type of surgery, aortic atheroma, and duration of CPB are predictors of neurologic complications following cardiac surgery.[43,45,46] Stroke is a devastating complication of cardiac surgery with a reported incidence ranging from 0.8% to 7%.[46] Prediction models can be used to estimate the perioperative risk of stroke.[32]

In patients undergoing CABG, the incidence of coexisting carotid artery disease more than 50% is 17% to 22% and more than 80% disease, 6% to 12%.[47,48] Approximately 30% of postoperative strokes are due to significant carotid artery stenosis.[49] Stroke risk increases with the severity of stenosis, and the stroke risk in patients with carotid stenoses of less than 50%, 50% to 80%, and more than 80% is approximately 2%, 10%, and 11% to 18.8%, respectively.[3,50,51] Even in the asymptomatic patient, carotid stenosis of 75% is an independent predictor of stroke risk after CABG.[52] ACC/AHA guidelines state that selective carotid screening should be considered in the following high-risk patient groups: older than 65 years, left main coronary artery stenosis, carotid bruit on examination, PVD, history of smoking, and history of transient ischemic attack or stroke.[3]

The goal of carotid revascularization before CABG is the prevention of cerebrovascular events. Carotid endarterectomy (CEA) and CABG can be performed as either a staged or combined procedure, and the combined incidence of stroke, MI, and death for either procedure is 10% to 12%.[53] In 1 review of 97 studies, there was a trend toward higher mortality, stroke, and MI in patients undergoing combined CEA-CABG relative to staged CEA-CABG.[53] According to the ACC/AHA guidelines, CEA should be considered before CABG or concomitant with CABG in patients with a symptomatic carotid stenosis or in asymptomatic patients with unilateral or bilateral internal carotid stenosis of 80% or more.[3] Carotid artery stenting (CAS) is a less invasive alternative than CEA for carotid revascularization. In a recent review by Guzman and colleagues[54] of 6 studies including 277 patients undergoing staged CAS and CABG, only 2.2% of patients suffered a stroke following CABG. However, the overall 30-day event rate after CABG (including events during CAS) for minor stroke, major stroke, death, and death or any stroke was 2.9%, 3.6%, 7.6%, and 12.3%, respectively. Although it is accepted that cerebral revascularization should take place before coronary revascularization unless it is a true emergency, future studies are necessary to clarify which carotid revascularization strategy is superior.

Nutrition

Preoperative assessment of nutritional status and body mass index (BMI) can identify patients at higher risk for cardiac surgery. Low BMI (<20 kg/m^2) and hypoalbuminemia (<2.5 g/dL) are predictors of increased mortality, postoperative RF, HLOS, and prolonged ventilatory support following CABG.[55,56] In malnourished patients undergoing elective cardiac surgery, nutritional status should be optimized before operation, if possible.

Obese patients undergoing cardiac surgery have increased incidence of infection of the sternal wound and saphenous vein graft harvest site, RF, prolonged ventilation, and HLOS.[56,57] Obesity and obstructive sleep apnea are independent risk factors for developing AF.[58] Obesity and the metabolic syndrome are associated with a higher risk of developing AF after CABG in patients older than 50 years and 50 years and under, respectively.[59] If clinically appropriate, cardiac surgery may be delayed while efforts at weight loss are attempted.

MEDICATIONS

After risk stratification is completed, the final phase of preoperative evaluation focuses on patient preparation to minimize complications. Perioperative medical therapy improves outcomes in patients undergoing noncardiac and cardiac surgery.[9,60–73] However, despite the potential benefit, these medications are likely underutilized in clinical practice. In patients undergoing CABG, Filion and colleagues[74] noted preoperative aspirin, β-blocker, ACEI, and statin use was 41.4%, 52.4%, 33.4%, and 30%, respectively. On the day of surgery, aspirin use remained stable at 43%, but β-blocker, ACEI, and statin use declined to 42.9%, 8.9%, and 8.9%, respectively. Cardiac surgical patients are also frequently exposed to a variety of antiplatelet agents and anticoagulants, which can potentiate surgical bleeding. Current medical therapy should be reviewed for all patients, keeping in mind which medications should be initiated, continued, and stopped before surgery.

Antiplatelet Therapy

Aspirin, plavix, and glycoprotein (GP) IIB/IIIA inhibitors are beneficial in the management of acute coronary syndrome and during percutaneous coronary intervention (PCI).[75] Early (<6 hours) postoperative administration of aspirin is associated with a reduced risk of saphenous vein graft thrombosis, mortality, MI, stroke, RF, and bowel infarction.[64,68] Preoperative use of aspirin is associated with an increased risk for postoperative bleeding and need for transfusion.[76] Concomitant use of other antiplatelet agents and anticoagulants and certain disease states (eg, aspirin hyperresponders, thrombocytopenia, and renal disease) may potentiate the bleeding risk of aspirin. The preoperative use of clopidogrel in the presence or absence of aspirin in patients undergoing CABG is associated with increased postoperative bleeding, transfusions, and reoperations.[77] In urgent or emergent CABG, aspirin administration should be continued or initiated in the preoperative period as the benefits outweigh the risk of bleeding. In elective CABG, the Society of Thoracic Surgeons (STS) and ACC/AHA recommend that it is reasonable to consider withholding aspirin before surgery for 3 to 5 days or 7 to 10 days, respectively. Aspirin should be resumed within 6 hours of a surgical revascularization procedure if there are no contraindications.[3,78] Clopidogrel should be stopped 5 to 7 days before CABG.[3,75,78]

Eptifibatide and tirofiban are short-acting GP IIB/IIIA inhibitors, and should be discontinued 4 to 6 hours before cardiac surgery. Abciximab is a longer-acting agent, and should be discontinued 12 to 24 hours before surgery.[75,78] After administration, there is little free abciximab circulating in the plasma but large quantities of eptifibatide and tirofiban. Platelet transfusion is an effective strategy to increase the circulating platelet population with available GP IIB/IIIA inhibitors for abciximab but not for eptifibatide and tirofiban.

Anticoagulant Therapy

UFH, LMWH, fondaparinux, and direct thrombin inhibitors are beneficial in the management of acute coronary syndromes and during PCI, and are used for prophylactic and therapeutic anticoagulation.[75] UFH has not been shown to increase postoperative blood loss after cardiac surgery when discontinued shortly before operation. Preoperative LMWH and fondaparinux administration are associated with increased bleeding, and based on expert opinion, LMWH and fondaparinux should be discontinued 24 hours before surgery and replaced with UFH (if anticoagulation is indicated).[75,78] There are limited data regarding the safety of preoperative administration of direct thrombin inhibitors before CABG. Bivalirudin, a short-acting direct thrombin inhibitor, should be discontinued 3 hours before surgery. Hirudin and argatroban, longer-acting agents, should be stopped earlier than bivalirudin and replaced with UFH before cardiac surgery.[75,78] Warfarin should be stopped at least 5 days before cardiac surgery to allow normalization of the INR.[23] If continued therapeutic anticoagulation is necessary, UFH or LMWH may be initiated preoperatively.

β-Blocker Therapy

β-Blocker therapy improves acute and long-term outcomes for patients with ischemic heart disease.[75,79] In addition, in high-risk patients undergoing major noncardiac and vascular therapy, β-blocker therapy reduces the rate of cardiovascular events.[60,62] There has been cautious extension of their application to cardiac surgical patients due to concerns regarding their negative inotropic effects and possible exacerbation of underlying reactive airway disease. Nearly 40% of patients undergoing CABG do not receive preoperative β-blocker therapy, and patients with higher-risk features (eg, DM, CHF, underlying lung disease, and older age) are less likely to be treated with β-blocker therapy. Preoperative β-blocker therapy is associated with a statistically significant lower rate of 30-day mortality. Although a similar effect is seen in women, the elderly, and patients with chronic lung disease, DM, or moderately depressed LV function during subgroup analysis, a trend toward higher mortality is present in patients with a LVEF less than 30%.[65]

β-Blocker therapy has also been shown to reduce the incidence of postoperative AF when administered pre-[66] and postoperatively.[9] Perioperative interruption of long-term β-blocker therapy increases susceptibility to postoperative arrhythmias.[6] In addition to lowering the incidence of AF, β-blocker therapy is associated with reduced risk of postoperative neurologic complications.[67] The ACC/AHA recommends the use of preoperative or early postoperative β-blocker therapy in patients undergoing cardiac surgery without contraindications to its use.[3]

Sotalol has β-blocker and class III antiarrhythmic drug effects. Sotalol has been found to be more effective in reducing the incidence of postoperative AF than β-blocker therapy[69] but its use is associated with more postoperative bradyarrhythmias and hypotension.[80] The ACC/AHA recommends that low-dose sotalol can be considered in patients who are not candidates for traditional β-blocker therapy to lower the incidence of postoperative AF.[3]

ACEI or Angiotensin-II Receptor Blocker Therapy

ACEI or angiotensin-II receptor blocker (ARB) therapy reduces the risk of developing AF, particularly in patients with systolic dysfunction or LV hypertrophy.[81] In patients undergoing CABG, postoperative withdrawal of ACEI therapy is associated with an increased incidence of new onset and recurrent AF, and perioperative treatment with ACEI is associated with a reduced risk of AF.[6] In an underpowered study of cardiac surgical patients, preoperative ACEI or ARB therapy was associated with a nearly 30% lower risk of developing AF, but this reduction was not statistically significant.[63] In addition, treatment with quinapril for 4 weeks preoperatively and 1 year postoperatively in patients undergoing CABG reduced clinical ischemic events.[70] The antiinflammatory properties of ACEI or ARB therapy likely contribute to these cardioprotective effects.[82] However, preoperative administration of ACEI or ARB therapy may increase the perioperative requirement for vasopressor drug administration.[83] Although there are no specific guidelines, it is probably reasonable to continue preoperative ACEI or ARB therapy in patients with underlying hypertension given their potential benefits but consider withholding therapy in patients with marginal blood pressure.

Statins

Preoperative administration of 3-hydroxy-3-methylglutaryl coenzyme A reductase inhibitor (statin) therapy in vascular and cardiac surgery is associated with 59% and 38% reductions in mortality, respectively.[61] Liakopoulos and colleagues[71] found that preoperative statin therapy in patients undergoing cardiac surgery was associated with a reduction in early all-cause mortality, AF, and stroke. Statin therapy may be protective through lipid-independent or pleiotropic effects including antiinflammatory, antithrombotic, and vasodilatory effects.[84,85] All patients undergoing cardiac surgery should receive statin therapy unless specifically contraindicated.[3]

Amiodarone

Preoperative administration of amiodarone is an effective, well-tolerated therapy for prevention of postoperative AF.[72] In the PAPABEAR trial, a 13-day perioperative course of oral amiodarone in patients undergoing cardiac surgery significantly reduced the overall incidence of atrial tachyarrhythmias regardless of concomitant preoperative β-blocker therapy and postoperative sustained ventricular tachyarrhythmias.[72] A single-day, preoperative loading dose of oral amiodarone did not reduce the incidence of postoperative AF in patients undergoing cardiac surgery.[86] Given that effective amiodarone prophylaxis requires a preoperative treatment period, loading protocols seem limited to elective cardiac surgery. Intravenous amiodarone given immediately after cardiac surgery is also effective in reducing the incidence of AF.[87] ACC/AHA guidelines recommend that preoperative administration of amiodarone should be considered for patients at high risk for developing AF with contraindications to β-blocker therapy.[3]

SUMMARY

Morbidity and mortality associated with cardiac surgery is significant to the patient and costly to the health care system. During preoperative evaluation, statistical risk models should be used to obtain objective estimates of operative mortality and morbidity. In patients with severe LV dysfunction, a cardiac imaging modality should be considered to help identify dysfunctional but viable myocardium. A recent MI, particularly if associated with LV thrombus formation or severe RV dysfunction, may prompt a delay in cardiac surgery. Patients at high risk for renal dysfunction need management strategies aimed at minimizing renal insults. Existing pulmonary conditions should be treated as best possible before initiation of mechanical ventilation. Carotid Doppler should be performed in patients at increased risk for coexistent carotid artery disease, and if significant carotid artery disease is present, CEA should be considered either before or concomitant with cardiac surgery. With regard to medical therapy, β-blocker, ACEI, and statin therapy should be used in the absence of contraindications, and amiodarone therapy instituted in patients at high risk for AF. Clopidogrel should be withheld 5 to 7 days before surgery, and the risk/benefit ratio of preoperative aspirin therapy assessed.

REFERENCES

1. Mangano DT. Cardiovascular morbidity and CABG surgery – a perspective: epidemiology, costs, and potential therapeutic solutions. J Cardiovasc Surg 1995;10:366–8.
2. Jones RH, Hannan EL, Hammermeister KE, et al. Identification of preoperative variables needed for risk adjustment of short-term mortality after coronary artery bypass graft surgery. The Working Group Panel on the Cooperative CABG Database Project. J Am Coll Cardiol 1996;28:1478–87.
3. Eagle KA, Guyton RA, Davidoff R, et al. ACC/AHA 2004 guideline update for coronary artery bypass graft surgery: a report of the American College of Cardiology/American Heart Association Task Force on Practice Guidelines (Committee to Update the 1999 Guidelines for Coronary Artery Bypass Graft Surgery). Circulation 2004;110:e340–437.
4. Albert MA. HNAE: preoperative evaluation for cardiac surgery. In: Cohn LH, editor. Cardiac surgery in the adult. 3rd edition. New York: McGraw-Hill; 2008. p. 261–80.
5. Mitchell LB. Incidence, timing, and outcome of atrial tachyarrhythmias. In: Steinberg JS, editor. Atrial fibrillation after cardiac surgery. Boston (MA): Kluwer Academic Publishers; 2000. p. 37–50.
6. Mathew JP, Fontes ML, Tudor IC, et al. A multicenter risk index for atrial fibrillation after cardiac surgery. JAMA 2004;291:1720–9.
7. Almassi GH, Schowalter T, Nicolosi AC, et al. Atrial fibrillation after cardiac surgery: a major morbid event? Ann Surg 1997;226:501–11.
8. Echahidi N, Pibarot P, O'Hara G, et al. Mechanisms, prevention, and treatment of atrial fibrillation after cardiac surgery. J Am Coll Cardiol 2008;51:793–801.
9. Andrews TC, Reimold SC, Berlin JA, et al. Prevention of supraventricular arrhythmias after coronary artery bypass surgery. A meta-analysis of randomized control trials. Circulation 1991;84:III236–44.
10. Alderman EL, Fisher LD, Litwin P, et al. Results of coronary artery surgery in patients with poor left ventricular function (CASS). Circulation 1983;68:785–95.
11. Topkara VK, Cheema FH, Kesavaramanujam S, et al. Coronary artery bypass grafting in patients with low ejection fraction. Circulation 2005;112:I344–50.
12. Christenson JT, Simonet F, Badel P, et al. Evaluation of preoperative intra-aortic balloon pump support in high risk coronary patients. Eur J Cardiothorac Surg 1997;11:1097–103.
13. Di Carli MF, Asgarzadie F, Schelbert HR, et al. Quantitative relation between myocardial viability and improvement in heart failure symptoms after revascularization in patients with ischemic cardiomyopathy. Circulation 1995;92:3436–44.
14. Bax JJ, Wijns W, Cornel JH, et al. Accuracy of currently available techniques for prediction of functional recovery after revascularization in patients with left ventricular dysfunction due to chronic coronary artery disease: comparison of pooled data. J Am Coll Cardiol 1997;30:1451–60.
15. Baer FM, Theissen P, Schneider CA, et al. Dobutamine magnetic resonance imaging predicts contractile recovery of chronically dysfunctional myocardium after successful revascularization. J Am Coll Cardiol 1998;31:1040–8.
16. Braxton JH, Hammond GL, Letsou GV, et al. Optimal timing of coronary artery bypass graft surgery after acute myocardial infarction. Circulation 1995;92:II66–8.
17. Kulier A, Levin J, Moser R, et al. Impact of preoperative anemia on outcome in patients undergoing coronary artery bypass graft surgery. Circulation 2007; 116:471–9.

18. Murphy GJ, Reeves BC, Rogers CA, et al. Increased mortality, postoperative morbidity, and cost after red blood cell transfusion in patients having cardiac surgery. Circulation 2007;116:2544–52.

19. Warkentin TE, Greinacher A, Koster A, et al. Treatment and prevention of heparin-induced thrombocytopenia: American College of Chest Physicians Evidence-Based Clinical Practice Guidelines (8th Edition). Chest 2008;133:340S–80S.

20. Everett BM, Yeh R, Foo SY, et al. Prevalence of heparin/platelet factor 4 antibodies before and after cardiac surgery. Ann Thorac Surg 2007;83:592–7.

21. Liu JC, Lewis BE, Steen LH, et al. Patency of coronary artery bypass grafts in patients with heparin-induced thrombocytopenia. Am J Correct 2002;89:979–81.

22. Kearon C, Crowther M, Hirsh J. Management of patients with hereditary hypercoagulable disorders. Annu Rev Microbiol 2000;51:169–85.

23. Dunning J, Versteegh M, Fabbri A, et al. Guideline on antiplatelet and anticoagulation management in cardiac surgery. Eur J Cardiothorac Surg 2008;34:73–92.

24. Hogan WJ, McBane RD, Santrach PJ, et al. Antiphospholipid syndrome and perioperative hemostatic management of cardiac valvular surgery. Mayo Clin Proc 2000;75:971–6.

25. Cooper WA, O'Brien SM, Thourani VH, et al. Impact of renal dysfunction on outcomes of coronary artery bypass surgery: results from the Society of Thoracic Surgeons National Adult Cardiac Database. Circulation 2006;113:1063–70.

26. Thakar CV, Worley S, Arrigain S, et al. Influence of renal dysfunction on mortality after cardiac surgery: modifying effect of preoperative renal function. Kidney Int 2005;67:1112–9.

27. Wang F, Dupuis JY, Nathan H, et al. An analysis of the association between preoperative renal dysfunction and outcome in cardiac surgery: estimated creatinine clearance or plasma creatinine level as measures of renal function. Chest 2003;124:1852–62.

28. Mangano CM, Diamondstone LS, Ramsay JG, et al. Renal dysfunction after myocardial revascularization: risk factors, adverse outcomes, and hospital resource utilization. The Multicenter Study of Perioperative Ischemia Research Group. Ann Intern Med 1998;128:194–203.

29. Ranucci M, Ballotta A, Kunkl A, et al. Influence of the timing of cardiac catheterization and the amount of contrast media on acute renal failure after cardiac surgery. Am J Cardiol 2008;101:1112–8.

30. Mehta RH, Grab JD, O'Brien SM, et al. Bedside tool for predicting the risk of postoperative dialysis in patients undergoing cardiac surgery. Circulation 2006;114:2208–16.

31. Burns KE, Chu MW, Novick RJ, et al. Perioperative N-acetylcysteine to prevent renal dysfunction in high-risk patients undergoing CABG surgery: a randomized controlled trial. JAMA 2005;294:342–50.

32. Charlesworth DC, Likosky DS, Marrin CA, et al. Development and validation of a prediction model for strokes after coronary artery bypass grafting. Ann Thorac Surg 2003;76:436–43.

33. Leavitt BJ, Sheppard L, Maloney C, et al. Effect of diabetes and associated conditions on long-term survival after coronary artery bypass graft surgery. Circulation 2004;110:II41–4.

34. Lauruschkat AH, Arnrich B, Albert AA, et al. Prevalence and risks of undiagnosed diabetes mellitus in patients undergoing coronary artery bypass grafting. Circulation 2005;112:2397–402.

35. Furnary AP, Zerr KJ, Grunkemeier GL, et al. Continuous intravenous insulin infusion reduces the incidence of deep sternal wound infection in diabetic patients after cardiac surgical procedures. Ann Thorac Surg 1999;67:352–60.

36. Furnary AP, Gao G, Grunkemeier GL, et al. Continuous insulin infusion reduces mortality in patients with diabetes undergoing coronary artery bypass grafting. J Thorac Cardiovasc Surg 2003;125:1007–21.

37. Albacker T, Carvalho G, Schricker T, et al. High-dose insulin therapy attenuates systemic inflammatory response in coronary artery bypass grafting patients. Ann Thorac Surg 2008;86:20–7.

38. Cohen A, Katz M, Katz R, et al. Chronic obstructive pulmonary disease in patients undergoing coronary artery bypass grafting. J Thorac Cardiovasc Surg 1995; 109:574–81.

39. Fuster RG, Argudo JA, Albarova OG, et al. Prognostic value of chronic obstructive pulmonary disease in coronary artery bypass grafting. Eur J Cardiothorac Surg 2006;29:202–9.

40. Spivack SD, Shinozaki T, Albertini JJ, et al. Preoperative prediction of postoperative respiratory outcome. Coronary artery bypass grafting. Chest 1996;109: 1222–30.

41. Filsoufi F, Rahmanian PB, Castillo JG, et al. Predictors and early and late outcomes of respiratory failure in contemporary cardiac surgery. Chest 2008; 133:713–21.

42. Hulzebos EH, Helders PJ, Favie NJ, et al. Preoperative intensive inspiratory muscle training to prevent postoperative pulmonary complications in high-risk patients undergoing CABG surgery: a randomized clinical trial. JAMA 2006; 296:1851–7.

43. Boeken U, Litmathe J, Feindt P, et al. Neurological complications after cardiac surgery: risk factors and correlation to the surgical procedure. Thorac Cardiovasc Surg 2005;53:33–6.

44. Shaw PJ, Bates D, Cartlidge NE, et al. Neurologic and neuropsychological morbidity following major surgery: comparison of coronary artery bypass and peripheral vascular surgery. Stroke 1987;18:700–7.

45. Roach GW, Kanchuger M, Mangano CM, et al. Adverse cerebral outcomes after coronary bypass surgery. Multicenter Study of Perioperative Ischemia Research Group and the Ischemia Research and Education Foundation Investigators. N Engl J Med 1996;335:1857–63.

46. Gardner TJ, Horneffer PJ, Manolio TA, et al. Stroke following coronary artery bypass grafting: a ten-year study. Ann Thorac Surg 1985;40:574–81.

47. Schwartz LB, Bridgman AH, Kieffer RW, et al. Asymptomatic carotid artery stenosis and stroke in patients undergoing cardiopulmonary bypass. J Vasc Surg 1995;21:146–53.

48. Berens ES, Kouchoukos NT, Murphy SF, et al. Preoperative carotid artery screening in elderly patients undergoing cardiac surgery. J Vasc Surg 1992;15: 313–21.

49. D'Agostino RS, Svensson LG, Neumann DJ, et al. Screening carotid ultrasonography and risk factors for stroke in coronary artery surgery patients. Ann Thorac Surg 1996;62:1714–23.

50. Salasidis GC, Latter DA, Steinmetz OK, et al. Carotid artery duplex scanning in preoperative assessment for coronary artery revascularization: the association between peripheral vascular disease, carotid artery stenosis, and stroke. J Vasc Surg 1995;21:154–60.

51. Wareing TH, Davila-Roman VG, Daily BB, et al. Strategy for the reduction of stroke incidence in cardiac surgical patients. Ann Thorac Surg 1993;55:1400–7.

52. Faggioli GL, Curl GR, Ricotta JJ. The role of carotid screening before coronary artery bypass. J Vasc Surg 1990;12:724–9.

53. Naylor AR, Cuffe RL, Rothwell PM, et al. A systematic review of outcomes following staged and synchronous carotid endarterectomy and coronary artery bypass. Eur J Vasc Endovasc Surg 2003;25:380–9.

54. Guzman LA, Costa MA, Angiolillo DJ, et al. A systematic review of outcomes in patients with staged carotid artery stenting and coronary artery bypass graft surgery. Stroke 2008;39:361–5.

55. Reeves BC, Ascione R, Chamberlain MH, et al. Effect of body mass index on early outcomes in patients undergoing coronary artery bypass surgery. J Am Coll Cardiol 2003;42:668–76.

56. Engelman DT, Adams DH, Byrne JG, et al. Impact of body mass index and albumin on morbidity and mortality after cardiac surgery. J Thorac Cardiovasc Surg 1999;118:866–73.

57. Wigfield CH, Lindsey JD, Munoz A, et al. Is extreme obesity a risk factor for cardiac surgery? An analysis of patients with a BMI > or = 40. Eur J Cardiothorac Surg 2006;29:434–40.

58. Gami AS, Hodge DO, Herges RM, et al. Obstructive sleep apnea, obesity, and the risk of incident atrial fibrillation. J Am Coll Cardiol 2007;49:565–71.

59. Echahidi N, Mohty D, Pibarot P, et al. Obesity and metabolic syndrome are independent risk factors for atrial fibrillation after coronary artery bypass graft surgery. Circulation 2007;116:I213–9.

60. Mangano DT, Layug EL, Wallace A, et al. Effect of atenolol on mortality and cardiovascular morbidity after noncardiac surgery. Multicenter Study of Perioperative Ischemia Research Group. N Engl J Med 1996;335:1713–20.

61. Hindler K, Shaw AD, Samuels J, et al. Improved postoperative outcomes associated with preoperative statin therapy. Anesthesiology 2006;105:1260–72.

62. Poldermans D, Boersma E, Bax JJ, et al. The effect of bisoprolol on perioperative mortality and myocardial infarction in high-risk patients undergoing vascular surgery. Dutch Echocardiographic Cardiac Risk Evaluation Applying Stress Echocardiography Study Group. N Engl J Med 1999;341:1789–94.

63. White CM, Kluger J, Lertsburapa K, et al. Effect of preoperative angiotensin converting enzyme inhibitor or angiotensin receptor blocker use on the frequency of atrial fibrillation after cardiac surgery: a cohort study from the atrial fibrillation suppression trials II and III. Eur J Cardiothorac Surg 2007;31:817–20.

64. Mangano DT. Aspirin and mortality from coronary bypass surgery. N Engl J Med 2002;347:1309–17.

65. Ferguson TB Jr, Coombs LP, Peterson ED. Preoperative beta-blocker use and mortality and morbidity following CABG surgery in North America. JAMA 2002; 287:2221–7.

66. Lamb RK, Prabhakar G, Thorpe JA, et al. The use of atenolol in the prevention of supraventricular arrhythmias following coronary artery surgery. Eur Heart J 1988; 9:32–6.

67. Amory DW, Grigore A, Amory JK, et al. Neuroprotection is associated with beta-adrenergic receptor antagonists during cardiac surgery: evidence from 2,575 patients. J Cardiothorac Vasc Anesth 2002;16:270–7.

68. Stein PD, Schunemann HJ, Dalen JE, et al. Antithrombotic therapy in patients with saphenous vein and internal mammary artery bypass grafts: the Seventh ACCP Conference on Antithrombotic and Thrombolytic Therapy. Chest 2004;126:600S–8S.

69. Burgess DC, Kilborn MJ, Keech AC. Interventions for prevention of post-operative atrial fibrillation and its complications after cardiac surgery: a meta-analysis. Eur Heart J 2006;27:2846–57.

70. Oosterga M, Voors AA, Pinto YM, et al. Effects of quinapril on clinical outcome after coronary artery bypass grafting (The QUO VADIS Study). QUinapril on Vascular Ace and Determinants of Ischemia. Am J Cardiol 2001;87:542–6.
71. Liakopoulos OJ, Choi YH, Haldenwang PL, et al. Impact of preoperative statin therapy on adverse postoperative outcomes in patients undergoing cardiac surgery: a meta-analysis of over 30,000 patients. Eur Heart J 2008;29: 1548–59.
72. Mitchell LB, Exner DV, Wyse DG, et al. Prophylactic oral amiodarone for the prevention of arrhythmias that begin early after revascularization, valve replacement, or repair: PAPABEAR: a randomized controlled trial. JAMA 2005;294: 3093–100.
73. Daoud EG, Strickberger SA, Man KC, et al. Preoperative amiodarone as prophylaxis against atrial fibrillation after heart surgery. N Engl J Med 1997;337:1785–91.
74. Filion KB, Pilote L, Rahme E, et al. Use of perioperative cardiac medical therapy among patients undergoing coronary artery bypass graft surgery. J Cardiovasc Surg 2008;23:209–15.
75. Anderson JL, Adams CD, Antman EM, et al. ACC/AHA 2007 guidelines for the management of patients with unstable angina/non ST-elevation myocardial infarction: a report of the American College of Cardiology/American Heart Association Task Force on Practice Guidelines (Writing Committee to Revise the 2002 Guidelines for the Management of Patients With Unstable Angina/Non ST-Elevation Myocardial Infarction): developed in collaboration with the American College of Emergency Physicians, the Society for Cardiovascular Angiography and Interventions, and the Society of Thoracic Surgeons: endorsed by the American Association of Cardiovascular and Pulmonary Rehabilitation and the Society for Academic Emergency Medicine. Circulation 2007;116:e148–304.
76. Sethi GK, Copeland JG, Goldman S, et al. Implications of preoperative administration of aspirin in patients undergoing coronary artery bypass grafting. Department of Veterans Affairs Cooperative Study on Antiplatelet Therapy. J Am Coll Cardiol 1990;15:15–20.
77. Hongo RH, Ley J, Dick SE, et al. The effect of clopidogrel in combination with aspirin when given before coronary artery bypass grafting. J Am Coll Cardiol 2002;40:231–7.
78. Ferraris VA, Ferraris SP, Moliterno DJ, et al. The Society of Thoracic Surgeons practice guideline series: aspirin and other antiplatelet agents during operative coronary revascularization (executive summary). Ann Thorac Surg 2005;79: 1454–61.
79. Hunt SA, Abraham WT, Chin MH, et al. ACC/AHA 2005 Guideline Update for the Diagnosis and Management of Chronic Heart Failure in the Adult: a report of the American College of Cardiology/American Heart Association Task Force on Practice Guidelines (Writing Committee to Update the 2001 Guidelines for the Evaluation and Management of Heart Failure): developed in collaboration with the American College of Chest Physicians and the International Society for Heart and Lung Transplantation: endorsed by the Heart Rhythm Society. Circulation 2005;112:e154–235.
80. Nystrom U, Edvardsson N, Berggren H, et al. Oral sotalol reduces the incidence of atrial fibrillation after coronary artery bypass surgery. Thorac Cardiovasc Surg 1993;41:34–7.
81. Healey JS, Baranchuk A, Crystal E, et al. Prevention of atrial fibrillation with angiotensin-converting enzyme inhibitors and angiotensin receptor blockers: a meta-analysis. J Am Coll Cardiol 2005;45:1832–9.

82. Brull DJ, Sanders J, Rumley A, et al. Impact of angiotensin converting enzyme inhibition on post-coronary artery bypass interleukin 6 release. Heart 2002;87: 252–5.
83. Raja SG, Fida N. Should angiotensin converting enzyme inhibitors/angiotensin II receptor antagonists be omitted before cardiac surgery to avoid postoperative vasodilation? Interact Cardiovasc Thorac Surg 2008;7:470–5.
84. Ray KK, Cannon CP. The potential relevance of the multiple lipid-independent (pleiotropic) effects of statins in the management of acute coronary syndromes. J Am Coll Cardiol 2005;46:1425–33.
85. Le Manach Y, Coriat P, Collard CD, et al. Statin therapy within the perioperative period. Anesthesiology 2008;108:1141–6.
86. Maras D, Boskovic SD, Popovic Z, et al. Single-day loading dose of oral amiodarone for the prevention of new-onset atrial fibrillation after coronary artery bypass surgery. Am Heart J 2001;141:E8.
87. Guarnieri T, Nolan S, Gottlieb SO, et al. Intravenous amiodarone for the prevention of atrial fibrillation after open heart surgery: the Amiodarone Reduction in Coronary Heart (ARCH) trial. J Am Coll Cardiol 1999;34:343–7.

Noncardiac Surgery in the Patient with Heart Disease

James B. Froehlich, MD, MPH[a],*, Lee A. Fleisher, MD[b]

KEYWORDS

• Perioperative • Pre-operative • Risk • Surgery

THE SHAPE OF PREOPERATIVE RISK ASSESSMENT

The clinical question of preoperative assessment for cardiac risk continues to be a vexing one for many clinicians, surgeons, and their patients despite the significant number of studies and guidelines that have been published to aid in the assessment of perioperative risk. More importantly, clinicians are increasingly asked what they can do to lower the risk of perioperative cardiac complications.

Perioperative risk assessment has gone through a significant evolution in the last few years. Beginning approximately 4 decades ago, there were few tools available to clinicians to guide the evaluation of perioperative risk. The American Society of Anesthesiology Classification System (ASA class) is an extremely crude tool and gave clinicians only the vaguest idea what sort of risk their patients faced during surgery. This system left most patients no better informed about their risks of surgery (**Box 1**). The more modern era of clinical risk assessment for perioperative complications began with the work of Lee Goldman at the Massachusetts General Hospital.[1] He identified factors associated with increased risk for perioperative cardiac complications among patients referred for preoperative evaluation. This approach represented the first time that a scientific effort was made to identify predictors of risk for perioperative cardiac complications. This work was followed by similar studies by Drs Eagle and Detsky,[2,3] who identified clinical factors associated with increased risk of cardiac complications during surgery. With these tools, clinicians could estimate risk, and providing surgeons and patients with important decision-making information.

The next significant advance in preoperative evaluation was the addition of stress testing in the form of treadmill exercise, treadmill thallium, and adenosine thallium testing. Subsequently, dobutamine stress and exercise stress echocardiography

[a] Department of Medicine, CVC Cardiovascular Medicine, University of Michigan Medical School, 1500 E. Medical Center Drive SPC 5853, Ann Arbor, Michigan 48109, USA
[b] University of Pennsylvania Health System, Department of Anesthesia, University of Pennsylvania School of Medicine, Philadelphia, PA 19104, USA
* Corresponding author.
E-mail address: jfroehli@umich.edu (J.B. Froehlich).

Med Clin N Am 93 (2009) 995–1016
doi:10.1016/j.mcna.2009.05.012   medical.theclinics.com
0025-7125/09/$ – see front matter © 2009 Elsevier Inc. All rights reserved.

were also added to tools for assessing perioperative risk. None of these tests, however, were designed to identify perioperative cardiac risk. Nonetheless, abnormalities on stress testing did show an association with perioperative cardiac risk. Combining stress testing with clinical evaluation proved to further refine the accuracy of perioperative risk assessment, and formed the basis of the American College of Cardiology (ACC)/American Heart Association (AHA) guidelines for assessing perioperative risk.[4]

Compared with the tremendous progress made in the treatment of acute and chronic coronary disease over the last 3 decades, little attention has been paid to interventions to decrease perioperative cardiac event rate. Only in the last 10 or 15 years have options to reduce perioperative risk been explored. Although operative and anesthetic techniques have improved significantly, thus decreasing perioperative cardiac event rates, operative mortality remains significant, especially among high-risk patients or those undergoing high-risk surgery. In addition, cardiac disease remains the leading cause of mortality in men and women, so cardiac risk assessment and prevention of cardiovascular events should be a high priority of any patient-physician encounter, including perioperative risk assessment.

This article reviews the literature of perioperative risk assessment and risk reduction in patients with cardiac disease. Testing modalities are reviewed with particular attention to what stress testing does (predicting perioperative risk versus finding coronary disease), which patients warrant stress testing, and what to do with the results. This article also reviews the role of perioperative angioplasty in light of recent studies, preoperative coronary angiography, and the current ACC/AHA guidelines.

PREOPERATIVE RISK ASSESSMENT IN THE LITERATURE

In decades past, the only classification system available to clinicians to stratify risk for their patients undergoing surgery was that used by the American Society of Anesthesiology. In this system, patients were given a score of between 1 and 5 (see **Box 1**). A patient received a 1 if they were "normal and healthy". Any patient with any systemic disease of any severity would be given a score of 2. Obviously, this could cover an extremely wide range from mere presence of mild hypertension up to and including diabetes or other systemic disease that significantly increased risk of perioperative events. Patients would only receive a score of 3 if they had systemic disease that limited activity. Patients were given a 4 if they were at constant threat of losing their life and 5 if they were not expected to survive 24 hours with or without any treatment.

Perhaps the biggest problem with this classification system was that almost every patient was a 2. Those with a score of 3, 4, or 5 were obviously at severe risk and

---

Box 1
ASA classification

1. Normal healthy patient

2. Mild systemic disease

3. Severe systemic disease that limits activity

4. Incapacitating systemic disease that is a constant threat to life

5. Moribund patient not expected to survive >24 hours, with or without operation

Data from American Society of Anesthesiology. New classification of physical status. Anesthesiology 1963;24:111.

patients with a score of 1 or 2 had an extremely wide range of risk. Therefore, the scoring system offered little information to the patient, surgeon, or the general care giver, to estimate the risk they faced during surgery.

The first attempt at a scientific quantification of risk during surgery in the modern era was performed by Lee Goldman at Massachusetts General Hospital. Reviewing the extensive medical records of 1001 patients who were referred for preoperative risk assessment, Dr Goldman and colleagues collected a wide range of demographic and clinical variables based mostly on the patient's history and examination.[1] A multivariable regression analysis identified those factors that were most strongly associated with subsequent perioperative cardiac complications. By doing so, Goldman and colleagues identified the risk factors most strongly associated with cardiac events, among which are active heart failure, recent myocardial infarction, severe or malignant arrhythmias, and aortic stenosis, or severe underlying comorbid medical disease. The Goldman investigators weighted each of the factors they identified that were associated with perioperative cardiac events, based on the strength of that association. These weights were then used to create a scoring system to identify the severity of risk. The resulting score was associated with the likelihood of subsequent perioperative cardiac complications (**Table 1**).

Subsequent studies refined this approach with further analysis in other patient groups. By evaluating patients at higher risk, such as those undergoing vascular surgery (who experience more perioperative cardiac events, therefore making it easier to identify predictors of risk retrospectively), Dr Eagle and colleagues identified 5 factors most strongly associated with subsequent perioperative cardiac events.[3] The 5 factors identified by these investigators were increased age, presence of diabetes requiring treatment, history of angina, a history of myocardial infarction (MI) or Q-waves on EKG, as well as a history of heart failure or a finding of heart failure on examination. This evaluation included symptoms as well as findings on medical history and physical examination. They showed an association between the presence of these factors and the likelihood of suffering a perioperative cardiac complication or death (**Table 2**) These investigators then went on to combine the clinical-risk evaluation with stress testing to further stratify risk. The role of stress testing is discussed later in this article.

More recently, a derivation and validation of perioperative cardiac risk assessment was performed by Lee and colleagues.[5] Evaluating patients who underwent noncardiac surgery, these investigators identified 6 factors that were associated with an increased rate of perioperative complications. For the first time, these investigators identified renal failure as a strong predictor of perioperative cardiac risk, and also identified the type of surgery in this analysis. Their subsequent validation study demonstrated that these 6 risk factors (including type of surgery, history of coronary

Table 1			
Complications and death during surgery according to Goldman risk score			
Risk Group (n)	Score	Complications (%)	Death (%)
I (537)	0–5	4 (0.7)	1 (0.2)
II (316)	6–12	16 (5)	5 (2)
III (130)	13–25	15 (12)	3 (2)
IV (18)	>25	4 (22)	10 (56)

Data from Goldman L, et al. Multifactorial index of cardiac risk in noncardiac surgical procedures. N Engl J Med 1977;297(16):845–50.

Table 2
Association between clinical markers of risk and rate of perioperative death or MI

Clinical Markers	Clinical Risk Groups Based on Number of Markers	Perioperative MI or Death (%)
• Age >70 y • Diabetes • Prior angina • MI by history or ECG (Q-waves) • Congestive heart failure	Low risk (no clinical markers) Intermediate risk (1 or 2 markers) High risk (≥3 markers)	3 8 18

Data from L'Italien GJ, et al. Development and validation of a Bayesian model for perioperative cardiac risk assessment in a cohort of 1,081 vascular surgical candidates. J Am Coll Cardiol 1996;27(4):779–86.

disease in any form, history of heart failure, history of cerebral vascular disease, diabetes, or renal failure with creatinine > 2.0 mg/dL) were each associated with a 2 to 3-fold increased risk in perioperative cardiac events (**Table 3**).

There are at least 2 things that are highly instructive about these studies. First is that they allow the identification of high-risk patients through a simple clinical evaluation, which in many cases can accurately predict risk of perioperative cardiac events. A clinical evaluation, based on an accurate history and physical, inclusive of exercise tolerance and ECG evaluation, is a potent predictor of perioperative cardiac event risk. Second, it is also important to note that all of these investigators found similar results in terms of the predictors of risk. A history of heart disease, other vascular disease, diabetes, and heart failure are logical associates of perioperative cardiac risk, and were identified as such by several investigators. It is also highly instructive to note what clinical factors were not found by any of these investigators. For example, none of the investigators reported that hypertension, a family history of coronary disease, tobacco use, or hypercholesterolemia were associated with perioperative risk of cardiac events. These are known to be risk factors for the development of coronary disease and strongly associated in populations with the development of coronary disease, but not, apparently, associated with the risk of perioperative cardiac events. It may be that prediction of perioperative cardiac events has less to do with finding coronary disease than with finding patients whose coronary disease is likely to become unstable with the stress of surgery. It is this conundrum, the identification of patients with potentially unstable coronary disease versus stable coronary disease,

Table 3
Revised cardiac risk index: factors associated with major cardiac complications

	Derivation Set, n = 2893 (%)	
	Crude Data	Adjusted or (95%) CI
Revised cardiac risk index		
1. High-risk type of surgery	27/894 (3)	2.8 (1.6, 4.9)
2. Ischemic heart disease	34/951 (4)	2.4 (1.3, 4.2)
3. History of congestive heart disease	23/434 (5)	1.9 (1.1, 3.5)
4. History of cerebrovascular disease	17/291 (6)	3.2 (1.8, 6.0)
5. Insulin therapy for diabetes	7/112 (6)	3.0 (1.3, 7.1)
6. Preoperative serum creatinine > 2.0 mg/dL	9/103 (9)	3.0 (1.4, 6.8)

Data from Lee TH, et al. Derivation and prospective validation of a simple index for prediction of cardiac risk of major noncardiac surgery. Circulation 1999;100(10):1043–9.

that may cause perioperative risk assessment to be such a vexing problem. The identification of patients with coronary disease may be a far easier task than identifying those with unstable or potentially unstable disease. This realization brings us to the subject of stress testing.

WHAT DO STRESS TESTS TELL US?

Practically since their development, stress tests (diagnostic and evaluative tests for coronary disease) have been applied to the clinical question of assessing perioperative risk. It is important to note how and why these tests were developed, however, as well as whether they should be applied to this use. Most stress tests were designed to diagnose coronary disease, not predict events. Most stress tests represent different ways to find coronary ischemia. Coronary ischemia is the result of hemodynamically significant atherosclerotic plaque, in most cases. Ischemia is not necessarily related to the stability of the plaque, but rather the degree of stenosis caused by the plaque. It is now generally believed that acute coronary syndromes are the result of plaque instability, plaque rupture, or coronary thrombosis. Stress tests may or may not predict which lesions are in fact unstable, and therefore may not be capable of predicting cardiac events, most of which are believed to be due to plaque instability.

A review of studies evaluating the performance of stress testing in assessing perioperative cardiac risk suggests a striking homogeneity of results. Despite being performed with different patient populations and looking at patients undergoing a variety of surgical procedures, these studies show remarkably consistent results. As can be seen in **Table 4**, these studies suggest that perioperative thallium testing is highly predictive of subsequent perioperative cardiac events. Specifically, almost all the patients who suffered a perioperative cardiac event had abnormal stress-testing results. Most of these studies were therefore interpreted as showing that perioperative thallium testing is useful in predicting perioperative events. A closer analysis of the data, however, suggests these test results are of limited clinical usefulness. As can be seen in the table, those patients with a negative or normal result on thallium testing had a low likelihood of suffering perioperative events. The negative predictive value of a normal thallium test is high, which means that for the clinician assessing perioperative risk, the finding of a normal stress test suggests a patient can safely undergo surgery with almost no risk of perioperative cardiac event.

The problem for the clinician, however, comes with interpreting an abnormal test. Because only a minority of patients with an abnormal stress test subsequently suffered a perioperative cardiac event, the positive predictive value of an abnormal thallium test is extremely low. On average, taken from many studies, a positive predictive value of only about 12% was seen after thallium testing for the prediction of perioperative cardiac events (see **Table 4**). This finding means that, for the clinician, many patients with coronary disease will be identified by thallium testing; only a few of whom will suffer a subsequent perioperative cardiac event. This finding undoubtedly stems from thallium testing having been designed to identify ischemia, and therefore coronary disease, but not necessarily unstable coronary disease or coronary lesions that are prone to rupture and the creation of cardiac events.

Dobutamine stress echocardiography has also been shown to be highly effective in identifying the presence of coronary disease, but, as can been seen from **Table 5**, it suffers from the same problem as perioperative thallium testing; it effectively identifies patients who will be free of cardiac events, but only poorly identifies those who go on to have perioperative cardiac events. Dobutamine stress echocardiograms identify the presence of coronary disease but not necessarily the likelihood of a near-term

Table 4 Thallium stress testing for preoperative risk assessment			
	N	Positive Predictive Value (%)	Negative Predictive Value (%)
Boucher 1985	48	19	100
Cutler 1987	116	20	100
Fletcher 1988	67	20	100
Sachs 1988	46	14	100
Eagle 1989	200	16	98
McEnroe 1990	95	9	96
Younis 1990	111	15	100
Mangano 1991	60	5	95
Strawn 1991	68	6	100
Watters 1991	26	20	100
Hendel 1992	327	14	99
Lette 1992	355	17	99
Madsen 1992	65	11	100
Brown 1993	231	13	99
Kresowik 1993	170	4	98
Baron 1994	457	4	96
Bry 1994	237	11	100
Koutelo 1995	106	6	100
Marshall 1995	117	16	97
Van Damme 1997	142	n/a	n/a
Huang 1998	106	13	100
Cohen 2003	153	4	100
Total	3303	12	99

or perioperative cardiac event. Among published studies, an average positive predictive value of only 20% was found for patients with an abnormal dobutamine stress echo. Like thallium testing, a strong negative predictive value was found, suggesting that both of these testing modalities, when normal, accurately predict a relative freedom from perioperative cardiac events.

WHO NEEDS A STRESS TEST PREOPERATIVELY?

Increasingly, the important work of Thomas Bayes is ignored in clinical medicine. Thomas Bayes was a British Presbyterian minister and mathematician who formulated a specific case of what has come to be known as Bayes' Theorem, which was published posthumously.[6] During his lifetime, he published only 1 mathematical work; a defense of the logical foundations of Sir Isaac Newton's calculus. Posthumously, however, he published a solution to the problem of "inverse probability" which describes a special case of what has come to be known as Bayes' Theorem. Mathematically, and in terms of logic formulation, Bayes' Theorem looks something like this:

$$Pr(A|B) = \frac{Pr(B|A)Pr(A)}{Pr(B)} \alpha L(A|B)Pr(A)$$

$$f(x|y) = \frac{f(x,y)}{f(y)} = \frac{f(y|x)f(x)}{f(y)}$$

Table 5 Dobutamine echo stress testing for preoperative risk assessment			
	N	Positive Predictive Value (%)	Negative Predictive Value (%)
Lane 1991	38	16	100
Lalka 1992	60	23	93
Eichenberger 1993	75	7	100
Langan 1993	74	17	100
Poldermans 1993	131	14	100
Davina-Roman 1993	88	10	100
Poldermans 1993	302	24	100
Shafritz 1997	42	NA	97
Plotkin 1998	80	33	100
Ballal 1999	233	0	96
Bossone 1999	46	25	100
Das 2000	530	15	100
Boersna 2001	1097	14	98
Morgan 2002	78	0	100
Torres 2002	105	18	98
Labib 2004	429	9	98
Total	466	20	99

Data from Fleischer LA, Beckman JA, Brown KA, et al. ACC/AHA 2007 guidelines on perioperative cardiovascular evaluation and care for noncardiac surgery. J Am Coll Cardiol 2007;50; 159–241.

For the clinician, however, Bayes' Theorem posits that the probability of a specific diagnosis is related to the prior probability (pretest probability) and the likelihood (the population prevalence of the disease). By combining a knowledge of the prevalence of the disease with the patient's presentation, a likelihood of diagnosis can be ascertained, which is then further refined, rather than definitively "ruled in" or "ruled out", by the results of further testing.

For the preoperative evaluation of cardiovascular risk, therefore, it should be understood that stress testing provides only a further refinement of the clinically determined pretest probability. This limitation was illustrated in work by L'Italien and colleagues that demonstrated the relationship between clinical risk assessment and stress test results in determining perioperative cardiovascular risk.[7] In a large population of 1081 subjects who underwent clinical preoperative evaluation, as well as preoperative thallium stress testing before vascular surgery, the investigators illustrated that patients with low clinical risk had good outcomes, regardless of thallium stress-test results preoperatively (**Fig. 1**). Likewise, those with high clinical risk had a high incidence of perioperative cardiovascular complications despite the results of thallium testing. Patients with a low pretest probability of perioperative cardiac events, based on clinical evaluation, remained low-risk patients despite thallium test results. The same was true for high-risk patients. It is only those of moderate or intermediate clinical risk whose risk was further stratified by thallium test results. In this way, the authors show that the widespread or universal application of stress testing before patients undergo even high-risk surgery will be of no use for most patients, and therefore should be applied selectively.

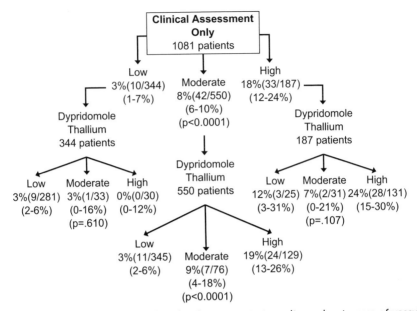

Fig. 1. Relationships among clinical evaluation, stress test results, and outcomes of vascular surgery: effect of pretest clinical risk probability on interpretation of stress testing. (*From* L'Italien GJ, et al. Development and validation of a Bayesian model for perioperative cardiac risk assessment in a cohort of 1,081 vascular surgical candidates. J Am Coll Cardiol 1996;27(4):779–86; with permission.)

Observational data from Boersma and colleagues further defends this concept. In their observational registry of patients undergoing vascular surgery, clinical risk score did an excellent job of predicting perioperative complications.[8] This group went on to demonstrate that with further follow-up, clinical risk assessment alone did an excellent job of predicting future perioperative events. Furthermore, randomizing patients to stress testing or no stress testing preoperatively had no significant effect on perioperative or even long-term cardiovascular events.[9]

In the DECREASE study, Poldermans and colleagues randomized patients to either preoperative testing or no testing.[9] For the purposes of this study, they focused on patients at intermediate risk, which they defined as patients having either 1 or 2 of the following risk factors: age greater than 70 years, angina, prior MI, compensated heart failure or history of heart failure, diabetes receiving treatment, renal dysfunction (defined as creatine monohydrate (CM) creatinine >160 μmol/L), or prior transient ischemic attack (TIA) or stroke. They randomized 770 such patients to either cardiac stress testing or no stress testing before surgery.

All patients were treated with perioperative β blockade, in the form of bisoprolol 2.5 mg once a day which was titrated to achieve resting heart rate 60 to 65 beats/minute. This dosage was continued postoperatively. At 30 days after surgery, the incidence of death or MI was not different between these 2 groups (1.8% versus. 2.3%; OR 0.78; 95% CI 0.28–2.1; $P = .62$). They found that whether or not patients underwent preoperative stress testing, in this group of intermediate risk patients, there was no difference in long-range outcomes (**Fig. 2**). The analysis of risk factors in the larger nonrandomized cohort, however, demonstrated that clinical risk factors were strongly associated with long-term incidence of death or MI (**Fig. 3**). The investigators

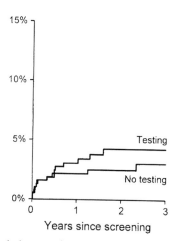

Fig. 2. Effect of stress testing in intermediate-risk patients undergoing vascular surgery with β blockade. (*From* Poldermans D, et al. Should major vascular surgery be delayed because of preoperative cardiac testing in intermediate-risk patients receiving beta-blocker therapy with tight heart rate control? [see comment]. J Am Coll Cardiol 2006;48(5):964–9; with permission.)

went on to observe that the heart rate control achieved was a predominant determinant of incidence of perioperative death or MI (**Fig. 4**). This finding suggests that the patient's sympathetic tone, or response to β-blocker therapy, is a potent predictor of perioperative events, which may obviate the need for preoperative stress testing.

An important factor to consider in determining who requires preoperative stress testing is how this information might be used or of benefit. Despite a widespread belief that coronary revascularization before noncardiac surgery can reduce perioperative cardiovascular events, this has been little studied. In the only randomized trial of preoperative coronary revascularization, McFalls and colleagues randomized 620

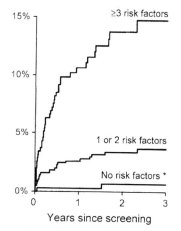

Fig. 3. Association between number of clinical risk factors and long-term outcomes after vascular surgery. (*From* Poldermans D, et al. Should major vascular surgery be delayed because of preoperative cardiac testing in intermediate-risk patients receiving beta-blocker therapy with tight heart rate control? [see comment]. J Am Coll Cardiol 2006;48(5):964–9; with permission.)

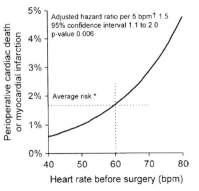

Fig. 4. Relationship between resting heart rate before surgery and perioperative death or MI. (*From* Poldermans D, et al. Should major vascular surgery be delayed because of preoperative cardiac testing in intermediate-risk patients receiving beta-blocker therapy with tight heart rate control? [see comment]. J Am Coll Cardiol 2006;48(5):964–9; with permission.)

patients who were scheduled for vascular surgery and had an indication for coronary revascularization to either medical therapy or coronary revascularization before noncardiac surgery.[10] Their results suggested no benefit at all from preoperative coronary revascularization (**Fig. 5**). This study is discussed in more detail in the section on lowering perioperative risk.

In the presence of medical therapy to prevent perioperative events, observations from Poldermans and colleagues suggest that stress testing may not add to clinical care.[8] In their observational registry of patients undergoing vascular surgery, all patients who received β-blockers had a lower perioperative event rate, regardless of the level of risk. This observation was true in their center, where β-blockers were begun preoperatively with titration to heart rate. This observation was also true regardless of stress test results. The marginal benefit of preoperative testing or coronary revascularization may also be reduced by other perioperative therapies that reduce cardiovascular risk. As discussed later in this article, HMG CoA reductase inhibitors,

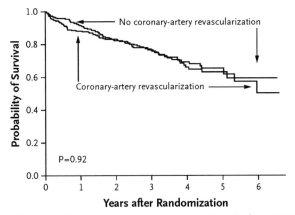

Fig. 5. Survival with and without coronary revascularization before noncardiac surgery. (*From* McFalls EO, et al. Coronary-artery revascularization before elective major vascular surgery [see comment]. N Engl J Med 2004;351(27):2795–804; with permission.)

or statins, have been shown to reduce cardiovascular events. Observation data would suggest this is true in the perioperative period as well.

WHO NEEDS PREOPERATIVE CARDIAC CATHETERIZATION?

The current ACC/AHA guidelines suggest that the indications for coronary angiography should be the same for patients who are facing preoperative evaluation as for those who are not.[11] Clearly, patients with unstable coronary syndromes or poorly controlled symptoms on medical therapy are recommended to undergo coronary angiography by the preoperative ACC/AHA guidelines as well as the guidelines for coronary angiography.[12] Among patients with stable coronary disease, only those with advanced multivessel or left main coronary disease and left ventricular (LV) dysfunction have been shown to benefit from coronary revascularization, and are recommended to undergo coronary angiography.

The presence of unstable or severe coronary conditions indicates the need for further evaluation before elective surgery according to current guidelines (**Box 2**).[13] This need would include patients with unstable angina or acute coronary syndromes. It has been well demonstrated that these patients benefit from coronary intervention. This need also includes patients with decompensated heart failure, as well as significant arrhythmias, such as ventricular tachycardia or any tachycardic rhythm with a rapid rate or clinical instability. Patients with severe valvular disease, specifically severe aortic stenosis and severe mitral stenosis, should undergo evaluation for valvular surgery. The indication for valvular surgery should be the same for those undergoing preoperative evaluation as for those who are not. In general, for aortic stenosis, surgical repair is indicated for those with symptoms or signs of decompensation.[14] In general, this is true regardless of the severity of the aortic stenosis. This indication for repair should be the same for those facing noncardiac surgery. Likewise, although the timing of surgery for severe mitral regurgitation is clinically challenging, the approach should be the same for all patients regardless of whether or not they are facing noncardiac surgery. This approach includes patients with symptoms, evidence of LV dilation or dysfunction, the presence of atrial arrhythmias, or, in some cases, severe mitral regurgitation or mitral stenosis by echocardiographic criteria.[14]

Percutaneous techniques for repairing or even replacing severe aortic and mitral valvular disease may change this equation in the near future. Percutaneous treatment of mitral stenosis is already well established and of proven efficacy. Percutaneous treatment of aortic stenosis is only in its infancy, but holds great promise for clinical usefulness in the near future.

Box 2
Active cardiac conditions for which evaluation is recommended before elective noncardiac surgery

- Unstable angina
- Decompensated heart failure
- Significant arrhythmias
- Severe valvular disease (AS < 1.0 cm²)

From Fleischer LA, Beckman JA, Brown KA, et al. ACC/AHA 2007 guidelines on perioperative cardiovascular evaluation and care for noncardiac surgery. J Am Coll Cardiol 2007;50; 159–241; with permission.

The question of who would benefit from coronary angiography before surgery depends largely on whether or not there would be any benefit to the patient. Certainly, as listed in **Box 2**, anyone who has an indication for coronary angiography, regardless of whether or not they face surgery, should have coronary angiography before elective noncardiac surgery. The question then becomes: Is there anyone else who would benefit from coronary angiography before noncardiac surgery?

A study that attempted to rigorously compare medical therapy with percutaneous coronary intervention (PCI) for coronary artery disease (CAD) was published recently by Boden and colleagues. For this study, called the COURAGE study, 2287 subjects with CAD that could be treated with revascularization were randomized to medical therapy alone or PCI plus medical therapy.[15] Roughly a third of subjects had single, double, and triple vessel coronary disease each, respectively. Roughly 20% in each group had Canadian angina class III symptoms. Follow-up failed to reveal any difference between the groups in terms of the end points of death or MI. As in the Coronary Artery Revascularization Prophylaxis (CARP) study, which randomized 620 patients with CAD to either revascularization or medical management before noncardiac surgery, this study also showed no difference in death, MI or stroke with coronary revascularization.

More recently, the DECREASE-5 study published by Poldermans and colleagues examined the question of a noninvasive approach to high-risk patients undergoing vascular surgery. In this study, high-risk patients (those with 3 or more risk factors and found to have stress-induced ischemia on testing) were randomly assigned to revascularization or no revascularization.[16] All patients received β-blocker in the form of bisoprolol titrated to achieve a heart rate between 60 and 65 beats/minute as well as antiplatelet therapy. For 430 such high-risk patients, 101 had extensive ischemia and were randomized to revascularization or no revascularization. Two thirds of the subjects had 3-vessel coronary disease. Two subjects died after coronary revascularization, but before surgery, because of ruptured aneurysm. There was no improvement in 30-day outcome, although there was a nonstatistically significant trend towards decreased end points of all-cause mortality or MI at 30 days and 1 year in the medically managed group.

WHAT CAN WE DO TO LOWER PERIOPERATIVE RISK FOR PATIENTS WITH CARDIAC DISEASE?

Little investigation was done into treatments that might lower perioperative risk until about 15 years ago. The first randomized trial to evaluate β blockade for perioperative risk reduction was published by Mangano and colleagues.[17] For this study the investigators randomized 200 subjects with or at risk for CAD to either atenolol or placebo. The medical therapy was continued for only 7 days perioperatively. At the time of discharge, there was no significant difference in outcomes between the groups. However, over the subsequent 2 years, the atenolol-treated group demonstrated an increased event-free survival, although therapy was not continued into the postoperative period. Most of this difference occurred in the first 6 months postoperatively. This study is somewhat difficult to interpret, as atenolol therapy was not continued, and other medical therapy was not controlled, beyond the perioperative period. It is difficult to draw a correlation between the brief perioperative treatment regimen and longer-term events.

Poldermans and colleagues performed a randomized trial of β-blocker therapy for patients undergoing major vascular surgery, which looked at the highest-risk patients. Among subjects facing major vascular surgery, these investigators identified those with clinical markers of risk, who also had evidence of ischemia on dobutamine stress echocardiography, and then randomized this cohort to bisoprolol or control. Bisoprolol was begun preoperatively and titrated to heart-rate control. In this high-risk cohort, managed with preoperatively titrated bisoprolol, there was a significant reduction in death and MI in patients undergoing major vascular surgery within the first month.[18] This group has also published observational data among all subjects at their center undergoing major vascular surgery. The investigators observed a significant reduction in cardiac complications associated with use of β-blockers, regardless of clinical risk score (**Fig. 6**). This reduction was far more significant for those subjects who had abnormal stress testing (**Fig. 7**). Poldermans and colleagues also analyzed their observational registry data to determine the effect of preoperative resting heart rate on outcomes among patients receiving β-blockers. They documented an event rate of 1.3% among subjects undergoing vascular surgery whose resting heart rate was less than 65 beats/minute preoperatively, versus 5.2% among those whose resting heart rate was greater than 65 beats/minute (**Fig. 8**).[9] These data suggest that, among high-risk patients (those with stress test abnormalities, multiple risk factors, and facing major vascular surgery) preoperative β blockade titrated to heart rate is associated with a reduced rate of perioperative cardiac complications.

Administrative data from Lindenauer and colleagues[19] further demonstrates that perioperative β blockade in high-risk patients is associated with decreased risk. Their data, however, also suggest that there may be no improvement, or even a worse outcome, associated with β-blocker use among patients with low or no clinical markers of risk. This group used a large administrative database with data from 782,969 patients, and identified those who received β blockade within 1 or 2 days

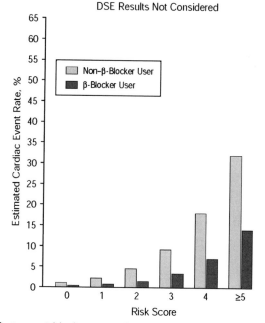

Fig. 6. Association between β-blocker use and cardiac events in patients undergoing vascular surgery. (*From* Boersma E, et al. Predictors of cardiac events after major vascular surgery: role of clinical characteristics, dobutamine echocardiography, and beta-blocker therapy. JAMA 2001;285(14):1865–73; with permission.)

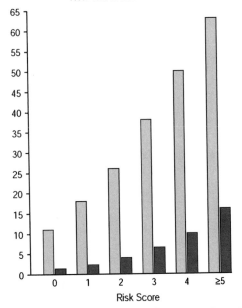

Fig. 7. Association between β-blocker use and cardiac events in patients with abnormal dobutamine echo test undergoing vascular surgery. (*From* Boersma E, et al. Predictors of cardiac events after major vascular surgery: role of clinical characteristics, dobutamine echocardiography, and beta-blocker therapy. JAMA 2001;285(14):1865–73; with permission.)

of surgery. These data do not allow determination of why β-blocker was given and patients were not randomized. Nonetheless, they suggest that patient clinical risk score correlates with benefit or harm associated with β-blocker use, suggesting that patients at high risk do receive some benefit from perioperative β blockade but that patients with little or no risk may actually suffer harm with the use of β blockade **(Fig. 9)**.

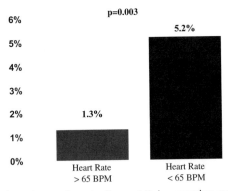

Fig. 8. Heart rate and perioperative death or MI in vascular surgery patients. (*From* Poldermans D, et al. Should major vascular surgery be delayed because of preoperative cardiac testing in intermediate-risk patients receiving beta-blocker therapy with tight heart rate control? [see comment]. J Am Coll Cardiol 2006;48(5):964–9; with permission.)

Propensity-Matched Cohort

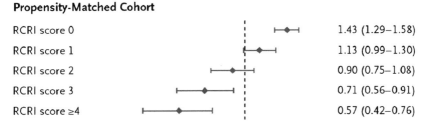

RCRI score 0	1.43 (1.29–1.58)
RCRI score 1	1.13 (0.99–1.30)
RCRI score 2	0.90 (0.75–1.08)
RCRI score 3	0.71 (0.56–0.91)
RCRI score ≥4	0.57 (0.42–0.76)

Fig. 9. Odds of in-hospital mortality during noncardiac surgery associated with β-blocker use stratified by patient clinical risk score. (*From* Lindenauer PK, et al. Perioperative beta-blocker therapy and mortality after major noncardiac surgery [see comment]. N Engl J Med 2005;353(4):349–61; with permission.)

Two other studies looked at outcomes of perioperative use of β blockade in a randomized fashion. The Diabetic Postoperative Mortality and Morbidity (DIPOM) study randomized 921 patients with diabetes who were undergoing major surgery to either 100 mg metroprolol extended release or placebo for up to 8 days (mean 4.6 days).[20] They found the end point of all-cause mortality, acute MI, unstable angina, or heart failure to be roughly similar numbers in both groups. In the β-blocker group, 21% of patients had an end point and 20% in the placebo group. The inclusion criterion was presence of diabetes, but not necessarily known coronary disease. Only 8% of this subject group had a history of prior MI.[20] In the Metoprolol after Vascular Surgery (MaVS) study, 496 patients undergoing vascular surgery, specifically, were randomized to a weight-based metroprolol dose (25–200 mg daily by mouth) versus placebo. Again, this was a heterogeneous group in terms of cardiac risk, with 60% of subjects having only 1 recognized coronary risk factor.[21] Prior MI rate among subjects before the study was 13.5%. The investigators found no difference in the primary composite end point of MI, unstable angina, heart failure, dysrhythmia, or cardiac death, which was 10.2% in the metroprolol group and 12.0% in the placebo group. They did observe significantly more hypotension or bradicardia requiring treatment in the group treated with β-blocker.

More recently, a much larger randomized trial of perioperative β blockade was performed. In the POISE trial, 8351 patients were randomized to either 200 mg of Troprol XL PO QD or placebo.[22] Subjects were more than 45 years of age, either with or at risk for atherosclerosis or with coronary disease or peripheral vascular disease overtly. The treatment regimen was 100 mg Troprol XL 2 to 4 hours preoperatively followed by another 100 mg in 6 hours if heart rate remained more than 45 and systolic blood pressure more than 100 mmHg. This regimen was followed by 200 mg a day subsequently. Specifically, the inclusion criteria were a history of coronary disease, peripheral artery disease, stroke, or heart failure within 3 years, undergoing major vascular surgery, or any 3 of the following risk factors: undergoing thoracic or abdominal surgery, history of heart failure, history of TIA, diabetes, chronically known sufficiency, age more than 70 years, or emergent surgery. With this regimen, the investigators observed a rate of cardiovascular death, MI, cardiac arrest of 5.8% versus 6.9% in the metroprolol and the placebo, respectively (*P* = .04). The primary outcome measure and the incidence of MI were significantly reduced with metroprolol. However, the stroke rate was significantly higher in the β-blocker group (1.0% versus 0.5%; *P* = .005), and the mortality rate after 30 days was also significantly increased. (Total mortality was 3.1% versus 2.3% with metroprolol versus placebo, respectively [*P* = .03].) Because of the unusual medical regimen and high dose of β-blocker used in the study, interpretation of the POISE trial is somewhat problematic. They clearly demonstrated that this regimen is associated with a decrease in cardiac end points. The investigators also demonstrated that this regimen is associated with increased incidence of stroke and death.

These studies suggest that the benefit from perioperative β blockade is proportional to the risk, showing a decrease in mortality and cardiac end points in the highest-risk patients. These studies also suggest that low-risk patients may not benefit from β blockade and could even be harmed. They also suggest that a high-dose β-blocker given on the day of surgery may be associated with an increased risk of perioperative hypotension, stroke, and death.

Perioperative statin use has unfortunately not been subjected to many randomized trials. One randomized trial reported by Durazzo and colleagues suggested benefit.[23] These investigators randomized 100 patients undergoing major vascular surgery to either atorvastatin 20 mg or placebo. In the follow-up in the immediate postoperative period and up to 180 days, the investigators demonstrated that the incidence of cardiac events was significantly higher with placebo (26.0%) compared with atorvastatin (8.0%) ($P = .031$). This finding was sustained up to 6 months ($P = .08$).

Observational data also suggest an association between statin use and improved outcomes. Lindenaeur and colleagues report the results from an administrative observational database of 780,591 patients undergoing surgery, among whom 77,082 (9.9%) received lipid-lowering therapy in the perioperative period.[24] There was a lower crude mortality rate (2.13% versus 3.05%, $P < 0.001$) as well as a significantly lower mortality after adjusting for covariates and matching for propensity score (odds ratio 0.62; 95% CI 0.58–0.67). In another observational study, Ward and colleagues reported results in 446 consecutive patients undergoing lower extremity vascular surgery. They observed that statin use was associated with fewer combined cardiovascular complications (6.9% versus 21.1%, $P = .008$), including all-cause mortality, cardiovascular mortality, MI, stroke, and major peripheral vascular complications.[25]

Kennedy and colleagues reported the association between statin use and outcomes in carotid endarterectomy. They reported the results in 3360 patients undergoing carotid endarterectomy in western Canada. Statin use was associated with a significant reduction in in-hospital outcomes in symptomatic patients undergoing carotid endarterectomy, even after adjusting for covariates, potential confounders, and propensity score and hospital type, with odds ratio for death 0.24 (95% CI 0.06–0.91).[26] This was not true for patients with asymptomatic carotid disease undergoing endarterectomy.

WHAT DO THE GUIDELINES SAY?

The first AHA/ACC guidelines on perioperative cardiovascular evaluation for noncardiac surgery, published in 1996, represented an initial attempt to organize and synthesize the extant knowledge about cardiovascular risk assessment.[4] It also provided clinicians with an algorithmic approach to the evaluation of cardiovascular risk in patients undergoing noncardiac surgery. In so doing, it helped identify clinical markers of risk, and demonstrate a method for integrating the clinical assessment of risk with selective testing and cardiac catheterization to assess the presence of coronary disease and, therefore, risk of perioperative cardiac events. Since that time, studies have further refined clinical risk prediction. More importantly, trials have attempted to identify methods for lowering perioperative cardiovascular risk. These methods have been shown to be of limited benefit, or beneficial for a limited number of patients facing noncardiac surgery.

The current guidelines, therefore, have shifted the paradigm to one of identifying the small group of patients facing noncardiac surgery who would benefit from stress testing, coronary angiography, coronary revascularization, or medical therapy to lower perioperative risk. Viewed in another way, current guidelines help identify the large number of patients facing noncardiac surgery who require no further evaluation or require no intervention to lower perioperative risk.

Not "Clearing" for Surgery

Internists and cardiologists are frequently asked by surgeons to "clear" patients for surgery. This system is an invalid paradigm for the perioperative evaluation of patients before noncardiac surgery. It is the job of the consultant in the perioperative period to provide a best estimate of the risk of a cardiovascular event during noncardiac surgery. This estimate of risk is essential for the patient and the surgeon to decide about the propriety of pursuing surgery. If, and only if, there is the need and the ability to better define cardiovascular risk, then it is also the role of the consultant to make that determination and recommend selective use of further testing. The overriding paradigm here, as with all medical testing, is that testing should be pursued if the results will alter patient care. As the best patient outcome is the ultimate goal of every encounter, it is also incumbent on the perioperative consultant to recommend intervention when, and only when, it will lower perioperative cardiovascular risk. Finally, and frequently overlooked, the perioperative consultation is an excellent opportunity for the assessment of long-term cardiovascular risk and recommendation of interventions to lower that risk. Cardiovascular disease remains the leading cause of death for Americans. It should be kept in mind that this whole process should occur with the understanding that the approach to evaluation and treatment of the perioperative patient should be no different than for the nonperioperative patient. The authors have no data to suggest that any testing or intervention is of benefit in perioperative evaluation of patients facing noncardiac surgery that would not be recommended for patients not facing surgery (**Box 3**).

As can be seen in the algorithm from the 2007 version of the ACC/AHA guidelines, an algorithmic approach is recommended to identify patients who require no further testing, which includes patients facing urgent or emergent surgery, those undergoing low-risk surgery, and those with a reasonable functional capacity without symptoms of coronary disease.[27] The algorithm further notes that those with active cardiac conditions, (which include uncompensated heart failure and unstable coronary syndromes), should have surgery deferred and undergo further evaluation.

The algorithm goes on to suggest that patients with no clinical risk factors probably do not warrant any further evaluation, and those with 1 or 2 risk factors should probably undergo further evaluation if, and only if, they are facing intermediate or high-risk surgery and noninvasive testing would change management. Finally, the algorithm suggests that those with 3 or more clinical risk factors and facing high-risk surgery, such as vascular surgery, should be considered for evaluations such as stress testing (**Fig. 10**).

Box 3
Perioperative cardiovascular evaluation paradigm

1. Estimate risk: thorough patient history, ECG, and examination

2. Better define risk: selective testing, if it will change patient care

3. Intervene to lower perioperative risk

4. Assess long-term cardiovascular risk: modify risk factors when possible

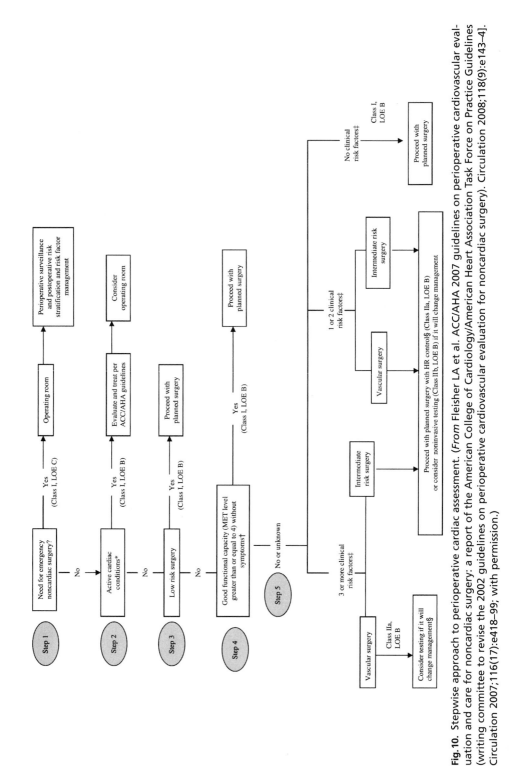

Fig. 10. Stepwise approach to perioperative cardiac assessment. (*From* Fleisher LA et al. ACC/AHA 2007 guidelines on perioperative cardiovascular evaluation and care for noncardiac surgery: a report of the American College of Cardiology/American Heart Association Task Force on Practice Guidelines (writing committee to revise the 2002 guidelines on perioperative cardiovascular evaluation for noncardiac surgery). Circulation 2008;118(9):e143–4]. Circulation 2007;116(17):e418–99; with permission.)

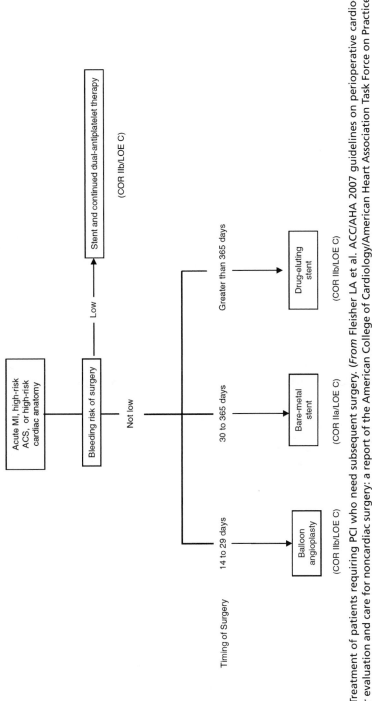

Fig. 11. Treatment of patients requiring PCI who need subsequent surgery. (*From* Fleisher LA et al. ACC/AHA 2007 guidelines on perioperative cardiovascular evaluation and care for noncardiac surgery: a report of the American College of Cardiology/American Heart Association Task Force on Practice Guidelines (writing committee to revise the 2002 guidelines on perioperative cardiovascular evaluation for noncardiac surgery). Circulation 2008;118(9):e143–4]. Circulation 2007;116(17):e418–99; with permission.)

The other 2 important questions that arise for the consultant are the use of perioperative medical therapy to lower risk, and the use of coronary revascularization. On the issue of perioperative medical therapy, guidelines suggest β-blocker use should be limited to those high-risk patients (having risk factors and abnormal stress testing), who are facing high-risk surgery such as vascular surgery. Those with lesser degrees of risk and facing lesser-risk surgery may benefit from perioperative β blockage, but the evidence is not strong (**Fig. 10**). The evidence detailed earlier makes drawing firm conclusions and identifying those who would clearly benefit somewhat problematic. Hopefully, future studies will further refine recommendations in this evolving science.

Coronary revascularization before noncardiac surgery will be indicated in some patients, which raises the question of timing of surgery after coronary revascularization. Several studies have raised concern about the risk of catastrophic stent thrombosis when subjecting patients who have undergone coronary angioplasty or stenting to the dual risks of discontinuing antiplatelet therapy and undergoing stressful surgery. The risk of coronary thrombosis is increased by the placement of a stent, and increased in duration by the placement of a drug-eluting stent. For this reason, the current guidelines recommend waiting after coronary angioplasty or stenting before elective noncardiac surgery and the cessation of antiplatelet therapy (**Fig. 11**). The recommendations for waiting period after angioplasty and stenting are generous, due to the paucity of data to better define the period of time at risk. Currently, it is recommended that antiplatelet therapy be continued and noncardiac surgery deferred for at least a month in the case of the placement of bare-metal stent, and preferably a year after placement of a drug-eluting stent. The longer the time period after coronary revascularization the lower the risk. In patients undergoing conventional ballooning angioplasty without stenting, noncardiac surgery should be delayed at least 2 to 4 weeks.

In conclusion, the perioperative evaluation of patients facing noncardiac surgery should closely resemble the evaluation of patients not facing surgery. Evaluation should be aimed at risk assessment, with selective further testing to better define risk, and selective application of interventions shown to lower perioperative risk for each patient. Factors to be included in this evaluation include the urgency of the noncardiac surgery, patient-specific risk factors, surgery-specific risk, and whether or not further testing will affect patient management and outcomes. The overall mission of the consultant is the same as for all our patients: evaluate cardiovascular risk, intervene to improve modifiable risk factors, and selectively test and intervene when it will improve cardiovascular risk.

REFERENCES

1. Goldman L, Caldera DL, Nussbaum SR, et al. Multifactorial index of cardiac risk in noncardiac surgical procedures. N Engl J Med 1977;297(16):845–50.
2. Detsky AS, Abrams HB, Forbath N, et al. Cardiac assessment for patients undergoing noncardiac surgery. A multifactorial clinical risk index. Arch Intern Med 1986;146(11):2131–4.
3. L'Italien GJ, Cambria RP, Cutler BS, et al. Comparative early and late cardiac morbidity among patients requiring different vascular surgery procedures. J Vasc Surg 1995;21(6):935–44.
4. Eagle KA, Brundage BH, Chaitman BR, et al. Guidelines for perioperative cardiovascular evaluation for noncardiac surgery. Report of the American College of Cardiology/American Heart Association Task Force on Practice Guidelines. Committee on Perioperative Cardiovascular Evaluation for Noncardiac Surgery. Circulation 1996;93(6):1278–317.

5. Lee TH, Marcantonio ER, Mangione CM, et al. Derivation and prospective validation of a simple index for prediction of cardiac risk of major noncardiac surgery.
   Circulation 1999;100(10):1043–9.
6. Bayes T. An essay towards solving a problem in the doctrine of chances. By the
   late Rev. Mr. Bayes, F.R.S. communicated by Mr. Price, in a letter to John Canton,
   A.M.F.R.S. Philos Trans 1763;53:370–418.
7. L'Italien GJ, Paul SD, Hendel RC, et al. Development and validation of a Bayesian
   model for perioperative cardiac risk assessment in a cohort of 1,081 vascular
   surgical candidates. J Am Coll Cardiol 1996;27(4):779–86.
8. Boersma E, Poldermans D, Bax JJ, et al. Predictors of cardiac events after major
   vascular surgery: Role of clinical characteristics, dobutamine echocardiography,
   and beta-blocker therapy. JAMA 2001;285(14):1865–73.
9. Poldermans D, Bax JJ, Schouten O, et al. Should major vascular surgery be delayed because of preoperative cardiac testing in intermediate-risk patients
   receiving beta-blocker therapy with tight heart rate control? J Am Coll Cardiol
   2006;48(5):964–9.
10. McFalls EO, Ward HB, Moritz TE, et al. Coronary-artery revascularization before
    elective major vascular surgery. N Engl J Med 2004;351(27):2795–804.
11. Fleisher LA, Beckman JA, Brown KA, et al. ACC/AHA 2007 guidelines on perioper-
    ative cardiovascular evaluation and care for noncardiac surgery: a report of the
    American College of Cardiology/American Heart Association Task Force on Prac-
    tice Guidelines (writing committee to revise the 2002 guidelines on perioperative
    cardiovascular evaluation for noncardiac surgery) developed in collaboration
    with the American Society of Echocardiography, American Society of Nuclear
    Cardiology, Heart Rhythm Society, Society of Cardiovascular Anesthesiologists,
    Society for Cardiovascular Angiography and Interventions, Society for Vascular
    Medicine and Biology, and Society for Vascular Surgery. [erratum appears in J
    Am Coll Cardiol. 2007;50(17):e242]. J Am Coll Cardiol 2007;50(17):e159–241.
12. Patel MR, Dehmer GJ, Hirshfeld JW, et al. ACCF/SCAI/STS/AATS/AHA/ASNC
    2009 Appropriateness Criteria for Coronary Revascularization: A Report by the
    American College of Cardiology Foundation Appropriateness Criteria Task Force,
    Society for Cardiovascular Angiography and Interventions, Society of Thoracic
    Surgeons, American Association for Thoracic Surgery, American Heart Associa-
    tion, and the American Society of Nuclear Cardiology Endorsed by the American
    Society of Echocardiography, the Heart Failure Society of America, and the
    Society of Cardiovascular Computed Tomography. J Am Coll Cardiol 2009;
    53(6):530–53.
13. Fleisher LA, Beckman JA, Brown KA, et al. ACC/AHA 2007 guidelines on perio-
    perative cardiovascular evaluation and care for noncardiac surgery: executive
    summary. A report of the American College of Cardiology/American Heart Asso-
    ciation Task Force on Practice Guidelines (writing committee to revise the 2002
    guidelines on perioperative cardiovascular evaluation for noncardiac surgery)
    developed in collaboration with the American Society of Echocardiography,
    American Society of Nuclear Cardiology, Heart Rhythm Society, Society of
    Cardiovascular Anesthesiologists, Society for Cardiovascular Angiography and
    Interventions, Society for Vascular Medicine and Biology, and Society for Vascular
    Surgery. [erratum appears in J Am Coll Cardiol 2008;52(9):794–7]. J Am Coll
    Cardiol 2007;50(17):1707–32.
14. American College of Cardiology and American Heart Association. ACC/AHA 2006
    guidelines for the management of patients with valvular heart disease: a report of
    the American College of Cardiology/American Heart Association Task Force on

Practice Guidelines (writing committee to revise the 1998 guidelines for the management of patients with valvular heart disease) developed in collaboration with the Society of Cardiovascular Anesthesiologists endorsed by the Society for Cardiovascular Angiography and Interventions and the Society of Thoracic Surgeons. [erratum appears in J Am Coll Cardiol. 2007;49(9):1014]. J Am Coll Cardiol 2006;48(3):e1–148.

15. Boden WE, O'Rourke RA, Teo KK, et al. Optimal medical therapy with or without PCI for stable coronary disease, N Engl J Med 2007;356(15):1503–16.

16. Poldermans D, Schouten O, Vidakovic R, et al. A clinical randomized trial to evaluate the safety of a noninvasive approach in high-risk patients undergoing major vascular surgery: the DECREASE-V pilot study. J Am Coll Cardiol 2007; 49(17):1763–9.

17. Mangano DT, Layug EL, Wallace A, et al. Effect of atenolol on mortality and cardiovascular morbidity after noncardiac surgery. Multicenter Study of Perioperative Ischemia Research Group. N Engl J Med 1996;335(23):1713–20.

18. Poldermans D, Boersma E, Bax JJ, et al. The effect of bisoprolol on perioperative mortality and myocardial infarction in high-risk patients undergoing vascular surgery. Dutch Echocardiographic Cardiac Risk Evaluation Applying Stress Echocardiography Study Group. N Engl J Med 1999;341(24):1789–94.

19. Lindenauer PK, Pekow P, Wang K, et al. Perioperative beta-blocker therapy and mortality after major noncardiac surgery. N Engl J Med 2005;353(4):349–61.

20. Juul AB, Wetterslev J, Gluud C, et al. Effect of perioperative beta blockade in patients with diabetes undergoing major non-cardiac surgery: randomised placebo controlled, blinded multicentre trial. BMJ 2006;332(7556):1482.

21. Yang H, Raymer K, Butler R, et al. The effects of perioperative beta-blockade: results of the Metoprolol after Vascular Surgery (MaVS) study, a randomized controlled trial. Am Heart J 2006;152(5):983–90.

22. POISE Study Group, Devereaux PJ, Yang H, et al. Effects of extended-release metoprolol succinate in patients undergoing non-cardiac surgery (POISE trial): a randomised controlled trial. Lancet 2008;371(9627):1839–47.

23. Durazzo AE, Machado FS, Ikeoka DT, et al. Reduction in cardiovascular events after vascular surgery with atorvastatin: a randomized trial. J Vasc Surg 2004; 39(5):967–75 [discussion: 975–6].

24. Lindenauer PK, Pekow P, Wang K, et al. Lipid-lowering therapy and in-hospital mortality following major noncardiac surgery. JAMA 2004;291(17):2092–9.

25. Ward RP, Leeper NJ, Kirkpatrick JN, et al. The effect of preoperative statin therapy on cardiovascular outcomes in patients undergoing infrainguinal vascular surgery. Int J Cardiol 2005;104(3):264–8.

26. Kennedy J, Quan H, Buchan AM, et al. Statins are associated with better outcomes after carotid endarterectomy in symptomatic patients. Stroke 2005; 36(10):2072–6.

27. Fleisher LA, Beckman JA, Brown KA, et al. ACC/AHA 2007 guidelines on perioperative cardiovascular evaluation and care for noncardiac surgery: a report of the American College of Cardiology/American Heart Association Task Force on Practice Guidelines (writing committee to revise the 2002 guidelines on perioperative cardiovascular evaluation for noncardiac surgery) developed in collaboration with the American Society of Echocardiography, American Society of Nuclear Cardiology, Heart Rhythm Society, Society of Cardiovascular Anesthesiologists, Society for Cardiovascular Angiography and Interventions, Society for Vascular Medicine and Biology, and Society for Vascular Surgery. [erratum appears in Circulation. 2008;118(9):e143–4]. Circulation 2007;116(17):e418–99.

Identification and Evaluation of the Patient with Lung Disease

Bobbie Jean Sweitzer, MD[a,b,c,]*, Gerald W. Smetana, MD[d]

KEYWORDS

- Postoperative pulmonary complications • Preoperative testing
- Asthma • Chronic obstructive lung disease
- Dyspnea • Cigarette use • Preoperative evaluation
- Obstructive sleep apnea

Preoperative pulmonary evaluation and optimization improves patient outcomes. Patients with pulmonary disease are at increased risk for pulmonary and nonpulmonary perioperative complications. Identification of diseases and risk stratification will inform discussion among anesthesiologists, surgeons, and hospitalists who care for patients in the perioperative period. Postoperative pulmonary complications (PPCs) occur frequently and increase costs, morbidity, and mortality. In addition, recent evidence indicates that patients who develop PPC have decreased long-term survival.[1] For example, in a study of patients older than 70 years undergoing noncardiac surgery, pulmonary complications predicted long-term mortality (hazard ratio = 2.41).[2] Somewhat unexpectedly, PPC are more costly than thromboembolic, cardiovascular, or infectious complications.[3] As the entire scope of pulmonary disease is too broad for a comprehensive review, this article focuses on the most common conditions encountered in the preoperative population, including unexplained dyspnea, asthma, chronic obstructive pulmonary disease (COPD), obstructive sleep apnea (OSA), smoking history, and risk factors for PPC (**Table 1**).[4] The evaluation of patients with these

[a] Department of Anesthesia and Critical Care, University of Chicago, MC 4028, 5841 S, Maryland Avenue, Chicago, IL 60637, USA
[b] Department of Medicine, University of Chicago, MC 4028, 5841 S, Maryland Avenue, Chicago, IL 60637, USA
[c] Anesthesia Perioperative Medicine Clinic, University of Chicago Medical Center, MC 4028, 5841 S, Maryland Avenue, Chicago, IL 60637, USA
[d] Division of General Medicine and Primary Care, Beth Israel Deaconess Medical Center, Harvard Medical School, Shapiro 621D, 330 Brookline Avenue, Boston, MA, USA
* Corresponding author. Department of Anesthesia and Critical Care, University of Chicago, MC 4028, 5841 S, Maryland Avenue, Chicago, IL 60637.
E-mail address: bsweitzer@dacc.uchicago.edu (B.J. Sweitzer).

Med Clin N Am 93 (2009) 1017–1030
doi:10.1016/j.mcna.2009.05.009
0025-7125/09/$ – see front matter © 2009 Elsevier Inc. All rights reserved.

medical.theclinics.com

conditions, risk stratification for PPC, and strategies to reduce PPC for high-risk patients are discussed.

A thorough history and physical examination are the foundation of preoperative assessment of patients who have known pulmonary disease, and others who are at risk for PPC. Important components of this history include age, a history of smoking, asthma, COPD, OSA, congestive heart failure (CHF), previous pulmonary complications during or after surgery, exercise tolerance, general health, and the type and urgency of the planned procedure. Symptoms such as cough, wheezing, sputum production, dyspnea, snoring, and orthopnea should be noted. The physical examination focuses on the cardiopulmonary system, looking for the presence of rales, wheezes, rhonchi, decreased breath sounds, prolonged expiratory phase, murmurs, S_3, S_4, and edema. Preoperative testing is necessary only in limited circumstances. There is no role for routine tests. The tests that may be valuable in specific conditions are discussed in this article.

DYSPNEA

Dyspnea, a common symptom, has been defined as the "subjective experience of breathing discomfort that consists of qualitatively distinct sensations that vary in intensity."[5] Dyspnea occurs in conditions in which the respiratory drive is increased or the respiratory system is subject to an increased mechanical load. The most common causes of acute dyspnea are COPD, asthma, and CHF (**Fig. 1**). In a group of patients with chronic dyspnea who were evaluated in a pulmonary clinic, two thirds of the patients had asthma, COPD, interstitial lung diseases, or a cardiomyopathy.[6] Generally, the 2 broad categories of cardiovascular dyspnea (ie, conditions of increased cardiac filling pressures or inadequate oxygen delivery) and pulmonary dyspnea (ie, conditions of increased respiratory drive, abnormal chest wall or pulmonary mechanics, muscle weakness, or gas exchange limitations) should be distinguished.[7] Dyspnea may be intermittent (eg, with asthma), recurrent (eg, with CHF), or persistent (eg, with COPD or interstitial lung disease) and may be influenced by body position (eg, supine, lateral, or upright). Nighttime orthopnea typically occurs in patients with CHF, OSA, gastroesophageal reflux disease (GERD), or asthma.

Clinicians should inquire about the quality of the respiratory discomfort by quantifying the intensity of the sensation, the frequency and duration of occurrence, and precipitating factors. These symptoms may provide clues to the cause of dyspnea. Chest tightness may indicate bronchospasm, rapid shallow breathing is associated with interstitial disease, and heavy breathing or fatigue suggests deconditioning.[7] Patient history alone is correct approximately two thirds of the time; and the negative predictive value of characteristic physical findings is higher than the positive predictive value of the same findings on examination.[6] Clinicians should obtain specific preoperative tests for patients with dyspnea based on results of the history and physical examination (see **Fig. 1**). Pulmonary function testing (PFT), including a methacholine challenge, can diagnose airflow obstruction. Chest radiography is useful to uncover acute disease such as pneumonia or to diagnose CHF or interstitial lung disease. Echocardiography may demonstrate reduced left ventricular ejection fraction, evidence of diastolic dysfunction, or pulmonary hypertension. Testing for anemia, hypothyroidism, or renal failure will occasionally establish the cause of the patient's dyspnea. Cardiopulmonary exercise testing (CET) may be helpful if the basis for dyspnea remains uncertain after clinical evaluation and initial diagnostic testing as noted above. In such cases, deconditioning may ultimately prove to be the basis for dyspnea.[6] CET is particularly useful in confirming deconditioning or psychogenic factors as the cause of dyspnea.

Table 1
Strength of the evidence for patient- and procedure-related risk factors for postoperative pulmonary complications

Factor	Strength of Recommendation[a]	Odds Ratio[b]
Potential patient-related risk factor		
Advanced age	A	2.09–3.04
ASA class ≥II	A	2.55–4.87
CHF	A	2.93
Functionally dependent	A	1.65–2.51
COPD	A	1.79
Weight loss	B	1.62
Impaired sensorium	B	1.39
Cigarette use	B	1.26
Alcohol use	B	1.21
Abnormal findings on chest examination	B	NA
Diabetes	C	
Obesity	D	
Asthma	D	
Obstructive sleep apnea	I	
Corticosteroid use	I	
HIV infection	I	
Arrhythmia	I	
Poor exercise capacity	I	
Potential procedure-related risk factor		
Aortic aneurysm repair	A	6.90
Thoracic surgery	A	4.24
Abdominal surgery	A	3.01
Upper abdominal surgery	A	2.91
Neurosurgery	A	2.53
Prolonged surgery	A	2.26
Head and neck surgery	A	2.21
Emergency surgery	A	2.21
Vascular surgery	A	2.10
General anesthesia	A	1.83
Perioperative transfusion	B	1.47
Hip surgery	D	
Gynecologic or urologic surgery	D	
Esophageal surgery	I	
Laboratory tests		
Albumin level <35 g/L	A	2.53
Chest radiography	B	4.81
BUN level >7.5 mmol/L (>21 mg/dL)	B	NA
Spirometry	I	

Abbreviations: ASA, American Society of Anesthesiologists; BUN, blood urea nitrogen; CHF, congestive heart failure; COPD, chronic obstructive pulmonary disease; NA, not available.

[a] Recommendation: A, good evidence to support the particular risk factor or laboratory predictor; B, at least fair evidence to support the particular risk factor or laboratory predictor; C, at least fair evidence to suggest that the particular factor is not a risk factor or that the laboratory test does not predict risk; D, good evidence to suggest that the particular factor is not a risk factor or that the laboratory test does not predict risk; I, insufficient evidence to determine whether the factor increases risk or whether the laboratory test predicts risk, and evidence is lacking, is of poor quality, or is conflicting.[12]

[b] For factors with A or B ratings. Odds ratios are trim-and-fill estimates. When these estimates were not possible, the pooled estimate is provided.

Reprinted from Smetana GW, Lawrence VA, Cornell JE. Preoperative pulmonary risk stratification for noncardiothoracic surgery: systematic review for the American College of Physicians. Ann Intern Med 2006;144:581; with permission.

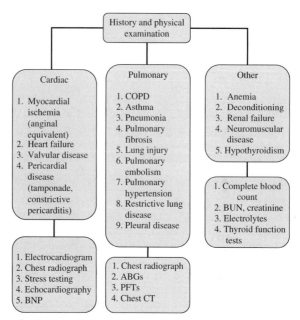

Fig.1. Evaluation of dyspnea. ABGs, arterial blood gases; BNP, brain natriuretic peptide; BUN, blood urea nitrogen; COPD, chronic obstructive pulmonary disease; CT, computerized tomography; PFTs, pulmonary function tests.

Most of the conditions that cause dyspnea, except for the psychogenic ones, increase the risk of PPC, especially if the condition is poorly controlled or unknown to the anesthesiologist. Therefore, preoperative evaluation that yields a proper diagnosis will allow for effective treatment and optimization of patient status.

ASTHMA

Well-controlled asthma does not seem to be a risk factor for either intraoperative or postoperative complications.[8,9] However, patients who are poorly controlled, as shown by wheezing at the time of anesthesia induction, have a higher risk of perioperative complications.[9] The medical history also provides clues that indicate higher risk. For example, in the study of Warner and colleagues, asthma severity, as determined by use of asthma medications and emergency room or office visits in the 30 days before surgery, influenced PPC rates. Tracheal intubation in patients with obstructive airways disease can trigger severe bronchospasm with hypoxia, rarely leading to brain damage or death.[10] The actual incidence of such events is unknown.

Preoperative corticosteroids and inhaled beta-agonists markedly decrease the incidence of bronchospasm after tracheal intubation.[8,9,11] The combination of corticosteroids and salbutamol attenuates intubation-induced bronchoconstriction to a greater degree than inhaled β_2 agonists alone.[8] Short courses of preoperative steroids (up to 1 week) are safe and do not seem to increase postoperative infections or delay wound healing.[12] The authors recommend prednisone 0.5 to 1 mg/kg orally for 1 to 4 days before surgery for patients who are likely to require endotracheal intubation and who have persistent airway obstruction despite use of inhaled medications. Before elective surgery, clinicians should treat patients with asthma according to a stepwise approach as outlined in a report by the National Asthma Education and Prevention

Program (NAEPP) Expert Panel Report.[13] This approach stratifies patients based on severity and provides guidance regarding the selection of specific agents and treatment intensity based on severity.

Before elective surgery, patients should be free of wheezes, cough, or dyspnea and have peak expiratory flows greater than 80% of predicted, or their personal best. Well-controlled asthma is characterized by daytime symptoms no more than twice per week and nighttime symptoms no more than twice per month.

CHRONIC OBSTRUCTIVE PULMONARY DISEASE

Unlike asthma, COPD does increase the risk of PPC (odds ratio = 1.79) (see **Table 1**).[4] The more severe the COPD, the greater the risk, but there is no prohibitive degree of severity that precludes surgery. If contemplating surgery in patients with COPD, clinicians should weigh the benefit of the proposed surgery against a lower risk procedure, or the natural course of the underlying condition. Alternatives to surgery and other risk factors need to be considered. Although COPD increases PPC, surprisingly the risk is less than that associated with other patient-related risk factors including CHF, advanced age, and poor general overall health status. Patients with COPD also have higher risk for nonpulmonary complications such as wound infections and atrial arrhythmias.[14]

In patients with COPD, preoperative spirometry may be useful to assess the disease severity and adequacy of bronchodilator therapy, but only in patients in whom it is difficult to determine this from the history and physical examination. Even before high-risk surgery, there is no role for routine PFTs. The rationale for this recommendation is that spirometry usually adds no information beyond that obtained by a careful history and physical examination. Patients with severe COPD as determined by spirometric values are unlikely to escape clinical detection.

As a general rule, the preoperative management of patients with COPD is the same as for patients with COPD who are not preparing for surgery. Routine preoperative antibiotics do not reduce PPC rates for patients with COPD; their use is restricted to patients with bacterial lower respiratory infections. Long-acting inhaled anticholinergics, long-acting β-agonists, and inhaled corticosteroids each can improve lung function in symptomatic patients.[15]

Patients with respiratory symptoms and significant airway obstruction benefit most from therapy. Combinations of inhaled agents have not been shown to have a distinct advantage over monotherapy. Long-acting bronchodilators are more effective and convenient than short-acting β-agonists.[16] Inhaled corticosteroids in addition to β-agonists are appropriate in symptomatic patients with airway obstruction. Chronic therapy with systemic steroids should be avoided because of long-term risks. Preoperative systemic corticosteroids for patients with COPD, when indicated, may shorten hospital and intensive care unit stays, and do not seem to adversely affect wound healing.[12,14] Clinicians should use preoperative corticosteroids in the same fashion as for patients with asthma. Patients with COPD can improve exercise tolerance, and reduce dyspnea and fatigue, by participating in exercise training programs.[16] Preoperative chest physiotherapy, including inspiratory muscle training, decreases PPC rates.[17,18]

OBSTRUCTIVE SLEEP APNEA

Sleep-disordered breathing affects up to 9% of women and 24% of men; most patients are unaware of their diagnosis.[19] During the preoperative assessment, one should question the patient about snoring and daytime somnolence, which may suggest undiagnosed obstructive sleep apnea (OSA). OSA has implications for anesthesia management and probably increases the risk of PPC. A history of snoring, daytime sleepiness, hypertension, obesity, and a family history of OSA are each risk factors for OSA (**Fig. 2**).[20] A large neck circumference (>17 inches in men, >16 inches in women or >60 cm in anyone) predicts a greater chance of OSA.[21] Various questionnaires have been developed to assist in identifying patients who may have sleep apnea but the only validated ones in the preoperative population are the STOP and STOP-Bang forms (**Boxes 1** and **2**).[22] The gold standard for diagnosis of OSA is sleep laboratory polysomnography, but this method is costly, time-consuming, and has limited availability.[23] Home nocturnal oximetry is a potential screening tool that is simpler, less costly, and more readily available.[24] To date, no studies have specifically evaluated the test characteristics of this more limited study in the preoperative setting.

Patients with OSA have increased rates of comorbidities including diabetes, hypertension, atrial fibrillation, bradyarrhythmias, ventricular ectopy, endothelial damage, stroke, heart failure, pulmonary hypertension, dilated cardiomyopathy, coronary artery disease, and myocardial infarction (see **Fig. 2**).[25,26] Mask ventilation, direct laryngoscopy, endotracheal intubation, and even fiber-optic visualization of the airway are more difficult in patients with OSA than in healthy patients. Potential postoperative complications in patients with OSA include airway obstruction, tachyarrhythmias, hypoxemia, atelectasis, ischemia, pneumonia, and prolonged hospitalizations.[27–30]

Preoperative evaluation should aim to identify patients at risk for OSA and optimize associated comorbid conditions. Echocardiography may be indicated if CHF or pulmonary hypertension is suspected, however no data suggest that this preoperative test improves perioperative outcomes. One should encourage patients to lose weight, as a decrease in body weight of as little as 10% can result in clinically significant improvements in the apnea-hypopnea index.[31,32] Whether continuous positive airway pressure (CPAP) or bilevel positive airway pressure (BPAP) therapy does more than improve daytime sleepiness is debatable, but some evidence suggests that it may reverse comorbid disease manifestations such as hypertension, CHF, and ischemia.[32,33] Patients should bring their CPAP devices to the hospital on the day of operation. Communication with the anesthesia team is important to improve patient outcomes. The American Society of Anesthesiologists has published recommendations for the perioperative care of patients with OSA.[34] Adherence to these guidelines will minimize practice variation and potentially improve patient outcomes.

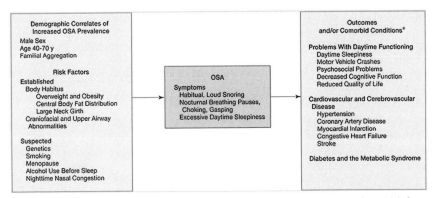

Fig. 2. Obstructive sleep apnea. (*Reprinted from* Young T, Skatrud J, Peppard PE. Risk factors for obstructive sleep apnea in adults. JAMA 2004;291:2014; with permission.)

Box 1
STOP questionnaire to screen for obstructive sleep apnea

1. Snoring
   Do you snore loudly (louder than talking or loud enough to be heard through closed doors)?

2. Tired
   Do you often feel tired, fatigued, or sleepy during the day?

3. Observed
   Has anyone observed you stop breathing during your sleep?

4. Blood pressure
   Do you have or are you being treated for high blood pressure?

- High risk of OSA: answering YES to 2 or more questions
- Low risk of OSA: answering YES to less than 2 questions

From Chung F, Yegneswaran B, Liao P, et al. STOP questionnaire. A tool to screen patients for obstructive sleep apnea. Anesthesiology 2008;108:812; with permission.

CIGARETTE USE

Patients who smoke are at risk for pulmonary and nonpulmonary perioperative complications even in the absence of chronic lung disease (see **Table 1**).[35–37] However, the absolute magnitude of risk for PPC is small (OR = 1.40).[4] A smoking history greater than 20 pack-years predicts greater risk than lesser amounts of smoking.[37]

Box 2
STOP-Bang questionnaire to screen for obstructive sleep apnea

1. Snoring
   Do you snore loudly (loud enough to be heard through closed doors)?

2. Tired
   Do you often feel tired, fatigued, or sleepy during daytime?

3. Observed
   Has anyone observed you stop breathing during your sleep?

4. Blood pressure
   Do you have or are you being treated for high blood pressure?

5. BMI
   BMI more than 35 kg/m^2?

6. Age
   Age greater than 50 years?

7. Neck circumference
   Neck circumference greater than 40 cm?

8. Gender
   Gender male?

High risk of OSA: answering YES to 3 or more items

Low risk of OSA: answering YES to less than 3 items

From Chung F, Yegneswaran B, Liao P, et al. STOP questionnaire. A tool to screen patients for obstructive sleep apnea. Anesthesiology 2008;108:812; with permission.

Smokers are more likely than nonsmokers to develop wound infections, oxygen desaturation, laryngospasm, and severe coughing with anesthesia.[38] Smoking decreases macrophage function, negatively affects coronary flow reserve, and causes vascular endothelial dysfunction, hypertension, tachycardia, and ischemia.[39,40] In one study, patients without a history of ischemic heart disease who smoked shortly before operation had significantly more episodes of rate-pressure, product-related, ST-segment depression than did nonsmokers, former smokers, or chronic smokers who did not smoke in the immediate preoperative period.[41] Although smoking increases the risk of postoperative intensive care admission (OR = 1.55),[42] it does not seem to be a risk factor for clinically significant cardiac complications such as postoperative myocardial infarction or cardiac death.[43]

Abstinence from smoking before surgery reduces PPC rates, but the ideal duration of preoperative abstinence remains the subject of study and controversy. The preponderance of the evidence suggests a need for at least 2 months of preoperative cessation to maximally reduce PPC risk. However, selection bias may have been a factor in studies that have reported greater perioperative risk in recent quitters. In contrast, PPC rates did *not* increase in patients who stopped smoking within weeks before thoracotomy for lung resection.[44] Within 12 hours after a patient quits smoking, carbon monoxide levels decrease, improving oxygen delivery and utilization.[45] Cyanide levels decrease, which benefits mitochondrial oxidative metabolism, and ciliary function improves. Quitting tobacco dramatically reduces surgical wound infections.[46] Sputum production increases in the first 1 to 2 months after cigarette cessation. This observation may contribute to the higher risk among recent quitters in some studies. The authors recommend that truly elective surgery be postponed for at least 8 weeks after smoking cessation to provide maximum reduction of PPC.[47]

The US Public Health Service recommends that physicians strongly advise smokers to quit because a physician's advice to quit smoking increases abstinence rates.[48] Effective interventions include medical advice and pharmacotherapy, such as nicotine-replacement therapy (NRT), which is safe in the perioperative period.[49] NRT is safe in patients with ischemic heart disease, and has been shown to decrease ischemia seen on stress testing in smokers with coronary artery disease.[50] Individual and group counseling may also increase rates of long-term abstinence. Varenicline is another option that has been proved to be even more effective than NRT as a strategy for smoking cessation. Excellent resources are available on the Internet and from the US Surgeon General.[51]

POSTOPERATIVE PULMONARY COMPLICATIONS

Postoperative pulmonary complications (PPC) occur in 6.8% of patients undergoing major noncardiac surgery.[4] Patient- and procedure-related risk factors influence PPC rates. Surgical factors that may affect risk are the site and duration of surgery and the type of anesthesia. PPC rates are higher after major abdominal, thoracic, and open abdominal aortic aneurysm (AAA) repair and surgeries longer than 3 hours (see **Table 1**). Head and neck procedures, neurosurgery and emergency surgeries confer greater risk than peripheral operations.[4,52] Recovery time, pain, and reduction in lung volumes are less after laparoscopic procedures, but it is unclear whether this translates into lower PPC rates.[4] In contrast, PPC risk is lower for percutaneous interventions. For example, in a study of patients undergoing endovascular versus open AAA repair, PPC rates were 3% and 16%, respectively.[53]

General anesthesia carries greater risk than peripheral nerve conduction blocks. Whether centroneuraxial (spinal or epidural) anesthesia is less risky is debatable.[54]

Two large meta-analyses, and retrospective and randomized trials, suggest that PPC rates are lower for patients who have spinal or epidural anesthesia for surgery or epidural analgesia postoperatively.[55–58] The ultimate choice of anesthesia is left to the anesthesiologist, but effective communication among medical, surgical, and anesthesia colleagues will help to guide this choice and reduce risk.

Patient-related predictors of PPCs include advanced age, COPD, smoking, general health status, OSA, and certain metabolic factors.[4,27] The 2006 review by Smetana and colleagues for the American College of Physicians (ACP) established for the first time that advanced age, regardless of other medical conditions, is an independent risk for PPC, and in fact, was the strongest patient-related predictor. When compared with patients younger than 50 years, those aged 50 to 59 years had an odds ratio (OR) of 1.50; those aged 60 to 69 years had an OR of 2.28, 70 to 79 years OR 3.90, and those 80 years or more had an OR of 5.63 for developing PPC. CHF (OR = 2.93) also proved to be a predictor of PPC in this same review. CHF is an especially important risk in the elderly.[59,60] Poor general health status, including impaired sensorium and functional dependency, increases PPC risk. In the American Society of Anesthesiologists (ASA) physical status classification, risk increases at each level, starting with ASA 2 patients (**Table 2**). Risks of PPC with COPD, smoking history, and OSA are discussed in the appropriate sections of this article.

Recently, Johnson and colleagues[61] updated and validated a previously published complex preoperative risk index for predicting postoperative respiratory failure (**Table 3**). Each risk factor receives a score of 1 to 4 based on the strength of the association between the factor and the risk of respiratory failure. A score less than 8 predicts low risk; 8 to 12, medium risk; and greater than 12, high risk. Age, general health status, COPD, and low albumin levels were found to be significant predictors. New risk factors not previously confirmed were sepsis, ascites, creatinine greater than or equal to 1.5 mg/dL, and dyspnea. The same group previously developed a risk index to predict postoperative pneumonia.[52] These helpful tools will be of use primarily to stratify risk and ensure accurate classification in research studies, as they are too complex for use in clinical practice.

Clinicians should not obtain routine preoperative spirometry, chest radiography, or arterial blood gas determination to predict PPC risk.[62] For most patients, these studies offer little more than can be determined by clinical evaluation. Results of spirometry and chest radiography can usually be predicted from clinical assessment and rarely change management.[63,64]

Many of the risk factors for PPC are nonmodifiable, so emphasis is on generic risk reduction strategies and postoperative surveillance. When possible, clinicians should also implement interventions that are specific to the particular risk factor. Pre- and postoperative pulmonary rehabilitation has been shown to decrease PPC in moderate

Table 2	
American Society of Anesthesiologists physical status classification	
Class 1	A normal healthy patient
Class 2	A patient with mild systemic disease
Class 3	A patient with severe systemic disease
Class 4	A patient with severe systemic disease that is a constant threat to life
Class 5	A moribund patient who is not expected to survive without the operation

Emergency cases are designated by the addition of "E" to the classification number.
Data from ASA Physical Status Classification System. 2008. Available at: http://www.asahq.org/clinical/physicalstatus.htm.

Table 3
Independent predictors of respiratory complications (development set)

Step no.	Factor	Odds Ratio (95% CI)	Score
1	ASA class (3 versus 1–2)	2.878 (2.463–3.362)	+3
1	ASA class (4–5 versus 1–2)	4.900 (4.105–5.849)	+5
2	Emergency	2.416 (2.170–2.690)	+2
3	Work RVU (10–17 versus <10)	2.299 (1.937–2.728)	+2
3	Work RVU (>17 versus <10)	4.445 (3.720–5.312)	+4
4	Preoperative albumin (≤3.5 versus >3.5)	1.485 (1.344–1.641)	+1
5	Integumentary versus hernia	1.144 (0.869–1.505)	+1
5	Respiratory and hemic versus hernia	3.116 (2.175–4.466)	+3
5	Heart versus hernia	2.310 (1.670–3.196)	+2
5	Aneurysm versus hernia	1.552 (1.203–2.002)	+2
5	Mouth, palate versus hernia	6.635 (4.782–9.206)	+7
5	Stomach, intestines versus hernia	2.126 (1.658–2.726)	+2
5	Endocrine versus hernia	1.537 (0.992–2.382)	+2
6	Preoperative sepsis	1.999 (1.707–2.341)	+2
7	Preoperative creatinine ≥1.5	1.651 (1.493–1.826)	+2
8	History of severe COPD	1.517 (1.362–1.689)	+2
9	Ascites	1.846 (1.496–2.278)	+2
10	Dyspnea (yes versus no)	1.318 (1.192–1.457)	+1
11	Impaired sensorium	1.498 (1.220–1.839)	+1
12	Preoperative bilirubin >1.0	1.205 (1.078–1.347)	+1
13	>2 alcoholic drinks/d in the 2 wk before admission	1.302 (1.135–1.494)	+1
14	Bleeding disorders	1.253 (1.074–1.462)	+1
15	Age (40–65 y versus <40 y)	1.704 (0.862–3.367)	+2
15	Age (>65 y versus <40 y)	2.062 (1.537–2.765)	+2
16	Preoperative white blood count (<2.5 versus 2.5–10)	1.480 (0.888–2.465)	+1
16	Preoperative white blood count (>10 versus 2.5–10)	1.204 (1.093–1.327)	+1
17	Preoperative serum sodium >145	1.564 (1.205–2.030)	+2
18	Weight loss >10%	1.255 (1.096–1.436)	+1
19	Preoperative acute renal failure	1.507 (1.171–1.939)	+2
20	Gender (male versus female)	1.193 (1.057–1.345)	+1
21	Congestive heart failure <30 d before operation	1.298 (1.089–1.547)	+1
22	Smoker	1.147 (1.049–1.255)	+1
23	Preoperative platelet count ≤150	1.211 (1.060–1.383)	+1
24	CVA/stroke with neurologic deficit	1.269 (1.095–1.471)	+1
25	Wound class (clean/contaminated versus clean)	1.156 (1.024–1.304)	+1
25	Wound class (contaminated versus clean)	1.361 (1.150–1.612)	+1
25	Wound class (infected versus clean)	1.249 (1.043–1.495)	+1
26	Preoperative SGOT >40	1.164 (1.041–1.301)	+1
27	Preoperative hematocrit ≤38	1.114 (1.014–1.225)	+1
28	CVA/stroke without neurologic deficit	1.228 (1.020–1.478)	+1

No. of records used = 90,055. The RRI score was divided into 3 discrete ranges based on the rate of RF: low (risk score <8; RF 0.1% to 0.2%), medium (risk score 8–12; RF 0.8% to 1.0%), and high (risk score >12; RF 6.5% to 6.8%). The scores accurately predicted the RF rate in each category. The c-indices (reflecting "discrimination," a measure of how well the scoring predicts the outcomes of RF) ranged from 0.8498 for the development set to 0.8594 for the validation data set, indicating good stability of the model.

Abbreviations: ASA, American Society of Anesthesiologists; COPD, chronic obstructive pulmonary disease; CVA, cerebrovascular accident; RRI, respiratory risk index; RVU, relative value unit; SGOT, serum glutamic-oxalacetic transaminase.

From Johnson RG, Arozullah AM, Neumayer L, et al. Multivariable predictors of postoperative respiratory failure after general and vascular surgery: results from the patient safety in surgery study. J Am Coll Surg 2007;204:1188–98; with permission.

to high-risk patients undergoing upper abdominal surgeries.[65] Lung expansion maneuvers including cough, deep breathing, incentive spirometry, positive end-expiratory pressure (PEEP), and CPAP reduce PPC rates. There does not seem to be a clear advantage for any particular modality. Preoperative inspiratory muscle training, a recently described modality that is an intensive multimodality intervention, reduces PPC rates in patients undergoing coronary bypass surgery.[14] Whether similar benefit exists for other high-risk surgeries is unknown, but this is an appealing and safe intervention that can be recommended pending further study.

SUMMARY

Evaluation of patients with pulmonary disease before surgery is a common activity for clinicians; this is an important undertaking as PPCs are as common and costly as cardiac complications. High-quality evidence from the literature has delineated those patient- and procedure-related factors that influence PPC rates. These risk factors are described in this article.

The evidence base for risk reduction strategies is not as robust. Further study will increase our understanding of which strategies reduce PPC risk to the greatest extent. Effective risk reduction strategies include maximizing airflow in obstructive disease, treating infections and CHF, and instituting preoperative pulmonary rehabilitation with deep breathing exercises or incentive spirometry. Clinicians should encourage patients to stop smoking at least 2 months before elective surgery, and lose weight if they have OSA. Communication among anesthesia, medical, and surgical colleagues is paramount to optimize perioperative care.

REFERENCES

1. Khuri SF, Henderson WG, DePalma RG, et al. Determinants of long-term survival after major surgery and the adverse effect of postoperative complications. Ann Surg 2005;242:326–41.
2. Manku K, Bacchetti P, Leung JM. Prognostic significance of postoperative in-hospital complications in elderly patients. I. Long-term survival. Anesth Analg 2003;96:583–9.
3. Dimick JB, Chen SL, Taheri PA, et al. Hospital costs associated with surgical complications: a report from the private-sector National Surgical Quality Improvement Program. J Am Coll Surg 2004;199:531–7.
4. Smetana GW, Lawrence VA, Cornell JE. Preoperative pulmonary risk stratification for noncardiothoracic surgery: systematic review for the American College of Physicians. Ann Intern Med 2006;144:581–95.
5. Dyspnea. Mechanisms, assessment, and management: a consensus statement. American Thoracic Society. Am J Respir Crit Care Med 1999;159:321–40.
6. Pratter MR, Curley FJ, Dubois J, et al. Cause and evaluation of chronic dyspnea in a pulmonary disease clinic. Arch Intern Med 1989;149:2277–82.
7. Manning HL, Schwartzstein RM. Pathophysiology of dyspnea. N Engl J Med 1995;333:1547–53.
8. Silvanus MT, Groeben H, Peters J. Corticosteroids and inhaled salbutamol in patients with reversible airway obstruction markedly decrease the incidence of bronchospasm after tracheal intubation. Anesthesiology 2004;100:1052–7.
9. Warner DO, Warner MA, Barnes RD, et al. Perioperative respiratory complications in patients with asthma. Anesthesiology 1996;85:460–7.
10. Caplan RA, Posner KL, Ward RJ, et al. Adverse respiratory events in anesthesia: a closed claims analysis. Anesthesiology 1990;72:823–33.

11. Maslow AD, Regan MM, Israel E, et al. Inhaled albuterol, but not intravenous lidocaine, protects against intubation-induced broncho-constriction in asthma. Anesthesiology 2000;93:1198–204.

12. Kabalin SC, Yarnold PR, Grammer LC. Low complication rate of corticosteroid-treated asthmatics undergoing surgical procedures. Arch Intern Med 1995;155: 1379–84.

13. National Asthma Education and Prevention Program: Expert panel report III. Guidelines for the diagnosis and management of asthma. Bethesda, MD: National Heart, Lung, and Blood Institute; 2007. (NIH publication no. 08-4051). Available at: www.nhlbi.nih.gov/guidelines/asthma/asthgdln.htm. Accessed October 15, 2008.

14. Starobin D, Kramer MR, Garty M, et al. Morbidity associated with systemic corticosteroid preparation for coronary artery bypass grafting in patients with chronic obstructive pulmonary disease: a case control study. J Cardiothorac Surg 2007;2:25–30.

15. Qaseem A, Snow V, Shekelle P, et al. Diagnosis and management of stable chronic obstructive pulmonary disease: a clinical practice guideline from the American college of Physicians. Ann Intern Med 2007;147:633–8.

16. Global initiative for chronic obstructive lung disease. Global strategy for the diagnosis, management, and prevention of chronic obstructive pulmonary disease. 2006. Available at: www.goldcopd.org. Accessed November 15, 2008.

17. Warner DO. Preventing postoperative pulmonary complications: the role of the anesthesiologist. Anesthesiology 2000;92:1467–72.

18. Hulzebos E, Helders P, Favie N, et al. Preoperative intensive inspiratory muscle training to prevent postoperative pulmonary complications in high-risk patients undergoing CABG surgery. A randomized clinical trial. JAMA 2006;296:1851–7.

19. Young T, Palta M, Dempsey J, et al. The occurrence of sleep disordered breathing among middle aged adults. N Engl J Med 1993;328:1230–5.

20. Young T, Skatrud J, Peppard PE. Risk factors for obstructive sleep apnea in adults. JAMA 2004;291:2013–6.

21. Katz I, Stradling J, Slutsjy AS, et al. Do patients with obstructive sleep apnea have thick necks? Am Rev Respir Dis 1990;141:1228–31.

22. Chung F, Yegneswaran B, Liao P, et al. STOP questionnaire. A tool to screen patients for obstructive sleep apnea. Anesthesiology 2008;108:812–21.

23. Practice parameters for the indications for polysomnography and related procedures. Polysomnography Task Force, American Sleep Disorders Association Standards of Practice Committee. Sleep 1997;20:406–22.

24. Whitelaw WA, Brant RF, Flemons WW. Clinical usefulness of home oximetry compared with polysomnography for assessment of sleep apnea. Am J Respir Crit Care Med 2005;171:188–93.

25. Caples SM, Gami AS, Somers VK. Obstructive sleep apnea. Ann Intern Med 2005;142:187–97.

26. Young T, Peppard PE, Gottlieb DJ. Epidemiology of obstructive sleep apnea. Am J Respir Crit Care Med 2002;165:1217–39.

27. Hwang D, Shakir N, Limann B, et al. Association of sleep-disordered breathing with postoperative complications. Chest 2008;133:1128–34.

28. Gupta RM, Parvizi J, Hanssen AD, et al. Postoperative complications in patients with obstructive sleep apnea syndrome undergoing hip or knee replacement: a case-control study. Mayo Clin Proc 2001;76:897–905.

29. Reeder MK, Muir AD, Foex P, et al. Postoperative myocardial ischaemia: temporal association with nocturnal hypoxaemia. Br J Anaesth 1991;67: 626–31.

30. Ballantyne GH, Svahn J, Capella RF, et al. Predictors of prolonged hospital stay following open and laparascopic gastric bypass for morbid obesity: body mass index, length of surgery, sleep apnea, asthma, and the metabolic syndrome. Obes Surg 2004;14:1042–50.

31. Smith PL, Gold AR, Meyers DA, et al. Weight loss in mildly to moderately obese patients with obstructive sleep apnea. Ann Intern Med 1985;103:850–5.

32. Crummy F, Piper AJ, Naughton MT. Obesity and the lung: 2. Obesity and sleep-disordered breathing. Thorax 2008;63:738–46.

33. Kaneko Y, Floras JS, Usui K, et al. Cardiovascular effects of continuous positive airway pressure in patients with heart failure and obstructive sleep apnea. N Engl J Med 2003;348:1233–41.

34. American Society of Anesthesiologists Task Force on Perioperative Management of Patients with Obstructive Sleep Apnea. Practice guidelines for the perioperative management of patients with obstructive sleep apnea. Anesthesiology 2006;104:1081–93.

35. Warner DO. Perioperative abstinence from cigarettes. Anesthesiology 2006;104: 356–67.

36. Wightman JA. A prospective survey of the incidence of postoperative pulmonary complications. Br J Surg 1968;55:85–91.

37. Warner MA, Divertie MB, Tinker JH. Preoperative cessation of smoking and pulmonary complications in coronary artery bypass patients. Anesthesiology 1984;60:380–3.

38. Myles PS, Iacono GA, Hunt JO, et al. Risk of respiratory complications and wound infection in patients undergoing ambulatory surgery: smokers versus nonsmokers. Anesthesiology 2002;97:842–7.

39. Kotani N, Kushikata T, Hashimoto H, et al. Recovery of intraoperative microbicidal and inflammatory functions of alveolar immune cells after a tobacco smoke-free period. Anesthesiology 2001;94:999–1006.

40. Benowitz NI, Gourlay SG. Cardiovascular toxicity of nicotine: implications for nicotine replacement therapy. J Am Coll Cardiol 1997;29:2422–31.

41. Woehlck HJ, Connolly LA, Cinquegrani MP, et al. Acute smoking increases ST depression in humans during general anesthesia. Anesth Analg 1999;89:856–60.

42. Moller AM, Maaloe R, Pedersen T. Postoperative intensive care admittance: the role of tobacco smoking. Acta Anaesthesiol Scand 2001;45:345–8.

43. Fleisher LA, Beckman JA, Brown KA, et al. ACC/AHA 2007 guidelines on perioperative cardiovascular evaluation and care for noncardiac surgery. J Am Coll Cardiol 2007;50:1707–32. Available at: www.acc.org. Accessed February 9, 2009.

44. Barrera R, Weiji S, Amar D, et al. Smoking and timing of cessation: impact on pulmonary complications after thoracotomy. Chest 2005;127:1977–83.

45. Akrawi W, Benumof JL. A pathophysiological basis for informed preoperative smoking cessation counseling. J Cardiothorac Vasc Anesth 1997;11:629–40.

46. Sorenson LT, Karlsmark T, Gottrup F. Abstinence from smoking reduces incisional wound infection: a randomized controlled trial. Ann Surg 2003;238:1–5.

47. Murin S. Smoking cessation before lung resection. Chest 2005;127:1873–5.

48. A clinical practice guideline for treating tobacco use and dependence. JAMA 2000;283:3244–54.

49. Warner DO. Helping surgical patients quit smoking: why, when and how? Anesth Analg 2005;101:481–7.

50. Mahmarian JJ, Moye LA, Nasser GA, et al. Nicotine patch therapy in smoking cessation reduces the extent of exercise-induced myocardial ischemia. J Am Coll Cardiol 1997;30:125–30.
51. Tobacco cessation – you can quit smoking now! Available at: http://www.sur geongeneral.gov/tobacco/. Accessed November 13, 2008.
52. Arozullah AM, Khuri SF, Henderson WG, et al. Development and validation of a multifactorial risk index for predicting postoperative pneumonia after major noncardiac surgery. Ann Intern Med 2001;135:847–57.
53. Elkouri S, Gloviczki P, McKusick MA, et al. Perioperative complications and early outcome after endovascular and open surgical repair of abdominal aortic aneurysms. J Vasc Surg 2004;39:497–505.
54. Lawrence VA, Cornell JE, Smetana GW. Strategies to reduce postoperative complications after noncardiothoracic surgery: systematic review for the American College of Physicians. Ann Intern Med 2006;144:596–608.
55. Ballantyne JC, Carr DB, deFerranti S, et al. The comparative effects of postoperative analgesic therapies on pulmonary outcome: cumulative meta-analyses of randomized, controlled trials. Anesth Analg 1998;86:598–612.
56. Rodgers A, Walker N, Schug S, et al. Reduction of postoperative mortality and morbidity with epidural or spinal anesthesia; results from overview of randomized trials. BMJ 2000;321:1493.
57. Park WY, Thompson JS, Lee KK. Effect of epidural anesthesia and analgesia on perioperative outcome: a randomized, controlled Veterans Affairs co-operative study. Ann Surg 2001;234:560–9.
58. Rigg JR, Jamrozik K, Myles PS, et al. Epidural anaesthesia and analgesia and outcome of major surgery: a randomized trial. Lancet 2002;359:1276–82.
59. Liu LL, Leung JM. Predicting adverse postoperative outcomes in patients aged 80 years or older. J Am Geriatr Soc 2000;48:405–12.
60. Leung JM, Dzankic S. Relative importance of preoperative health status versus intraoperative factors in predicting postoperative adverse outcomes in geriatric surgical patients. J Am Geriatr Soc 2001;49:1080–5.
61. Johnson RG, Arozullah AM, Neumayer L, et al. Multivariable predictors of postoperative respiratory failure after general and vascular surgery: results from the patient safety in surgery study. J Am Coll Surg 2007;204:1188–98.
62. Qaseem A, Snow V, Fitterman N, et al. Risk assessment for and strategies to reduce perioperative pulmonary complications for patients undergoing noncardiothoracic surgery: a guideline from the American College of Physicians. Ann Intern Med 2006;144:575–80.
63. Smetana GW, Macpherson DS. The case against routine preoperative laboratory testing. Med Clin North Am 2003;87:7–40.
64. Archer C, Levy AR, McGregor M. Value of routine preoperative chest x-rays: a meta-analysis. Can J Anaesth 1993;40:1022–7.
65. Chumillas S, Ponce JL, Delgado F, et al. Prevention of postoperative pulmonary complications through respiratory rehabilitation: a controlled clinical study. Arch Phys Med Rehabil 1998;79:5–9.

Surgery in the Patient with Endocrine Dysfunction

Benjamin A. Kohl, MD[a],*, Stanley Schwartz, MD[b]

KEYWORDS

- Endocrine • Perioperative • Diabetes • Hyperthyroidism
- Hypothyroidism • Adrenal insufficiency • Pheochromocytoma

Patients with preoperative endocrinopathies represent a particular challenge not only to anesthesiologists but also to surgeons and perioperative clinicians. The "endocrine axis" is complex and has multiple feedback loops, some of which are endocrine and paracrine related, and others that are strongly influenced by the surgical stress response. Familiarity with several of the common endocrinopathies facilitates management in the perioperative period. This review focuses on four of the most common endocrinopathies: diabetes mellitus, hyperthyroidism, hypothyroidism, and adrenal insufficiency. Perioperative challenges in patients presenting with pheochromocytoma are also discussed.

DIABETES MELLITUS

Diabetes, by far the most common endocrinopathy, affects almost 20 million Americans. Roughly 90% of these patients are classified as type 2, and the remainder are type 1. It is estimated that upwards of 50% of this entire population will require surgery at some point during their lifetime.[1] Likewise, from a resource use standpoint, the average patient with diabetes spends up to 50% more time in the hospital postoperatively than a patient without diabetes undergoing the same procedure.[2] It is often the complications that are a direct result of this disease (neuropathy, retinopathy, nephropathy, and vasculopathy) that culminate in the need for surgery. Type 1 diabetes mellitus (T1DM) is a consequence of the destruction and loss of pancreatic β-cells (insulin producing). This destruction is believed to be mediated by autoimmune processes and is likely T cell mediated. Patients with T1DM will

---

[a] Department of Anesthesiology and Critical Care, University of Pennsylvania School of Medicine, 3400 Spruce Street, Dulles Building, Suite 680, Philadelphia, PA 19104, USA
[b] Department of Medicine, University of Pennsylvania Health System, 51 N. 39th Street, Suite 400, Philadelphia Heart Institute, Philadelphia, PA 19104, USA
* Corresponding author.
E-mail address: benjamin.kohl@uphs.upenn.edu (B.A. Kohl).

Med Clin N Am 93 (2009) 1031–1047
doi:10.1016/j.mcna.2009.05.003
0025-7125/09/$ – see front matter © 2009 Elsevier Inc. All rights reserved.

often have other autoimmune processes, most commonly thyroid disease.[3] On the contrary, type 2 diabetes mellitus (T2DM) is a disease characterized by the interaction of genetic and environmental factors (stress, diet, and amount of exercise) culminating in insulin resistance, abnormal b cell function and, ultimately, the development of overt T2DM. T2DM results when compensatory increases in insulin secretion can no longer keep plasma glucose levels within normal limits because of abnormal β cell mass and function and inappropriate release of glucagon by pancreatic α cells.

These 2 classes effectively discriminate most patients with diabetes, but it is important for the perioperative clinician to understand that other pathologies may result in a similar phenotype, such as pancreatitis and pancreatic cancer. It should also be recognized that patients destined to develop T2DM will have a prediabetic state of impaired glucose tolerance diagnosed by a fasting blood glucose greater than 100 mg/dL or 2-hour postprandial glucose greater than or equal to 140 mg/dL after a standard glucose challenge. This situation is critical as it has been shown that patients coming into the hospital with previously unrecognized abnormal glucose tolerance, or overt diabetes, have worse outcomes and a greater number of complications during the hospitalization, often in association with surgical procedures.[4] Major efforts should be instituted to identify these patients before or on admission, and criteria for those at special risk have recently been delineated.[5]

The ability of perioperative clinicians to appropriately risk stratify these patients and develop an interventional strategy is dependent on the individual patient and the associated pathology. Although anesthesiologists are rarely involved in the long-term care of these patients, the consequences of uncontrolled diabetes (ie, electrolyte imbalances, dehydration, wound infection) in the perioperative period can be life threatening.[6–9] Therefore, appropriate risk stratification and an optimal interventional strategy are necessary.

It is imperative to do a careful preoperative assessment for all patients. The patient with diabetes requires a systematic approach as the disease affects numerous organ systems (**Table 1**). Furthermore, although the surgical stress response is similar for a given procedure, patients with diabetes (particularly T1DM) are less able to counteract the effects of the gluconeogenic and glycolytic hormones (ie, cortisol, epinephrine, glucagon, growth hormone) that are released, all of which counteract the effect of insulin and may contribute to hyperglycemia.

Before examining the patient, there are several laboratory values that can help discern the severity of disease. Glycosylated hemoglobin (Hb_{A1C}) values can reflect the degree of hyperglycemia to which red blood cells have been exposed. Because the average lifespan of an red blood cell is 120 days, the Hb_{A1C} level is an indicator of glycemic levels over that period of time (although it is more strongly related to the prior 8–12 weeks). A normal value is up to 6%, but some patients with values greater than 5.5% may have impaired glucose tolerance. The goal of the American Diabetes Association (ADA) for control of diabetes is an Hb_{A1C} level less than 7%; this can be considered as adequate control. Values more than 8% correspond to average blood glucose levels greater than 180 mg/dL and indicate poor glycemic control.[10]

Because diabetes is a leading cause of renal failure, measurement of renal function can give insight into the severity of disease. Furthermore, of particular concern to the perioperative clinician, diabetic patients with renal insufficiency are at greater risk for hypoglycemia given the prolonged half-life of insulin and sulfonylureas. By identifying these patients preoperatively, more frequent (every 30–60 minutes) monitoring of blood glucose can be anticipated. Although a serum creatinine value does not

Table 1	
Perioperative considerations in the diabetic patient	
Complications	**Perioperative Considerations**
Neuropathies Peripheral sensory	Heel pads, avoid heating pads
Cystopathy	Inability to urinate, overflow incontinence, UTIs, consider straight catheterization
Gastroparesis	Watch for medications that slow gastric motility; reflux esophagitis/gastritis
Hypoglycemic unawareness	Frequent monitoring
CV autonomic neuropathy	Arrhythmias, telemetry
Silent ischemia, angina without chest pain	Watch for unexplained dyspnea, hypotension, arrhythmias
Retinopathy Lens	Blurred vision with either worse control or with sudden improvement in chronic DMOOC
Proliferative retinopathy	Rule out preoperatively if no routine eye examination in past year
Nephropathy	Careful decision on the use of intravenous iodinated contrast
Hyporenin, hypoaldosterone state	Watch for hyperkalemia Avoid hypotension
Macrophage dysfunction with blood sugar >150	Increased risk of infections; increased risk of fungal disease with parenteral nutrition Delayed wound healing
Other conditions Hyperlipidemia	Statins valuable in hospital
Hypertension	Treat, watch potassium level, edema, pulse rate

Abbreviations: CV, cardiovascular; DMOOC, diabetes mellitus out of control; UTI, urinary tract infection.

diagnose renal impairment, in the steady state it gives a good estimate of the glomerular filtration rate (GFR) using the Cockcroft-Gault equation:[11]

$$GFR = \frac{(140 - age) \times weight\ (kg) \times (0.85\ if\ female)}{72 \times serum\ creatinine}$$

Finally, preoperative evaluation of patients with diabetes mellitus should focus on some of the more common associations and sequelae of the disease process (see **Table 1**). These patients are at increased risk for cerebrovascular accidents, myocardial infarctions, acute renal failure, and postoperative wound complications. This risk may be mitigated with control of perioperative hyperglycemia. Musculoskeletal manifestations are common and may predict difficulties with laryngoscopy and endotracheal intubation.[12] A positive "prayer sign" (inability to approximate fingers and palms with fingers extended) may be an indicator of joint rigidity.[13] Such complications are important to note in the perioperative period and provisions should be made to minimize further exacerbation.

The major goals for these patients pertinent to their endocrinopathy should be minimizing hyperglycemia and avoiding hypoglycemia, hypovolemia, and hypo or hyperkalemia. In addition, minimizing the length of time these patients remain "nil by mouth" (NPO) is important. Surgery and anesthesia invoke a "stress response" in patients that is characterized by hypersecretion of counterregulatory hormones (eg, glucagon, norepinephrine, cortisol, and growth hormone). This response culminates in increased gluconeogenesis, glycogenolysis, and peripheral insulin resistance. Indeed, endogenous insulin levels are dramatically increased in the face of injury despite often profound hyperglycemia (ie, relative insulin deficiency). The effect of this altered hormonal milieu may culminate in diabetic ketoacidosis (DKA) in patients with T1DM and hyperosmolar hyperglycemic nonketosis (HHNK) in patients with T2DM.[14] Understanding this hormonal imbalance is fundamental to appreciating the fine endocrine balance these patients withstand in the perioperative period (**Fig. 1**). On the one hand, the surgical stress response initiates counterregulatory hormone secretion and relative insulin deficiency culminating in hyperglycemia. On the other hand, perioperative fasting with increased endogenous and exogenous insulin can easily cause profound hypoglycemia. Thus, a perioperative strategy that anticipates such pathology and aims to restore normoglycemia should be undertaken.

Although the approach to outpatient diabetic management is to aim for the lowest sugar possible without undue hypoglycemia, a similar perioperative goal is less realistic and potentially dangerous.[15,16] There are no current guidelines on perioperative glycemic control, but the American College of Endocrinology has released a position statement on inpatient glycemic control.[17] Understanding that the perioperative period is unique, a reasonable approach would be to maintain blood glucose at less than 200 mg/dL intraoperatively and less than 150 mg/dL postoperatively, but avoid levels less than 80 mg/dL.[18,19] This strategy would avoid severe hyperglycemia and minimize hypoglycemia. Recent data suggests that extremely tight glycemic control (eg, 80–110 mg/dL) in critically ill patients may be detrimental.[20] Patients who are insulin dependent often require a change in their scheduled dosing, dependent on how long they are NPO before surgery, the frequency of their insulin administration, and when the case is scheduled (**Box 1**). Thiazoladinediones (TZD) can be held on the morning of surgery, and secretagogues must be held preoperatively. However,

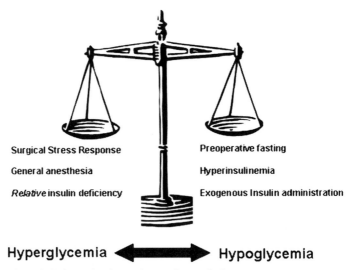

Surgical Stress Response

General anesthesia

Relative insulin deficiency

Preoperative fasting

Hyperinsulinemia

Exogenous Insulin administration

Hyperglycemia ⬅➡ Hypoglycemia

Fig. 1. The glycemic balance in the perioperative period.

Box 1

Perioperative management of patients with insulin-dependent diabetes

Need basal insulin at all times to avoid diabetic ketoacidosis

Night before procedure

Continue usual dose of p.m. glargine/NPH or a mixture (can recommend two thirds of usual dose if tightly controlled) the night before surgery (as long as taking usual oral intake the night before surgery)

For insulin pump users, continue usual overnight basal rate

Morning of procedure

No boluses of short-acting hypoglycemics unless blood sugar is greater than 200 mg/dL and greater than 3 hours preoperatively

May place on insulin drip OR give usual dose of glargine if routinely taken in morning

For insulin pump users, continue usual basal rate and infuse D5 throughout operation

If on NPH or other insulin mixture:

> No short-acting insulin within 3 to 4 hours of procedure (ie, no mixture preoperatively)
>
> Give half the usual intermediate-acting insulin, with D5, at controlled rate throughout procedure
>
> If doing operation without continuous D5, give no insulin preoperatively

Special situations

Emergency surgery

> No bolus of short-acting hypoglycemics preoperatively. Frequent (every 30–60 minutes) monitoring of blood sugar throughout operation. Start insulin infusion if blood sugar is greater than 200 mg/dL

Cardiac surgery

> Continue insulin infusion as needed to maintain blood glucose at 100 to 150 mg/dL in first 3 postoperative days

Abbreviations: D5–5%, dextrose containing solution; NPH, neutral protamine Hagedorn.

---

the biguanide, metformin, which has been associated with the development of lactic acidosis, should be withheld 24 hours preoperatively and restarted 48 to 72 hours postoperatively once normal renal function has been documented.[21,22] Long-acting sulfonylureas (ie, chlorpropramide), although rarely used, are best withheld 48 to 72 hours preoperatively to avoid potential hypoglycemia.[23] Incretins may be given (incretin mimetics subcutaneously and dipeptidyl peptidase (DPP)-IV inhibitors by mouth with a sip of water on the morning of surgery); in the absence of insulin or secretagogues, they do not cause hypoglycemia and seem particularly effective in reducing perioperative hyperglycemia as they counteract the effect of steroids on decreasing β cell function, best demonstrated in a murine model.[24–26] Antihyperglycemic agents (TZDs and incretins) and secretagogues may be restarted once enteral intake is permitted, although metformin is commonly avoided postoperatively in the hospital in case intercurrent events ensue that might change renal function acutely (hypotension, iodine dye induced renal dysfunction, sepsis, and so forth) and lead to the risk of lactic acidosis. **Box 1** summarizes perioperative insulin therapy recommendations in those patients (T1DM and T2DM) who routinely require insulin. In general, all of these patients should be scheduled as first case of the day to minimize a significant endocrine imbalance.

There are a paucity of data to guide the clinician on intraoperative glycemic control. Those undergoing cardiac surgery have been most heavily scrutinized. Unfortunately, there remains significant clinical uncertainty regarding the potential benefit of tight intraoperative glycemic control even in this subset of patients.[27–32] However, although no formal recommendations have been made, most clinicians would agree that maintaining plasma glucose below 200 mg/dL intraoperatively is reasonable. Similar consensus exists for the noncardiac surgical population.[33]

Postoperatively, attempts should be made to initiate enteral intake as soon as possible. Enteral intake should be started carefully and in consultation with a nutritionist familiar with the needs of diabetic patients.[34] Postoperative glycemic control has been (and continues to be) investigated thoroughly. Although there seems to be benefit with glycemic control in relation to postoperative surgical site infection,[6,35,36] there continues to be significant discussion on how this treatment modality relates to other morbidities and mortality.[37,38]

HYPERTHYROIDISM

The causes of hyperthyroidism are myriad. However, by far the most common cause is Graves disease. Graves disease is an autoimmune disorder caused by antibody generation directed at thyroid stimulating hormone (TSH) receptors causing an increase in thyroid hormone production. Clinical signs and symptoms of hyperthyroidism include tachycardia, atrial fibrillation, fever, tremor, goiter, and ophthalmopathy. Other manifestations include gastrointestinal symptoms such as diarrhea, nausea, and emesis. It is important to recognize that not all patients present with the classic symptomatology or laboratory findings. Patients with subclinical ("masked") hyperthyroidism are often asymptomatic and frequently have normal free thyroid hormone levels with suppressed TSH. This entity is more common in the geriatric population. In clinically overt hyperthyroidism, free thyroid hormone (T_4 and T_3) levels are frequently mildly elevated, however TSH is usually suppressed. In states of thyrotoxicosis, free T_4 levels can be dramatically increased. T_3 and T_4 have direct inotropic and chronotropic effects on the heart. In addition, thyroid hormones have a direct effect on vascular smooth muscle causing a decrement in systemic vascular resistance and blood pressure. As a result, the renin-angiotensin-aldosterone system is activated, enhancing sodium reabsorption and increasing circulating blood volume, increasing cardiac output by 50% to 300% (**Fig. 2**).[39,40] Chronically elevated levels of these hormones may limit the ability of patients to respond to the stress of surgery and can culminate in cardiovascular collapse.[41–43] The perioperative clinician must be familiar with the diagnosis and treatment of hyperthyroidism as failure to identify and treat appropriately can drastically increase mortality.

Patients with hyperthyroidism should take their antithyroid medications on the morning of surgery.[44] For those patients with uncontrolled hyperthyroidism who are presenting for elective surgery, their surgical procedure should be postponed until they are on a stable medical regimen to reduce their risk of thyroid storm.[45] For those patients presenting for urgent or emergent surgery, it is incumbent on the anesthesiologist to have ready access to drugs that block the systemic effects of excess thyroid hormone. Such drugs include β-blockers, antithyroid medications (including propylthiouracil and methimazole), and iodine. β-Blockers not only directly inhibit sympathetic activation but also inhibit the peripheral conversion of T_4 to T_3 (the most active thyroid

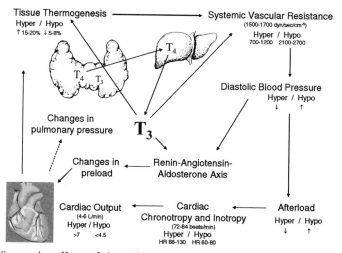

Fig. 2. Cardiovascular effects of thyroid hormone. (*Reprinted from* Klein I. Thyroid disease and the heart. Circulation 2007;116:1725; with permission.)

hormone). Thionamides, such as propylthiouracil (PTU) and methimazole, are actively transported into the thyroid gland and inhibit further production of hormone. Furthermore, PTU inhibits peripheral conversion of T_4 to T_3.[46] Finally, although necessary for normal thyroid function, inorganic iodide in excess will manifest an antithyroid action known as the Wolff-Chaikoff effect.[47] Potassium iodide is given enterally as either Lugol solution (8 mg iodide per drop) or saturated solution of potassium iodide (SSKI) and is usually administered preoperatively for thyroid surgery as it decreases the vascularity of the gland.[48] Inorganic iodide should not be administered before thionamide treatment as it may initially increase the amount of thyroid hormone released and precipitate thyroid storm (Jod-Basedow effect). Anesthetic agents that are vagolytic or sympathomimetic (eg, pancuronium, ephedrine, epinephrine, norepinephrine, atropine) are best avoided in patients with thyrotoxicosis.[21]

The most feared perioperative complication that usually arises from undiagnosed or undertreated hyperthyroidism is thyroid storm. Thyroid storm can occur anytime in the perioperative period, although it usually occurs either intraoperatively or in the first 48 hours postoperatively. The mortality of thyroid storm is 10% to 75% and the patient must be monitored in a critical care environment.[49] Symptoms are nonspecific and include hyperpyrexia (up to 41.1°C [106°F]), tachycardia, and delirium.[50] Other conditions that should be considered in the differential diagnosis include malignant hyperthermia, neuroleptic malignant syndrome, and pheochromocytoma. As the mortality of this entity is high if left untreated and the diagnosis is purely clinical (supported by laboratory data), it is often necessary to treat empirically before confirmation.[51] Treatment of thyroid storm includes thionamides, β-blockers (goal heart rate <90 bpm), and antipyretics (or external cooling measures).[21] Acetaminophen is preferred over salicylates as the latter may exacerbate thyrotoxicosis by decreasing thyroid protein binding and increasing free T_3 and T_4.[51] A search for the precipitating cause of thyroid storm should be undertaken immediately. The most common cause in the perioperative period is infection (sepsis). Blood, urine, and sputum cultures should be obtained, however empiric antibiotics are not recommended.[52] Finally, for those patients who are volume depleted, particularly if chronic hyperthyroidism exists, volume resuscitation with the addition of dextrose should be administered to replace depleted glycogen stores.[53]

HYPOTHYROIDISM

Hypothyroidism is a common endocrinopathy in the United States affecting about 1% of all patients and is more prevalent in women.[49] Primary hypothyroidism accounts for 95% of all cases and is characterized by low thyroid hormone levels (free T_4 <5 pmol/L) in the face of normal or elevated TSH (often >10 mU/L). Common signs and symptoms of hypothyroidism include lethargy, fatigue, anorexia, headaches, hoarse voice, depression, and cold intolerance. The most common noniatrogenic cause is chronic autoimmune thyroiditis (Hashimoto thyroiditis). There are many iatrogenic causes that the perioperative clinician needs to be familiar with. Surgical thyroid resection or radioactive ablations are common causes that can frequently be anticipated. Less obvious, however, include treatment of hyperthyroidism or other pituitary and hypothalamic disorders (Sheehan syndrome, pituitary dysfunction after head trauma).[54] A variety of drugs can induce hypothyroidism including lithium, amiodarone, iron, and cholestyramine. The surgical stress response in addition to general anesthesia may also incite hypothyroidism or, more commonly, the classic euthyroid sick syndrome.[55] After induction of general anesthesia, total T_3 levels decrease and remain low for at least 24 hours.[56] Understanding the implications of hypothyroidism on the morbidity and mortality of surgical patients may allow the perioperative clinician to anticipate complications and manage preemptively.[57]

Similar to hyperthyroidism, hypothyroidism affects multiple organ systems and encompasses a wide clinical spectrum. The most clinically important of these is the cardiovascular system. Whereas plasma catecholamine levels are generally within normal limits, β-adrenergic receptor function is depressed and results in an imbalance of α and β adrenergic activity, with α predominating. In general, a deficiency in thyroid activity culminates in depressed cardiac function (inotropy and chronotropy) and increased systemic vascular resistance. The pulmonary system is affected as there may be depressed responses to hypercarbia and hypoxemia[58] and, in more severe cases, decreased lung diffusion capacity.[59] The renin-angiotensin-aldosterone complex responds to this by excreting sodium (greater than free water) culminating in hyponatremia and intravascular volume depletion.

The preferred treatment of hypothyroidism is tetraiodothyronine (T_4, levothyroxine) replacement and patients should preferably be rendered euthyroid before surgery. The more active hormone (T_3) is less stable but is converted in vivo intracellularly. The half-life of levothyroxine is approximately 1 week and therefore it is not imperative that patients take their dose the morning of surgery.[44] If intravenous dosing is necessary, one half the enteral dose is equivalent. There is controversy about hypothyroid patients with known ischemic heart disease or presenting for coronary revascularization. Rapid replenishment of thyroid function risks increasing myocardial oxygen demand causing ischemia. However, delay in therapy may place the patient at risk of developing myxedema coma.[60] Currently, the consensus is that if a patient needs urgent cardiac revascularization, they should undergo the procedure before replacement therapy,[61,62] however many endocrinologists will recommend starting at least low dose T_4 in consultation with the cardiologist.

Patients presenting for surgery with hypothyroidism can be grouped into three broad categories: (1) hypothyroid patients well controlled on thyroid medications; (2) mild to moderately hypothyroid patients; (3) patients presenting with or developing severe hypothyroidism (myxedema coma) perioperatively. There is little to do with the first group other than be aware of their thyroid replacement dosing and be hyper-acute to signs and symptoms of worsening hypothyroidism postoperatively including delirium, prolonged ileus, infection without fever, and myxedema coma. Preoperative sedation in this group should be minimized as these patients can be exquisitely sensitive to narcotics and benzodiazepines. Most patients with mild to moderate hypothyroidism can undergo surgery without a disproportionate increase in perioperative risk.[57,62,63] Close attention to airway patency in the postoperative period is necessary as there are reports of airway obstruction in hypothyroid patients.[64] Intraoperative fluid replacement should be with dextrose containing normal saline. Controlled ventilation is recommended as these patients are at risk for hypoventilation. In those patients who present for surgery with severe hypothyroidism (depressed mental status, pericardial effusion, and heart failure) or in whom treatment is deemed necessary before urgent/emergent surgery (severely depressed T_4 and T_3), intravenous levothyroxine (200–500 mg given over 30 minutes) should be administered, followed by a daily dose of 50–100 mg intravenously.[65] As many patients with hypothyroidism also have adrenal insufficiency (and thyroid replacement may precipitate adrenal crisis), glucocorticoids should be administered concurrently.[21]

Myxedema coma is rare and usually presents postoperatively. It is commonly precipitated by additional insults such as infection, cold exposure, sedatives and analgesics, and a variety of other medications. Although the mortality of this entity has been reported to be as high as 80%, it seems to be decreasing in recent years likely due to an increased awareness and improved diagnostic testing.[61,66,67] Myxedema coma is characterized by severely depressed mental status (sometimes coma or seizure), hypothermia, bradycardia, hyponatremia, heart failure, and hypopnea. Although maintenance of normothermia is tempting, the resulting vasodilatation may cause cardiovascular collapse in someone with intravascular volume depletion, cardiac insufficiency, and pericardial effusion/tamponade; normothermia should be performed extremely carefully, if at all.[61] Myxedema coma is a medical emergency and necessitates urgent administration of levothyroxine. An initial intravenous bolus of 200 to 500 μg should be given followed by 50 to 100 μg/d. Dehydration is frequently present and aggressive volume resuscitation with dextrose and normal saline should be instituted. Intravenous glucocorticoids should be administered (eg, hydrocortisone 50 mg four times a day) because concomitant adrenal insufficiency is not uncommon. Resolution of symptoms, if properly treated, should be seen within 24 hours.

ADRENAL INSUFFICIENCY

The hypothalamic-pituitary-adrenal (HPA) axis is central to a patient's ability to generate a surgical stress response. A defect anywhere in this cycle has dramatic consequences in the perioperative period. Tuberculosis used to be the main cause of primary adrenal insufficiency (AI), but autoimmune adrenalitis is now the most common cause. Other causes of primary AI include infections, adrenalectomy, and sepsis.[68,69] However, of greater importance to perioperative clinicians is secondary AI. Secondary AI is characterized by atrophy of the adrenal cortex and occurs when insufficient adrenocorticotropic hormone (ACTH) is released to stimulate the adrenal cortex. It is most commonly caused by exogenous glucocorticoid administration, which suppresses hypothalamic corticotrophin releasing hormone (CRH) and pituitary ACTH. Although there is remarkable variability in individual response to a particular dose and length of treatment with steroids, in general any patient who has received the equivalent of 20 mg/d of prednisone for greater than 5 days is at risk for suppression of the HPA axis, and if they have been on therapy for approximately 1 month, they may have HPA suppression for up to 6 to 12 months after stopping therapy.[70–72] Similarly, an equivalent dose of prednisone 5 mg (or less) for any period of time will usually not significantly suppress the HPA axis.[73] Other modes of steroid administration should be noted preoperatively as topical, inhaled, and regional administration of glucocorticoids may cause adrenal suppression.[74] In addition, these generalizations pertain to the patient taking steroids in the morning. A lower dose of steroids in the evening may inhibit the normal diurnal ACTH release and affect the way that patient is able to respond to a surgical stress.[74]

Although glucocorticoids alone are not vasoactive, they mediate vascular tone by increasing responsiveness to catecholamines. This effect occurs at a local tissue level (ie, not centrally mediated) and likely is mediated by inhibition of prostacyclin production.[75,76] It is important to understand that mineralocorticoid deficiency does not have the same effect. Mineralocorticoid (ie, aldosterone) secretion is primarily regulated by the renin-angiotensin system. A deficiency in ACTH (by glucocorticoid administration) will not result in aldosterone deficiency.[74]

Tests to detect perioperative adrenal suppression or, perhaps more importantly, identify patients who will respond to supplemental glucocorticoids have been neither sensitive nor specific.[74,77–79] However, the short ACTH stimulation test is able to reliably assess adrenocortical function.[77,80] If this test is abnormal preoperatively, supplemental perioperative glucocorticoid administration is justified. If the risk for perioperative adrenal suppression is significant a systematic approach should be taken to determine if steroid supplementation is necessary (**Fig. 3**). The decision should be based on suspicion (from history and physical examination), acuity of the operation and anticipated severity of the procedure. It is our opinion that if there is a high suspicion for the presence or development of AI and the procedure is emergent, steroids should be administered. If there is less urgency and time allows, an ACTH stimulation test should be performed to see if the adrenal gland responds appropriately to supraphysiologic doses of ACTH. Finally, even if a preoperative ACTH stimulation test is normal and the patient is at high risk for perioperative AI, if unexplained hypotension persists despite volume repletion, steroids should be administered in a dose consistent with the level of injury. Postoperatively, steroids should be continued until the stress response diminishes (usually 48 hours).[81] The presence of unexplained nausea, vomiting, hypotension, orthostasis, change in mental status, hyponatremia, or hyperkalemia, should warrant checking T_4, TSH, random plasma cortisol and, depending on the urgency of the situation, may require empiric therapy with stress-dose steroids and possibly T_4. In addition, recrudescence of a stressor (eg, postoperative infection) may warrant reinstitution of supplemental glucocorticoids.

One drug that warrants mention for patients suspected of or at high risk of AI is etomidate. Etomidate is a frequently used anesthetic induction agent. Although it is a particularly attractive option for patients who are hemodynamically unstable, its effect of inhibiting steroid synthesis may precipitate acute AI and is best avoided in this population.[82,83]

PHEOCHROMOCYTOMA

Pheochromocytomas are rare neuroendocrine tumors, usually located in the adrenal medulla (although they may occur in extraadrenal tissues) originating in catecholamine-producing chromaffin cells. The "10-10-10" rule is a reminder that 10% of these tumors are bilateral, 10% are extraadrenal and less than 10% are malignant.

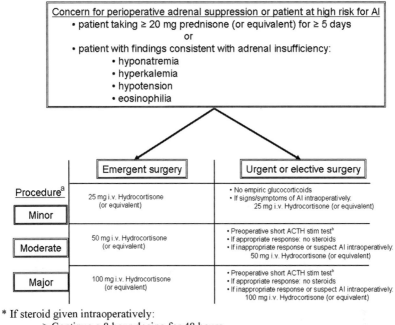

* If steroid given intraoperatively:
  --> Continue q 8 hour dosing for 48 hours
  --> If continued need, consider endocrine consultation

Fig. 3. Algorithm for perioperative steroid administration. ACTH, adrenocorticotrophic hormone; AI, adrenal insufficiency; i.v., intravenous; stim, stimulation. [a] Minor procedures include those performed under local anesthesia or those less than 1 hour in duration; moderate procedures include most vascular surgeries or orthopedic procedures; major procedures include larger, prolonged operations such as esophagectomy or those using cardiopulmonary bypass. [b] The short ACTH stimulation involves administration of 250 µg i.v. synthetic ACTH (Cortrosyn, Cosyntropin) followed by a plasma cortisol collection in 30 minutes. A plasma cortisol concentration of more than 18 to 20 µg/dL is consistent with normal adrenal function.

Most pheochromocytomas synthesize and secrete norepinephrine, although hypersecretion of epinephrine can also be seen. Signs and symptoms include periodic flushing, palpitations, sweating, headaches, and hypertension. Patients usually present perioperatively for (not despite) their pheochromocytoma. However, some patients may present with their first catecholamine crisis during routine surgery and thus familiarity with this syndrome is critical.

If a diagnosis of pheochromocytoma is suspected, the initial recommended test is measurement of plasma free metanephrines, as the sensitivity is reportedly 99%.[84] Thus, a negative test essentially excludes this diagnosis. Urinary vanillylmandelic acid (VMA) levels have much higher specificity (95%). Once there is biochemical evidence of a catecholamine secreting tumor, radiographic imaging studies are performed to localize the tumor (usually MRI or nuclear imaging).[85]

Not surprisingly, the end organ that is most negatively impacted in this syndrome is the cardiovascular system. Chronic, often severe, hypertension can frequently be corroborated with abnormal ECG findings (repolarization abnormalities, ventricular hypertrophy, nonspecific ST-T wave changes, and QTc interval prolongation). Some of these abnormalities will resolve after removal of the tumor.[86] The most common pathology seen in these patients is a hypertrophic cardiomyopathy secondary to norepinephrine-induced hypertension. As most of these tumors are nonmalignant, surgery may be curative in more than 90% of cases.[87]

Careful preoperative preparation of the patient with pheochromocytoma is necessary. Failure to properly premedicate can increase perioperative mortality dramatically.[87] The goal entails adequate α- and β-adrenergic blockade. Current recommendations are that phenoxybenzamine (a long-acting noncompetitive α-adrenergic antagonist) be initiated roughly 1 to 2 weeks preoperatively.[88,89] Because the half-life of this drug is 24 to 36 hours, patients often require large amounts of intravenous fluid postoperatively and may be somnolent during this time due to central α_2-adrenoceptor blockade. Roizen and colleagues[90] recommended the following criteria for establishing adequate preoperative α-adrenergic blockade: (1) blood pressure should be no higher than 160/90 mmHg in the 24 hours preoperatively; (2) orthostatic hypotension *should* be present; (3) no ST-T wave changes on ECG for 1 week preoperatively; and (4) no more than one premature ventricular contraction every 5 minutes. For those patients with persistent tachycardia or hypertension, a β-blocker can be initiated 3 to 5 days before surgery.[61] There is a theoretical risk of inciting unopposed α-agonism if β-antagonists are started first, culminating in severely increased vascular resistance. Metyrosine (a competitive inhibitor of tyrosine hydroxylase) has also been used successfully preoperatively. Tyrosine hydroxylase facilitates conversion of tyrosine to dihydroxyphenylalanine (DOPA), and is the rate-limiting step in catecholamine synthesis. Metyrosine depletes tumor stores of catecholamines. Institution of early α antagonism in addition to realization that these patients are frequently severely hypovolemic has dramatically decreased perioperative mortality in these patients.[91] Echocardiography can be extremely valuable in detecting overall systolic and diastolic function. Left ventricular hypertrophy is present in most of these patients; however, ventricular dilatation is a more ominous sign. For this reason, some have suggested obtaining a preoperative echocardiogram regardless of blood pressure.[92]

Attempts to minimize hemodynamic fluctuations pre- and intraoperatively are advisable. Sufficient preoperative anxiolysis is warranted. In addition to standard monitors, careful hemodynamic monitoring is necessary and an intraarterial catheter should be placed before anesthetic induction. Furthermore, several large-bore intravenous catheters should be placed (rapid volume administration is often necessary) and serious consideration should be given to central intravenous access for administration of vasoactive medications.[93] Placement of a pulmonary artery catheter is not necessary, although may be helpful in the presence of significant cardiac disease.[94,95] Agents that directly or indirectly increase catecholamine levels, such as ketamine and ephedrine, should be avoided. In addition, morphine (which causes histamine release) has been associated with and felt to be a trigger of pheochromocytoma crisis.[96] Meperidine and droperidol have also been associated with severe hypertension and are best avoided.[97] Intraoperative hypertensive crises are best treated with rapid-acting direct vasodilators (eg, nitroprusside, nitroglycerine, nicardipine).

Postoperatively these patients may continue to be hypertensive for up to 1 week due to elevated catecholamine levels in adrenergic nerve endings. Alternatively, aggressive preoperative adrenergic blockade may render the patient hypotensive postoperatively, usually for 24 to 48 hours at which point most of the phenoxybenzamine has been eliminated. With improved understanding of the pathophysiology of this disease in addition to numerous investigations studying various techniques, perioperative outcome has improved dramatically.[88]

SUMMARY

Patients with endocrine dysfunction present unique challenges to perioperative clinicians. Diabetes mellitus is the most common endocrinopathy in patients presenting for surgery. Numerous investigations have shown that the increased mortality formerly seen in these patients can be dramatically minimized (to the level of their nondiabetic counterparts) with careful glycemic management. It is always advisable to normalize, as best as possible, the endocrinopathy or hemodynamic consequences before surgery, particularly in cases of hypo- and hyperthyroidism and pheochromocytoma. Adrenal insufficiency often presents intra- or postoperatively and thus, being familiar with the signs and symptoms allows the perioperative clinician to be acutely aware and institute immediate therapy if necessary.

REFERENCES

1. Glister BC, Vigersky RA. Perioperative management of type 1 diabetes mellitus. Endocrinol Metab Clin North Am 2003;32:411–36.
2. Gavin LA. Perioperative management of the diabetic patient. Endocrinol Metab Clin North Am 1992;21:457–75.
3. Olson OC. The immunology, genetics, and etiology of diabetes mellitus. 2nd edition. New York: Raven Press; 1988.
4. Umpierrez GE, Isaacs SD, Bazargan N, et al. Hyperglycemia: an independent marker of in-hospital mortality in patients with undiagnosed diabetes. J Clin Endocrinol Metab 2002;87:978–82.
5. Kim KS, Kim SK, Lee YK, et al. Diagnostic value of glycated haemoglobin for the early detection of diabetes in high-risk subjects. Diabet Med 2008;25:997–1000.
6. Furnary AP, Zerr KJ, Grunkemeier GL, et al. Continuous intravenous insulin infusion reduces the incidence of deep sternal wound infection in diabetic patients after cardiac surgical procedures. Ann Thorac Surg 1999;67:352–60 [discussion: 60–2].
7. Zerr KJ, Furnary AP, Grunkemeier GL, et al. Glucose control lowers the risk of wound infection in diabetics after open heart operations. Ann Thorac Surg 1997;63:356–61.
8. Pozzilli P, Leslie RD. Infections and diabetes: mechanisms and prospects for prevention. Diabet Med 1994;11:935–41.
9. Latham R, Lancaster AD, Covington JF, et al. The association of diabetes and glucose control with surgical-site infections among cardiothoracic surgery patients. Infect Control Hosp Epidemiol 2001;22:607–12.
10. Nathan DM, Singer DE, Hurxthal K, et al. The clinical information value of the glycosylated hemoglobin assay. N Engl J Med 1984;310:341–6.
11. Stevens LA, Coresh J, Greene T, et al. Assessing kidney function – measured and estimated glomerular filtration rate. N Engl J Med 2006;354:2473–83.
12. Reissell E, Orko R, Maunuksela EL, et al. Predictability of difficult laryngoscopy in patients with long-term diabetes mellitus. Anaesthesia 1990;45:1024–7.
13. Hogan K, Rusy D, Springman SR. Difficult laryngoscopy and diabetes mellitus. Anesth Analg 1988;67:1162–5.
14. Monk TG, Mueller M, White PF. Treatment of stress response during balanced anesthesia. Comparative effects of isoflurane, alfentanil, and trimethaphan. Anesthesiology 1992;76:39–45.

15. American Diabetes Association. Standards of medical care in diabetes – 2007. Diabetes Care 2007;30(Suppl 1):S4–41.
16. American Association of Clinical Endocrinologists medical guidelines for clinical practice for the management of diabetes mellitus. Available at: http://www.aace.com/pub/pdf/guidelines/DMGuidelines2007.pdf. Accessed September 27, 2008.
17. Garber AJ, Moghissi ES, Bransome ED Jr, et al. American College of Endocrinology position statement on inpatient diabetes and metabolic control. Endocr Pract 2004;10(Suppl 2):4–9.
18. Kosiborod M, Inzucchi SE, Krumholz HM, et al. Glucometrics in patients hospitalized with acute myocardial infarction: defining the optimal outcomes-based measure of risk. Circulation 2008;117:1018–27.
19. Pinto DS, Skolnick AH, Kirtane AJ, et al. U-shaped relationship of blood glucose with adverse outcomes among patients with ST-segment elevation myocardial infarction. J Am Coll Cardiol 2005;46:178–80.
20. NICE-SUGAR Study Investigators, Finfer S, Chittock DR, et al. Intensive versus conventional glucose control in critically ill patients. N Engl J Med 2009; 360(13):1283–97.
21. Mercado DL, Petty BG. Perioperative medication management. Med Clin North Am 2003;87:41–57.
22. Metchick LN, Petit WA Jr, Inzucchi SE. Inpatient management of diabetes mellitus. Am J Med 2002;113:317–23.
23. Marks JB. Perioperative management of diabetes. Am Fam Physician 2003;67: 93–100.
24. Lambillotte C, Gilon P, Henquin JC. Direct glucocorticoid inhibition of insulin secretion. An in vitro study of dexamethasone effects in mouse islets. J Clin Invest 1997;99:414–23.
25. Chia CW, Egan JM. Special features: incretin-based therapies in type 2 diabetes mellitus. J Clin Endocrinol Metab 2008;93:3703–16.
26. Gautier JF, Choukem SP, Girard J. Physiology of incretins (GIP and GLP-1) and abnormalities in type 2 diabetes. Diabetes Metab 2008;34(Suppl 2):S65–72.
27. Doenst T, Wijeysundera D, Karkouti K, et al. Hyperglycemia during cardiopulmonary bypass is an independent risk factor for mortality in patients undergoing cardiac surgery. J Thorac Cardiovasc Surg 2005;130:1144. e1–1144.e8.
28. Gandhi GY, Nuttall GA, Abel MD, et al. Intensive intraoperative insulin therapy versus conventional glucose management during cardiac surgery: a randomized trial. Ann Intern Med 2007;146:233–43.
29. Gandhi GY, Nuttall GA, Abel MD, et al. Intraoperative hyperglycemia and perioperative outcomes in cardiac surgery patients. Mayo Clin Proc 2005;80:862–6.
30. Lazar HL, Chipkin SR, Fitzgerald CA, et al. Tight glycemic control in diabetic coronary artery bypass graft patients improves perioperative outcomes and decreases recurrent ischemic events. Circulation 2004;109:1497–502.
31. Ouattara A, Lecomte P, Le Manach Y, et al. Poor intraoperative blood glucose control is associated with a worsened hospital outcome after cardiac surgery in diabetic patients. Anesthesiology 2005;103:687–94.
32. Puskas F, Grocott HP, White WD, et al. Intraoperative hyperglycemia and cognitive decline after CABG. Ann Thorac Surg 2007;84:1467–73.
33. Fleisher LA, Beckman JA, Brown KA, et al. ACC/AHA 2007 guidelines on perioperative cardiovascular evaluation and care for noncardiac surgery: a report of the American College of Cardiology/American Heart Association Task Force on Practice Guidelines (Writing Committee to Revise the 2002 Guidelines on

Perioperative Cardiovascular Evaluation for Noncardiac Surgery): developed in collaboration with the American Society of Echocardiography, American Society of Nuclear Cardiology, Heart Rhythm Society, Society of Cardiovascular Anesthesiologists, Society for Cardiovascular Angiography and Interventions, Society for Vascular Medicine and Biology, and Society for Vascular Surgery. Circulation 2007;116:e418–99.

34. Swift CS, Boucher JL. Nutrition therapy for the hospitalized patient with diabetes. Endocr Pract 2006;12(Suppl 3):61–7.

35. van den Berghe G, Wouters P, Weekers F, et al. Intensive insulin therapy in the critically ill patients. N Engl J Med 2001;345:1359–67.

36. Golden SH, Peart-Vigilance C, Kao WH, et al. Perioperative glycemic control and the risk of infectious complications in a cohort of adults with diabetes. Diabetes Care 1999;22:1408–14.

37. Treggiari MM, Karir V, Yanez ND, et al. Intensive insulin therapy and mortality in critically ill patients. Crit Care 2008;12:R29.

38. De La Rosa GD, Donado JH, Restrepo AH, et al. Strict glycemic control in patients hospitalized in a mixed medical and surgical intensive care unit: a randomized clinical trial. Crit Care 2008;12:R120.

39. Klein I, Danzi S. Thyroid disease and the heart. Circulation 2007;116:1725–35.

40. Biondi B, Palmieri EA, Lombardi G, et al. Effects of thyroid hormone on cardiac function: the relative importance of heart rate, loading conditions, and myocardial contractility in the regulation of cardiac performance in human hyperthyroidism. J Clin Endocrinol Metab 2002;87:968–74.

41. Forfar JC, Muir AL, Sawers SA, et al. Abnormal left ventricular function in hyperthyroidism: evidence for a possible reversible cardiomyopathy. N Engl J Med 1982;307:1165–70.

42. Woeber KA. Thyrotoxicosis and the heart. N Engl J Med 1992;327:94–8.

43. Klein I, Ojamaa K. Thyroid hormone and the cardiovascular system. N Engl J Med 2001;344:501–9.

44. Spell NO 3rd. Stopping and restarting medications in the perioperative period. Med Clin North Am 2001;85:1117–28.

45. Prescott PT. Disorders of the thyroid. In: Lubin MF, Smith RB, Dodson TF, et al, editors. Medical management of the surgical patient. 4th edition. New York: Cambridge University Press; 2006. p. 367–73.

46. Farwell AP, Braverman LE. Thyroid and antithyroid drugs. In: Hardman JG, Limberd LE, editors. Goodman and Gilman's: the pharmacological basis of therapeutics. 10th edition. New York: McGraw-Hill; 2001. p. 1563–96.

47. Markou K, Georgopoulos N, Kyriazopoulou V, et al. Iodine-induced hypothyroidism. Thyroid 2001;11:501–10.

48. Streetman DD, Khanderia U. Diagnosis and treatment of Graves disease. Ann Pharmacother 2003;37:1100–9.

49. Ringel MD. Management of hypothyroidism and hyperthyroidism in the intensive care unit. Crit Care Clin 2001;17:59–74.

50. Howton JC. Thyroid storm presenting as coma. Ann Emerg Med 1988;17:343–5.

51. McKeown NJ, Tews MC, Gossain VV, et al. Hyperthyroidism. Emerg Med Clin North Am 2005;23:669–85, viii.

52. Burch HB, Wartofsky L. Life-threatening thyrotoxicosis. Thyroid storm. Endocrinol Metab Clin North Am 1993;22:263–77.

53. Nayak B, Burman K. Thyrotoxicosis and thyroid storm. Endocrinol Metab Clin North Am 2006;35:663–86, vii.

54. Benvenga S, Campenni A, Ruggeri RM, et al. Clinical review 113: hypopituitarism secondary to head trauma. J Clin Endocrinol Metab 2000;85:1353–61.

55. Wellby ML, Kennedy JA, Barreau PB, et al. Endocrine and cytokine changes during elective surgery. J Clin Pathol 1994;47:1049–51.

56. Stathatos N, Wartofsky L. Perioperative management of patients with hypothyroidism. Endocrinol Metab Clin North Am 2003;32:503–18.

57. Ladenson PW, Levin AA, Ridgway EC, et al. Complications of surgery in hypothyroid patients. Am J Med 1984;77:261–6.

58. Zwillich CW, Pierson DJ, Hofeldt FD, et al. Ventilatory control in myxedema and hypothyroidism. N Engl J Med 1975;292:662–5.

59. Wilson WR, Bedell GN. The pulmonary abnormalities in myxedema. J Clin Invest 1960;39:42–55.

60. O'Connor CJ, March R, Tuman KJ. Severe myxedema after cardiopulmonary bypass. Anesth Analg 2003;96:62–4.

61. Connery LE, Coursin DB. Assessment and therapy of selected endocrine disorders. Anesthesiol Clin North America 2004;22:93–123.

62. Schiff RL, Welsh GA. Perioperative evaluation and management of the patient with endocrine dysfunction. Med Clin North Am 2003;87:175–92.

63. Weinberg AD, Brennan MD, Gorman CA, et al. Outcome of anesthesia and surgery in hypothyroid patients. Arch Intern Med 1983;143:893–7.

64. Benfari G, de Vincentiis M. Postoperative airway obstruction: a complication of a previously undiagnosed hypothyroidism. Otolaryngol Head Neck Surg 2005; 132:343–4.

65. Bennett-Guerrero E, Kramer DC, Schwinn DA. Effect of chronic and acute thyroid hormone reduction on perioperative outcome. Anesth Analg 1997;85:30–6.

66. Wartofsky L. Myxedema coma. Endocrinol Metab Clin North Am 2006;35:687–98, vii–viii.

67. Dutta P, Bhansali A, Masoodi SR, et al. Predictors of outcome in myxoedema coma: a study from a tertiary care centre. Crit Care 2008;12:R1.

68. Arlt W, Allolio B. Adrenal insufficiency. Lancet 2003;361:1881–93.

69. Shenker Y, Skatrud JB. Adrenal insufficiency in critically ill patients. Am J Respir Crit Care Med 2001;163:1520–3.

70. Nicholson G, Burrin JM, Hall GM. Peri-operative steroid supplementation. Anaesthesia 1998;53:1091–104.

71. Henzen C, Suter A, Lerch E, et al. Suppression and recovery of adrenal response after short-term, high-dose glucocorticoid treatment. Lancet 2000; 355:542–5.

72. Hopkins RL, Leinung MC. Exogenous Cushing's syndrome and glucocorticoid withdrawal. Endocrinol Metab Clin North Am 2005;34:371–84, ix.

73. Jabbour SA. Steroids and the surgical patient. Med Clin North Am 2001;85: 1311–7.

74. Axelrod L. Perioperative management of patients treated with glucocorticoids. Endocrinol Metab Clin North Am 2003;32:367–83.

75. Axelrod L. Inhibition of prostacyclin production mediates permissive effect of glucocorticoids on vascular tone. Perturbations of this mechanism contribute to pathogenesis of Cushing's syndrome and Addison's disease. Lancet 1983;1: 904–6.

76. Rascher W, Dietz R, Schomig A, et al. Reversal of corticosterone-induced supersensitivity of vascular smooth muscle to noradrenaline by arachidonic acid and prostacyclin. Eur J Pharmacol 1980;68:267–73.

77. Kehlet H, Binder C. Value of an ACTH test in assessing hypothalamic-pituitary-adrenocortical function in glucocorticoid-treated patients. Br Med J 1973;2: 147–9.
78. Knudsen L, Christiansen LA, Lorentzen JE. Hypotension during and after operation in glucocorticoid-treated patients. Br J Anaesth 1981;53:295–301.
79. Plumpton FS, Besser GM, Cole PV. Corticosteroid treatment and surgery. 1. An investigation of the indications for steroid cover. Anaesthesia 1969;24:3–11.
80. Lindholm J, Kehlet H. Re-evaluation of the clinical value of the 30 min ACTH test in assessing the hypothalamic-pituitary-adrenocortical function. Clin Endocrinol (Oxf) 1987;26:53–9.
81. Salem M, Tainsh RE Jr, Bromberg J, et al. Perioperative glucocorticoid coverage. A reassessment 42 years after emergence of a problem. Ann Surg 1994;219: 416–25.
82. Thomas Z, Fraser GL. An update on the diagnosis of adrenal insufficiency and the use of corticotherapy in critical illness. Ann Pharmacother 2007;41: 1456–65.
83. Wagner RL, White PF, Kan PB, et al. Inhibition of adrenal steroidogenesis by the anesthetic etomidate. N Engl J Med 1984;310:1415–21.
84. Lenders JW, Pacak K, Walther MM, et al. Biochemical diagnosis of pheochromocytoma: which test is best? JAMA 2002;287:1427–34.
85. Pacak K, Linehan WM, Eisenhofer G, et al. Recent advances in genetics, diagnosis, localization, and treatment of pheochromocytoma. Ann Intern Med 2001; 134:315–29.
86. Liao WB, Liu CF, Chiang CW, et al. Cardiovascular manifestations of pheochromocytoma. Am J Emerg Med 2000;18:622–5.
87. Plouin PF, Duclos JM, Soppelsa F, et al. Factors associated with perioperative morbidity and mortality in patients with pheochromocytoma: analysis of 165 operations at a single center. J Clin Endocrinol Metab 2001;86:1480–6.
88. Bravo EL. Pheochromocytoma. Curr Ther Endocrinol Metab 1997;6:195–7.
89. Newell KA, Prinz RA, Brooks MH, et al. Plasma catecholamine changes during excision of pheochromocytoma. Surgery 1988;104:1064–73.
90. Roizen MF, Schreider BD, Hassan SZ. Anesthesia for patients with pheochromocytoma. Anesthesiol Clin North America 1987;5:269–75.
91. Geoghegan JG, Emberton M, Bloom SR, et al. Changing trends in the management of phaeochromocytoma. Br J Surg 1998;85:117–20.
92. Bravo EL. Evolving concepts in the pathophysiology, diagnosis, and treatment of pheochromocytoma. Endocr Rev 1994;15:356–68.
93. Kinney MA, Warner ME, vanHeerden JA, et al. Perianesthetic risks and outcomes of pheochromocytoma and paraganglioma resection. Anesth Analg 2000;91: 1118–23.
94. Prys-Roberts C. Phaeochromocytoma – recent progress in its management. Br J Anaesth 2000;85:44–57.
95. Young JB, Landsberg L. Catecholamines and the adrenal medulla. In: Wilson JD, Foster DW, Kronenberg HM, et al, editors. Williams textbook of endocrinology. Philadelphia: Saunders; 1998. p. 705–28.
96. Jovenich JJ. Anesthesia in adrenal surgery. Urol Clin North Am 1989;16:583–7.
97. Kinney MA, Narr BJ, Warner MA. Perioperative management of pheochromocytoma. J Cardiothorac Vasc Anesth 2002;16:359–69.

Obesity, Metabolic Syndrome, and the Surgical Patient

Phillip D. Levin, MB, BChir, Charles Weissman, MD*

KEYWORDS

- Metabolic syndrome • Obesity • Preoperative evaluation
- Bariatric surgery • Obstructive sleep apnea
- Cardiovascular disease

Contemporary life, with its sedentary lifestyles, fast foods, processed foodstuff, and desk-bound service employment, is beset by an epidemic of overweight and obese individuals. The World Health Organization reported that worldwide a billion adults are overweight and at least 30% of them are obese. Moreover, increasing numbers of children are obese. In the United States, two National Health and Nutrition Examination Surveys of adults aged 20 to 74 years showed that the prevalence of obesity increased from 15% in the 1976 to 1980 survey to 34% in the 2003 to 2004 survey. This epidemic has been associated with significant increases in the prevalence of glucose intolerance and/or type 2 diabetes mellitus, hypertension, dyslipidemia, and cardiovascular diseases. This constellation of conditions has piqued the interest of the medical community, which has dubbed it the metabolic syndrome and developed formal definitions (**Box 1**). Patients with the metabolic syndrome have increased risks for developing coronary artery disease, stroke, peripheral vascular disease, and type 2 diabetes mellitus, and greater mortality from coronary disease and other causes.[1] Furthermore, such patients have a proinflammatory and prothrombotic state. Whether this syndrome is a disease in and of itself, is merely a list of obesity-induced complications, or is composed of discrete disorders is the subject of much investigation and controversy.[2] For example, although individuals with the metabolic syndrome have a cardiovascular risk 50% to 60% higher than others, the absolute cardiovascular risk of the metabolic syndrome is not higher than those of its individual components.[3]

The reason that abdominal or central obesity is associated with the development of hypertension, hypercholesterolemia, and insulin resistance is partially attributed to abdominal (or visceral) fat being more metabolically active than subcutaneous fat.

Department of Anesthesiology and Critical Care Medicine, Hebrew University Medical Center, Hebrew University-Hadassah School of Medicine, Kiryat Hadassah, POB 12000, Jerusalem 91120, Israel
* Corresponding author.
E-mail address: charles@hadassah.org.il (C. Weissman).

Med Clin N Am 93 (2009) 1049–1063
doi:10.1016/j.mcna.2009.05.004
0025-7125/09/$ – see front matter © 2009 Elsevier Inc. All rights reserved.

medical.theclinics.com

Box 1
Obesity and metabolic syndrome definitions

Overweight—body mass index (BMI) >25–29.9 kg/m^2

Obesity—BMI $\geq$ 30 kg/m^2

Extreme (morbid) obesity—BMI $\geq$ 40 kg/m^2

Central (abdominal) obesity—Waste/hip ratio >0.9 (men) or >0.85 (women)

Metabolic syndrome

Definition # 1—American Heart Association—National Heart, Lung and Blood Institute (presence of 3 or more criteria)

1. Elevated waist circumference

   Men: $\geq$ 40 in (102 cm)

   Women: $\geq$ 35 in (88 cm)

2. Elevated triglycerides

   $\geq$ 150 mg/dL

3. Reduced HDL cholesterol

   Men: <40 mg/dL

   Women: <50 mg/dL

4. Elevated blood pressure

   $\geq$ 130/85 mm Hg

5. Elevated fasting glucose

   $\geq$ 100 mg/dL

Definition # 2—International Diabetes Federation—(central obesity plus 2 of the other 4 criteria)

1. Central Obesity—waist circumference

   Men: Europids $\geq$ 94 cm; South Asians, Japanese, Chinese $\geq$ 90 cm

   Women: Europids, South Asians, Japanese, Chinese $\geq$ 80 cm

2. Elevated triglycerides:

   $\geq$ 150 mg/dL or treatment for this lipid abnormality

3. Reduced HDL cholesterol

   Men: <40 mg/dL

   Women: <50 mg/dL

   Or treatment for this lipid abnormality

4. Elevated blood pressure

   $\geq$ 130/85 mm Hg

   Or treatment of previously diagnosed hypertension

5. Elevated fasting glucose

   $\geq$ 100 mg/dL or previously diagnosed type 2 diabetes mellitus

Visceral fat releases nonesterified fatty acids, which contribute to a proinflammatory state.[4] This plays a prominent role in mediating all stages of atherosclerosis, including the atherosclerotic progression and destabilization that precedes clinical events such as myocardial infarction. The proinflammatory state also induces a hypercoagulable state by promoting increases in fibrinogen and plasminogen activator inhibitor (inhibiting fibrinolysis). The visceral adipose tissue also secretes the adipokine adiponectin, which has potent vasculoprotective, angiogenic, antiinflammatory, and antiatherogenic properties. However, in obesity adiponectin secretion is decreased. Whether the proinflammatory and hypercoagulable states found in the obese and those with metabolic syndrome exacerbate the proinflammatory and hypercoagulable states caused by the stress of surgery is unclear. However, it is possible to speculate that the increased perioperative complication rate among patients with obesity or metabolic syndrome reported by some (but not all) investigators might represent an additive effect from the two entities.[5,6]

The adverse effects of obesity and the metabolic syndrome on the outcomes of surgery have been described for a wide range of surgical procedures. In a retrospective study of 5304 consecutive patients undergoing coronary artery bypass grafting (CABG), 49% met criteria for the metabolic syndrome. Among patients with the metabolic syndrome, mortality was 2.4%, as opposed to 0.9% without ($P<.001$). Obesity was not a significant independent risk factor for mortality;[7] however, presence of the metabolic syndrome has been shown to be a risk factor for vein graft occlusion within 5 years of CABG and for cardiac events during the 12 years after percutaneous coronary intervention.[8,9] The metabolic syndrome has also been associated with increased all-cause and cardiovascular mortality 10 years after CABG in nondiabetic patients.[10] Among patients undergoing percutaneous nephrolithotomy, the presence of the metabolic syndrome, as well as its individual components (diabetes mellitus, hypertension, and obesity), was associated with greater complication rates and the need for additional interventions.[11] Women with the metabolic syndrome and its components had an increased likelihood of undergoing cataract extraction.[12] Obesity was found to be a risk factor for wound infection and dehiscence, incisional hernia, and stoma complications after colorectal surgery. Similarly, the risk for complications after lumbar or thoracic spine surgery has been correlated with increasing body mass index (BMI),[13] and in a study of major intra-abdominal cancer surgery, obesity was found to be a risk factor for postoperative wound problems, but not for mortality or major complications.[14]

Since there is a 35% to 40% prevalence of the metabolic syndrome in the US population, it is encountered on a daily basis during preoperative evaluations.[15] Indeed, among 312 patients scheduled for cardiovascular and thoracic surgery, the metabolic syndrome was found in 54%, with 33% having three contributing conditions, 14% having four contributing conditions, and 7% having five contributing conditions.[16] Patients with obesity or metabolic syndrome may have complicated medical histories and occult (and thus untreated) diseases such as coronary artery disease or heart failure. Given that the metabolic syndrome and obesity are associated with a 1.4- to 4.5-fold increase in cardiovascular morbidity and mortality from myocardial infarctions and ischemic strokes,[17] the concept of the metabolic syndrome may direct physicians to search for obesity-related conditions (such as potentially problematic atherosclerotic diseases) and may assist in estimating the potential risks for surgery. It is important to realize that the metabolic syndrome framework, as opposed to the Framingham Risk Score, does not include many of the traditional risk factors for coronary artery disease, such as age, smoking, family history, and male gender.[18]

Beyond atherosclerotic disease, the metabolic syndrome and obesity are associated with other conditions (such as obstructive sleep apnea [OSA]), which themselves are further risk factors for anesthetic difficulty. Thus the "average" patient with obesity or metabolic syndrome, who may also have diabetes mellitus and sleep apnea, will have multiple risk factors for perioperative morbidity. Preoperative patient assessment therefore has to be directed at evaluating specific conditions often found in association with the metabolic syndrome or obesity in addition to evaluation of the general medical condition. This includes assessment of airway and respiratory problems (relating to the likelihood of difficult intubation, OSA, and postoperative respiratory complications), the presence of liver disease (nonalcoholic fatty liver disease and cirrhosis), and increased thrombotic risk plus an assessment of cardiac status and risk for perioperative cardiac events. Beyond perioperative evaluation, these patients also require specific attention to management of concurrent medications and the applicability of day surgery. These issues will be considered later in further detail.

CARDIOVASCULAR DISEASE

The metabolic syndrome and obesity are associated with cardiac disease. Evaluating perioperative cardiovascular risk and the need for cardiac investigation is based on a balance between the extent of surgery, cardiac history, symptoms, and timing of previous investigations. As extent of surgery increases, cardiac reserve must be greater. The recent guidelines from the American Heart Association (AHA)/American College of Cardiology (ACC) review protocols for diagnosis.[19] In practice, approximately 35% of patients planned for bariatric surgery (considered a moderate cardiac risk procedure) underwent cardiac investigation.[20] Difficulty arises when evaluating obese patients, since exercise tolerance (a cardinal marker in the assessment of cardiac risk) may be severely limited and the efficacy of diagnostic test (such as thallium scans) may be reduced.

OBSTRUCTIVE SLEEP APNEA

OSA is defined as periodic, partial, or complete upper airway obstruction during sleep occurring at least five times per hour associated with daytime somnolence.[21] In the general population, disturbed breathing during sleep occurs in 9% of women and 24% of men, whereas overt OSA is found in 2% of women and 4% of men.[22,23] Obesity is a major risk factor with up to 71% of the morbidly obese suffering from OSA. Amongst surgical patients OSA has been identified in up to 24%[24–26] with the majority being undiagnosed.[27]

The recurrent airway obstruction of OSA occurs mainly during rapid eye movement (REM) sleep[28,29] and can lead to hypoxia, hypercarbia, pulmonary hypertension, and right heart failure in the most severe cases. OSA is also associated with an inflammatory condition remarkably similar to that of the metabolic syndrome, including increased cytokines,[30,31] hypertension, insulin resistance,[32,33] and an increased risk for cardiovascular events (coronary artery disease, heart failure, and stroke).[34] Whether these outcomes result from OSA or concomitant metabolic syndrome is difficult to determine, because 87% of individuals with sleep apnea may also have the metabolic syndrome.[35]

Perioperative screening questionnaires for OSA have been suggested; however, comparison of three such tools[36] showed only moderate sensitivity for the detection of OSA (66% to 87%), low specificity, and reasonable ability to predict postoperative complications. The simplest questionnaire (based on 8 questions relating to snoring, daytime tiredness, observed airway obstruction, presence of high blood pressure,

BMI, age, neck circumference, and gender [STOP-BANG[37]]) was associated with the highest odds ratio (OR) for predicting perioperative complications (OR 3.0, 95% CI 1.2–7.5).[36] Whether screening has an effect on perioperative outcome (either from altered perioperative management or institution of specific therapy) has yet to be shown.

Surgery disrupts sleep patterns with a decrease in REM sleep during the first postoperative nights, and a subsequent rebound increase.[38] As airway obstruction in OSA occurs particularly during REM sleep, the finding that hypoxia is more common in OSA patients on the second and third postoperative nights[39,40] is not surprising, and parallels an increase in cardiovascular events during this period.[41,42]

Detecting OSA is important. Patients with OSA show increased sensitivity to the respiratory depressant effects of benzodiazepines and opiates[43] mandating caution with their use in the pre- and postoperative periods. Obesity and OSA are also associated with an increased incidence of difficult endotracheal intubation.[44] As continuous positive airway pressure (CPAP) is considered to be one of the mainstays of treatment of OSA, patients who use CPAP should be encouraged to bring their CPAP machines to the hospital for use during the pre- and postoperative periods. Chronic CPAP use (>1 month) has been shown to reverse the respiratory and cardiac effects of OSA and thus in patients with severe OSA, deferring nonurgent surgery until the establishment of CPAP use may be of benefit (although not proven in studies). Finally patients undergoing extensive surgery may require postoperative observation in an ICU.

Regional (spinal and epidural) anesthesia may offer benefits for the OSA patient, because use of opiates can be reduced and airway interventions prevented. However, epidural opiates have been associated with respiratory arrest in OSA patients,[45] and obesity can obscure anatomic landmarks, leading to technical difficulties in performing regional anesthesia. Regional anesthesia also has potential side effects including block failure, hypotension, respiratory depression, and local anesthetic toxicity (principally seizures and cardiac arrhythmias). These may mandate emergency interventions, which may be difficult to perform in the severely obese patient, and which may have a detrimental outcome. An observational study of 9038 regional anesthetic administrations performed on 6920 patients, including 31% obese patients, showed that the obese patients were 1.6 times more likely to have a failed block, and potentially more likely to have complications.[46] However, the study also showed that satisfaction was similar to that in the nonobese patients.[46]

Regarding the requirement for postoperative admission to hospital rather than day surgery, the American Society of Anesthesiologists guidelines for the management of patients with OSA[22] suggest that day surgery can be considered for patients at risk for OSA, particularly when local or regional anesthesia is administered. The recommendations for patients with severe OSA or requiring more extensive surgery are equivocal. Severe OSA, invasive surgery, parenteral opiates, obstructive episodes in the recovery room, hypoxia, and drowsiness may all represent indications for hospital admission.[47]

Unfortunately the effects of obesity on the respiratory system are not limited to OSA. The supine position, anesthesia, and pharmacologic muscle paralysis all decrease the functional residual capacity (FRC), even in the absence of obesity. Increasing BMI exacerbates these reductions and obesity is exponentially related to decreases particularly in FRC and expiratory reserve volume.[48,49] The clinical effects of these changes result from the decreased oxygen reserve (smaller FRC) following induction of anesthesia. This increases the likelihood of hypoxia in the period between induction of anesthesia and commencement of ventilation following intubation and also increases the risk for developing perioperative atelectasis. Although preoperative lung function tests can quantify these changes, and may possibly predict the likelihood of perioperative respiratory complications in the obese, their effect on patient management is not established and they are not recommended as a routine preoperative test.[50] Obesity is associated with an increased risk for difficult intubation. If predicted preoperatively this indicates awake fiber optic intubation. Difficulty in intubation encountered after induction of anesthesia may lead to a situation of inadequate ventilation in a patient with limited oxygen reserves, and the danger of significant hypoxia.

Blood gas levels (to detect carbon dioxide retention or baseline hypoxia), hemoglobin concentration (high in chronic hypoxia), and cardiac echo (to establish the presence of pulmonary hypertension) may indicate the extent of pulmonary disease in the obese patient. These tests may also be useful in risk stratification; however, they are usually indicated only by the patient's clinical condition and extent of surgery. Weight reduction can lead to improvement in many of these parameters; however, this is not usually possible in the short term.

NONALCOHOLIC FATTY LIVER DISEASE

This is the commonest form of chronic liver disease present in the United States today, occurring in approximately 30% of the general US population.[51,52] Its prevalence increases to 62% in diabetics[53] and to 91% in those undergoing bariatric surgery.[54] Nonalcoholic fatty liver disease (NAFLD) explains 90% of cases with raised alanine transaminase (ALT) when other common causes of liver damage have been excluded.[55] The condition's name arises from pathologic findings that are similar to the findings resulting from alcohol damage, but occurring in individuals without a history of alcohol consumption. These include steatosis, lobular inflammation, and ballooning degeneration.[56] NAFLD represents part of a spectrum of nonalcoholic liver damage, ranging in clinical severity from asymptomatic raised liver enzyme levels, through nonalcoholic steatohepatitis (present in 5.7% of the population), to liver fibrosis and cirrhosis.

The long-term hepatic implications of NAFLD are not entirely clear. Patients with bland steatosis were shown to have minimally increased liver related mortality or incidence of cirrhosis over 17 years.[57] However, in contrast, approximately 40% of patients with NAFLD referred to a hepatology clinic and having two liver biopsies showed increased fibrosis on the follow-up biopsy.[58] As these patients are those who presented to a hepatology clinic and had two biopsies, the findings from this study may reflect selection bias, and may not reflect the general population. Patients who do develop cirrhosis, however, have 33% mortality over a 7 year follow-up period[59] and may develop hepatocellular carcinoma.

NAFLD is strongly associated with the presence of diabetes mellitus (78% of NAFLD patients also have diabetes[53,58]) and is a predictor of increased cardiovascular morbidity,[60] possibly mediated by a direct effect on vascular endothelium.[60] Indeed in population based studies (using unexplained elevation of ALT as the indicator of NAFLD) the presence of NAFLD has been independently associated with increased all-cause and cardiovascular mortality, particularly in the 45 to 55 age group.[55] NAFLD is also found very frequently in combination with other elements of the metabolic syndrome, and has been referred to as the hepatic expression of the metabolic syndrome. Separating the mortality effects (and particularly cardiovascular effects) of NAFLD from those associated with diabetes or the metabolic syndrome is thus complex.

What significance does this have in the perioperative period? Cirrhosis (as measured by the Child Pugh or Model for End-Stage Liver Disease [MELD] scores), is a major risk factor for complications in the perioperative period,[61,62] increasing mortality from 1.1% in noncirrhotic patients to 8.3% to 25% in cirrhotic patients under-going different types of surgery.[63] As patients with the metabolic syndrome or obesity are at very high risk for NAFLD, and a proportion of NAFLD patients might have undi-agnosed cirrhosis, clinical and biochemical signs of cirrhosis should be sought before surgery. Further, the association of NAFLD with cardiovascular disease should be considered when evaluating perioperative cardiac risk. Unfortunately to date the peri-operative risk of NAFLD has not been systematically explored.

THROMBOTIC RISK

Obesity is a well established risk factor for deep vein thrombosis (DVT) and pulmonary emboli (PE) in the healthy population,[64,65] hospitalized medical patients, and hospital-ized surgical patients.[66] The mechanisms proposed to explain the increased risk include an imbalance among three elements related to obesity and/or the metabolic syndrome: procoagulant and anticoagulant mechanisms, endothelial dysfunction, and platelet hyperreactivity.[67] In addition, increased weight is associated with decreased mobility and physical pressure on large veins.

In contrast to obesity-related venous thrombosis, the metabolic syndrome (including obesity) is a risk factor for arterial thrombosis (ischemic heart disease and stroke). Debate has arisen as to whether there is a common etiology between arterial thrombosis and venous thrombosis.[68] The largest study to address common risk factors for venous and arterial thrombosis is a meta-analysis of 63,000 patients. This study showed that obesity was associated with an OR for venous thromboem-bolic disease of 2.33 (95%CI 1.68–2.34), whereas hypertension, diabetes mellitus, and triglyceride levels were also significant predictors.[69] This indicates that elements of the metabolic syndrome beyond obesity may indeed increase the risk of venous thromboembolism. Smaller case–control studies investigating the link between the metabolic syndrome and venous thromboembolism have shown varied results.[14,70,71]

The estimated risks for perioperative DVT and PE for patients undergoing general surgery without specific DVT prophylaxis is 14% for DVT and 0.5% for PE.[72] Perioper-ative use of low-molecular-weight heparin reduces this risk by 72%.[72] In the obese population (patients undergoing bariatric surgery) the risk for DVT and/or PE has been estimated to be 3.4 per 1000 discharges[73] or 0.2% for DVT and 0.1% for PE.[66] The risk for perioperative DVT and/or PE is significantly influenced by both intrinsic factors (such as obesity, patient age,[66,73,74] prior venous thromboembo-lism,[66,74,75] and preexisiting comorbidities such as cancer) and extrinsic factors (type and extent of surgery, type of anesthesia, and use of DVT prophylaxis). For example, lower limb orthopedic surgery is associated with one of the highest DVT risks (up to 60% without prophylaxis[66]), whereas regional anesthesia has a protective effect, decreasing DVT risk by up to 50%.[76]

DVT prophylaxis can include physical devices such as pneumatic compression devices[76] or pharmacologic anticoagulants, principally heparins. Dose, route, and timing of heparin administration remain controversial.[66] Subcutaneous administration of low-molecular-weight heparins in the obese leads to variable anti-X levels,[66,77] and some have even suggested the use of low-dose IV unfractionated heparin.[66,78,79] Extensive guidelines have been published discussing perioperative DVT prophylaxis.[66]

BARIATRIC SURGERY AND THE METABOLIC SYNDROME

One of the more common surgeries encountered in the obese is bariatric surgery, per-formed after the failure of conventional treatment (diet and exercise programs) to provide long-term sustained weight loss.[80] Such surgery should be considered for all patients with a BMI of more than 40 kg/m[2] and for those with a BMI of more than 35 kg/m[2] with obesity related problems, and/or after failure of nonsurgical approaches to long-term weight loss (less than a 30%–50% loss of excess body weight). Patients considering bariatric surgery should be well motivated to change their lifestyle to one of exercise and strict compliance with diet, and they should be psychologically stable and have a supportive family and/or social environment. The presence of metabolic syndrome features beyond obesity makes such surgery even more essential despite increased surgical morbidity (but not mortality).[81]

The extent of the preoperative evaluation required before bariatric surgery is controversial. Some advocate no special testing, but a thorough history, physical examination, ECG, pulse oximetry, and laboratory tests are considered routine, and most recommendations agree that patients should have a psychological assessment and, if found suitable, education on postsurgery lifestyle changes. Other potential preoperative tests for consideration include endoscopy of the upper gastrointestinal tract to exclude hiatus hernia, reflux esophagitis, and Helicobacter pylori infection;[82] ultrasonography to rule out gallstone disease; and polysomnography to exclude OSA. Many investigators consider the latter especially important because of the potential postoperative and long-term complications of OSA. In a group of relatively young patients (mean age 39 years), ECG abnormalities and obstructive apnea were detected before bariatric surgery in 62% and 40%, respectively. None were a contraindication to surgery.[83] Others reported a prevalence of sleep apnea in 77% of patients scheduled for bariatric surgery with its presence related to the metabolic syndrome.[84,85] In patients with pulmonary problems, spirometry and arterial blood gas measurements may be considered.[83] It is generally suggested that the ACC/AHA guidelines be used to assess the degree of cardiovascular workup required. Routine dobutamine stress testing was not found to be useful before bariatric surgery.[86] In a study of a limited number of patients, short-term postoperative complications were greater in patients with reduced cardiorespiratory fitness (peak VO_2 <15.8 mL/kg/min), leading to the recommendation that such fitness be optimized before bariatric surgery.[87] Postoperative morbidity is greater in men, patients older than 45 years, hypertensives, diabetics, patients with OSA, asthmatics, and among those with risk factors for pulmonary embolus and cirrhosis.[88]

Bariatric surgery results in a weight loss of up to 75% of excess body weight, with most of the weight loss occurring within 6 to 12 months of surgery, as well as a reduction in long-term (10 years) mortality.[89] This weight loss, especially the reduction in visceral adiposity, is associated with improvement in many aspects of the metabolic syndrome, such as hypertension, type 2 diabetes mellitus, C-reactive protein (CRP) concentrations, and dyslipidemia.[89–91] The reversibility of the metabolic syndrome is dependent on the amount of weight lost, with 1 case of the metabolic syndrome being reversed for every 2.1 surgeries.[92] In contrast to bariatric surgery, there is controversy as to whether removing abdominal fat in obese subjects, by either liposuction or lipectomy, improves the metabolic syndrome. Patients examined 10 to 12 weeks after liposuction had unchanged insulin resistance and plasma concentrations of CRP, tumor necrosis factor (TNF), and adiponectin.[93] However, among women who maintained a stable body weight for 6 months following abdominal liposuction, the incidence of insulin resistance decreased, as did concentrations of TNF and CRP, whereas adiponectin and HDL-cholesterol levels were higher than before surgery.[94] Forty days after abdominal dermolipectomy similar results were observed.[95] Whether these possible beneficial effects of abdominal fat removal result in sustained weight reduction, fewer detrimental metabolic effects, and improved outcome needs further study.

PERIOPERATIVE DRUG THERAPY

Many patients with obesity or metabolic syndrome receive therapy for glucose intolerance (reviewed elsewhere[96]), dyslipidemia, and hypertension.

Lipid Lowering Drugs

Statins (3-hydroxy-3-methyl glutaryl coenzyme A inhibitors) decrease serum cholesterol and are widely used in primary and secondary prevention of cardiovascular disease. Above 50% of cardiac and vascular surgery patients are receiving a statin.[97,98] Statins also have effects unrelated to lipid levels that are principally antiinflammatory, vasodilatory, and antithrombotic.[99] Large observational studies[100,101] and meta-analyses[102] have shown that perioperative statin use is associated with reduced morbidity and mortality; however, large prospective trials have yet to be reported. Observational trials of statins are limited as (1) statin therapy might reflect overall more aggressive therapy for the management of existing cardiovascular disease, (2) they do not relate to the length of time statins were administered before surgery, and (3) they do not deal with the possibly deleterious effect of statin cessation immediately before surgery.

Abrupt cessation of statins is associated with deleterious effects in vitro and in vivo. For example, among patients with acute coronary syndromes, event rate and mortality were higher in those whose statins were stopped.[103] Although there is currently insufficient evidence to recommend the initiation of statin therapy as a specific intervention to decrease perioperative morbidity or mortality, continuing existing statin therapy through the perioperative period seems logical and has been recommended.[99]

Beta-blockers

Until recently, beta-blockers were widely recommended to reduce surgery-related cardiovascular morbidity and mortality.[19] The recent Perioperative Ischemic Evaluation (POISE) trial[104] complicated these recommendations. This 8331 patient prospective trial compared perioperative metoprolol to placebo. Although the metoprolol group showed decreased perioperative myocardial infarction, it also showed an overall increase in mortality (mortality 3.1% versus 2.3%, $P = .03$) and an increased incidence of stroke.[104] Although questions regarding the precise study methodology (choice of metoprolol, dose, administration protocol, etc[105]) have been raised, this study has led to the recommendation that beta-blockers be continued and not be stopped in the perioperative period if already prescribed; that they not be routinely started before surgery, even in patients with increased cardiovascular risk; and that consideration be given to strict intraoperative heart rate control, if needed.[105]

SUMMARY

Obesity and the metabolic syndrome are unfortunately becoming increasingly common perioperative issues. Their presence often portends the existence of cardiovascular and metabolic derangements that can affect the convalescence and outcome of surgery. Further investigation is indicated to better understand the etiology, extent, and perioperative consequences of these conditions, especially as they interact with the metabolic and cardiovascular responses to the stresses of surgery. The ultimate aim of such research is to find ways to minimize the untoward effects of surgery in patients with obesity or metabolic syndrome.

REFERENCES

1. Isomaa B, Almgren P, Tuomi T, et al. Cardiovascular morbidity and mortality associated with the metabolic syndrome. Diabetes Care 2001;24:683–9.
2. Kahn R. Metabolic syndrome – what is the clinical usefulness? Lancet 2008;371: 1892–3.
3. Qiao Q, Gao W, Zhang L, et al. Metabolic syndrome and cardiovascular disease. Ann Clin Biochem 2007;44:232–63.
4. Grundy SM, Brewer HB, Cleeman JI, et al. Lenfant C for the conference participants' definition of metabolic syndrome: report of the National Heart, Lung, and Blood Institute/American Heart Association conference on scientific issues related to definition. Circulation 2004;109:433–8.
5. Gendall KA, Raingia S, Kennedy R, et al. The impact of obesity on outcome after major colorectal surgery. Dis Colon Rectum 2007;50:2223–37.
6. Mullen JT, Davenport DL, Hutter MM, et al. Impact of body mass index on perioperative outcomes in patients undergoing major abdominal cancer surgery. Ann Surg Oncol 2008;15(8):2164–72.
7. Echahidi N, Pibarot P, Despres JP, et al. Metabolic syndrome increases operative mortality in patients undergoing coronary artery bypass grafting surgery. J Am Coll Cardiol 2007;50:843–51.
8. Yilmaz MB, Guray U, Guray Y, et al. Metabolic syndrome negatively impacts early patency of saphenous vein grafts. Coron Artery Dis 2006;17:41–4.
9. Kasai T, Miyauchi K, Kurata T, et al. Prognostic value of the metabolic syndrome for long-term outcomes in patients undergoing percutaneous coronary intervention. Circ J 2006;70:1531–7.
10. Kajimoto K, Kasai T, Miyauchi K, et al. Metabolic syndrome predicts 10-year mortality in non-diabetic patients following coronary artery bypass surgery. Circ J 2008;72:1481–6.
11. Tefekli A, Kertoglu H, Tepler K, et al. Does the metabolic syndrome or its components affect the outcome of percutaneous nephrolithotomy? J Endourol 2008;22:35–40.
12. Lindblad BE, Hakabsson N, Phillipson B, et al. Metabolic syndrome components in relation to risk of cataract extraction: a prospective cohort study of women. Ophthalmology 2008;115(10):1687–92.
13. Patel N, Bagan B, Vadera S, et al. Obesity and spine surgery: relation to perioperative complications. J Neurosurg Spine 2007;6:291–7.
14. Ray JG, Lonn E, Yi Q, et al. Venous thromboembolism in association with features of the metabolic syndrome. QJM 2007;100:679–84.
15. Ford ES. Prevalence of the metabolic syndrome defined by the International Diabetes Federation among adults in the U.S. Diabetes Care 2005;28:2745–9.
16. Vijayaraghavan K, Jeffries M, Windsor ML, et al. Metabolic syndrome and postoperative complications in cardiothoracic and vascular surgical and percutaneous interventions. J Am Osteopath Assoc 2005;105:27.
17. Boden-Albala B, Sacco RL, Lee HS, et al. Metabolic syndrome and ischemic stroke risk. Stroke 2008;39:30–5.
18. Wannamethee SG, Shaper AG, Lennon L, et al. Metabolic syndrome vs Framingham Risk Score for prediction of coronary heart disease, stroke, and type 2 diabetes mellitus. Arch Intern Med 2005;165:2644–50.
19. Fleisher LA, Beckman JA, Brown KA, et al. ACC/AHA 2007 guidelines on perioperative cardiovascular evaluation and care for noncardiac surgery: executive summary: a report of the American College of Cardiology/American

Heart Association Task Force on practice guidelines (Writing Committee to revise the 2002 guidelines on perioperative cardiovascular evaluation for noncardiac surgery): developed in collaboration with the American Society of Echocardiography, American Society of Nuclear Cardiology, Heart Rhythm Society, Society of Cardiovascular Anesthesiologists, Society for Cardiovascular Angiography and Interventions, Society for Vascular Medicine and Biology, and Society for Vascular Surgery. Circulation 2007;116:1971–96.

20. Kuruba R, Koche LS, Murr MM. Preoperative assessment and perioperative care of patients undergoing bariatric surgery. Med Clin North Am 2007;91:339–51, ix.

21. Flemons WW. Clinical practice: Obstructive sleep apnea. N Engl J Med 2002; 347:498–504.

22. Gross JB, Bachenberg KL, Benumof JL, et al. Practice guidelines for the perioperative management of patients with obstructive sleep apnea: a report by the American Society of Anesthesiologists Task Force on perioperative management of patients with obstructive sleep apnea. Anesthesiology 2006;104:1081–93.

23. Young T, Peppard PE, Gottlieb DJ. Epidemiology of obstructive sleep apnea: a population health perspective. Am J Respir Crit Care Med 2002;165:1217–39.

24. Fidan H, Fidan F, Unlu M, et al. Prevalence of sleep apnoea in patients undergoing operation. Sleep Breath 2006;10:161–5.

25. Yegneswaran B, Chung F. The importance of screening for obstructive sleep apnea before surgery. Sleep Med 2008;107(3):915–20.

26. Chung F, Ward B, Ho J, et al. Preoperative identification of sleep apnea risk in elective surgical patients, using the Berlin questionnaire. J Clin Anesth 2007; 19:130–4.

27. Young T, Evans L, Finn L, et al. Estimation of the clinically diagnosed proportion of sleep apnea syndrome in middle-aged men and women. Sleep 1997;20: 705–6.

28. Strollo PJ Jr, Rogers RM. Obstructive sleep apnea. N Engl J Med 1996;334: 99–104.

29. Cherniack NS. Respiratory dysrhythmias during sleep. N Engl J Med 1981;305: 325–30.

30. Vgontzas AN, Papanicolaou DA, Bixler EO, et al. Sleep apnea and daytime sleepiness and fatigue: relation to visceral obesity, insulin resistance, and hypercytokinemia. J Clin Endocrinol Metab 2000;85:1151–8.

31. Punjabi NM, Polotsky VY. Disorders of glucose metabolism in sleep apnea. J Appl Physiol 2005;99:1998–2007.

32. Punjabi NM, Shahar E, Redline S, et al. Sleep-disordered breathing, glucose intolerance, and insulin resistance: the Sleep Heart Health Study. Am J Epidemiol 2004;160:521–30.

33. Harsch IA, Schahin SP, Radespiel-Troger M, et al. Continuous positive airway pressure treatment rapidly improves insulin sensitivity in patients with obstructive sleep apnea syndrome. Am J Respir Crit Care Med 2004;169:156–62.

34. Jean-Louis G, Zizi F, Clark LT, et al. Obstructive sleep apnea and cardiovascular disease: role of the metabolic syndrome and its components. J Clin Sleep Med 2008;4:261–72.

35. Coughlin SR, Mawdsley L, Mugarza JA, et al. Obstructive sleep apnoea is independently associated with an increased prevalence of metabolic syndrome. Eur Heart J 2004;25:735–41.

36. Chung F, Yegneswaran B, Liao P, et al. Validation of the Berlin questionnaire and American Society of Anesthesiologists checklist as screening tools for obstructive sleep apnea in surgical patients. Anesthesiology 2008;108:822–30.

37. Chung F, Yegneswaran B, Liao P, et al. STOP questionnaire: a tool to screen patients for obstructive sleep apnea. Anesthesiology 2008;108:812–21.

38. Gogenur I, Wildschiotz G, Rosenberg J. Circadian distribution of sleep phases after major abdominal surgery. Br J Anaesth 2008;100:45–9.

39. Knill RL, Moote CA, Skinner MI, et al. Anesthesia with abdominal surgery leads to intense REM sleep during the first postoperative week. Anesthesiology 1990; 73:52–61.

40. Rosenberg J, Wildschiodtz G, Pedersen MH, et al. Late postoperative nocturnal episodic hypoxaemia and associated sleep pattern. Br J Anaesth 1994;72: 145–50.

41. Gill NP, Wright B, Reilly CS. Relationship between hypoxaemic and cardiac ischaemic events in the perioperative period. Br J Anaesth 1992;68:471–3.

42. Reeder MK, Muir AD, Foex P, et al. Postoperative myocardial ischaemia: temporal association with nocturnal hypoxaemia. Br J Anaesth 1991;67:626–31.

43. Mickelson SA. Preoperative and postoperative management of obstructive sleep apnea patients. Otolaryngol Clin North Am 2007;40:877–89.

44. Kim JA, Lee JJ. Preoperative predictors of difficult intubation in patients with obstructive sleep apnea syndrome. Can J Anaesth 2006;53:393–7.

45. Ostermeier AM, Roizen MF, Hautkappe M, et al. Three sudden postoperative respiratory arrests associated with epidural opioids in patients with sleep apnea. Anesth Analg 1997;85:452–60.

46. Nielsen KC, Guller U, Steele SM, et al. Influence of obesity on surgical regional anesthesia in the ambulatory setting: an analysis of 9038 blocks. Anesthesiology 2005;102:181–7.

47. Kaw R, Michota F, Jaffer A, et al. Unrecognized sleep apnea in the surgical patient: implications for the perioperative setting. Chest 2006;129:198–205.

48. Jones RL, Nzekwu MM. The effects of body mass index on lung volumes. Chest 2006;130:827–33.

49. Pelosi P, Croci M, Ravagnan I, et al. The effects of body mass on lung volumes, respiratory mechanics, and gas exchange during general anesthesia. Anesth Analg 1998;87:654–60.

50. Hamoui N, Anthone G, Crookes PF. The value of pulmonary function testing prior to bariatric surgery. Obes Surg 2006;16:1570–3.

51. Nugent C, Younossi ZM. Evaluation and management of obesity-related nonalcoholic fatty liver disease. Nat Clin Pract Gastroenterol Hepatol 2007;4:432–41.

52. Angulo P, Hui JM, Marchesini G, et al. The NAFLD fibrosis score: a noninvasive system that identifies liver fibrosis in patients with NAFLD. Hepatology 2007;45: 846–54.

53. Jimba S, Nakagami T, Takahashi M, et al. Prevalence of nonalcoholic fatty liver disease and its association with impaired glucose metabolism in Japanese adults. Diabet Med 2005;22:1141–5.

54. Machado M, Marques-Vidal P, Cortez-Pinto H. Hepatic histology in obese patients undergoing bariatric surgery. J Hepatol 2006;45:600–6.

55. Dunn W, Xu R, Wingard DL, et al. Suspected nonalcoholic fatty liver disease and mortality risk in a population-based cohort study. Am J Gastroenterol 2008;103: 2263–71.

56. Kleiner DE, Brunt EM, Van Natta M, et al. Design and validation of a histological scoring system for nonalcoholic fatty liver disease. Hepatology 2005;41: 1313–21.

57. Dam-Larsen S, Franzmann M, Andersen IB, et al. Long term prognosis of fatty liver: risk of chronic liver disease and death. Gut 2004;53:750–5.

58. Ekstedt M, Franzen LE, Mathiesen UL, et al. Long-term follow-up of patients with NAFLD and elevated liver enzymes. Hepatology 2006;44:865–73.

59. Adams LA, Lymp JF, St Sauver J, et al. The natural history of nonalcoholic fatty liver disease: a population-based cohort study. Gastroenterology 2005;129: 113–21.

60. Targher G, Arcaro G. Nonalcoholic fatty liver disease and increased risk of cardiovascular disease. Atherosclerosis 2007;191:235–40.

61. Teh SH, Nagorney DM, Stevens SR, et al. Risk factors for mortality after surgery in patients with cirrhosis. Gastroenterology 2007;132:1261–9.

62. Hoteit MA, Ghazale AH, Bain AJ, et al. Model for end-stage liver disease score versus Child score in predicting the outcome of surgical procedures in patients with cirrhosis. World J Gastroenterol 2008;14:1774–80.

63. Millwala F, Nguyen GC, Thuluvath PJ. Outcomes of patients with cirrhosis undergoing nonhepatic surgery: risk assessment and management. World J Gastroenterol 2007;13:4056–63.

64. Hansson PO, Eriksson H, Welin L, et al. Smoking and abdominal obesity: risk factors for venous thromboembolism among middle-aged men: "the study of men born in 1913". Arch Intern Med 1999;159:1886–90.

65. Goldhaber SZ, Savage DD, Garrison RJ, et al. Risk factors for pulmonary embolism: The Framingham Study. Am J Med 1983;74:1023–8.

66. Geerts WH, Bergqvist D, Pineo GF, et al. Prevention of venous thromboembolism: American College of Chest Physicians Evidence-Based Clinical Practice Guidelines (8th Edition). Chest 2008;133:381S–453S.

67. Franchini M, Targher G, Montagnana M, et al. The metabolic syndrome and the risk of arterial and venous thrombosis. Thromb Res 2008;122(6):727–35.

68. Prandoni P, Bilora F, Marchiori A, et al. An association between atherosclerosis and venous thrombosis. N Engl J Med 2003;348:1435–41.

69. Ageno W, Becattini C, T' Brighton, et al. Cardiovascular risk factors and venous thromboembolism: a meta-analysis. Circulation 2008;117:93–102.

70. Ay C, Tengler T, Vormittag R, et al. Venous thromboembolism–a manifestation of the metabolic syndrome. Haematologica 2007;92:374–80.

71. Ageno W, Prandoni P, Romualdi E, et al. The metabolic syndrome and the risk of venous thrombosis: a case-control study. J Thromb Haemost 2006;4:1914–8.

72. Mismetti P, Laporte S, Darmon JY, et al. Meta-analysis of low molecular weight heparin in the prevention of venous thromboembolism in general surgery. Br J Surg 2001;88:913–30.

73. Poulose BK, Griffin MR, Zhu Y, et al. National analysis of adverse patient safety for events in bariatric surgery. Am Surg 2005;71:406–13.

74. Gonzalez R, Haines K, Nelson LG, et al. Predictive factors of thromboembolic events in patients undergoing Roux-en-Y gastric bypass. Surg Obes Relat Dis 2006;2:30–5.

75. Prystowsky JB, Morasch MD, Eskandari MK, et al. Prospective analysis of the incidence of deep venous thrombosis in bariatric surgery patients. Surgery 2005;138:759–63.

76. Roderick P, Ferris G, Wilson K, et al. Towards evidence-based guidelines for the prevention of venous thromboembolism: systematic reviews of mechanical methods, oral anticoagulation, dextran and regional anaesthesia as thromboprophylaxis. Health Technol Assess 2005;9:iii–x, 1.

77. Frederiksen SG, Hedenbro JL, Norgren L. Enoxaparin effect depends on body weight and current doses may be inadequate in obese patients. Br J Surg 2003; 90:547–8.

78. Shepherd F, Rosborough TK, Schwartz ML. Unfractionated heparin infusion for thromboprophylaxis in highest risk gastric bypass surgery. Obes Surg 2004; 14:601–5.
79. Quebbemann B, Akhondzadeh M, Dallal R. Continuous intravenous heparin infusion prevents peri-operative thromboembolic events in bariatric surgery patients. Obes Surg 2005;15:1221–4.
80. Bult MJF, van Dalen T, Muller AF. Surgical treatment of obesity. Eur J Endocrinol 2008;158:135–45.
81. Estaban-Varela J, Hinojosa MW, Nguyen NT. Bariatric surgery outcomes in morbidly obese with the metabolic syndrome at US academic medical centers. Obes Surg 2008;18(10):1273–7.
82. Munoz R, Ibanez L, Salinas J, et al. Importance of routine preoperative upper GI endoscopy: why all patients should be evaluated? Obes Surg 2009;19(4): 427–31.
83. Catheline JM, Bihan H, Le Quang T, et al. Preoperative cardiac and pulmonary assessment in bariatric surgery. Obes Surg 2008;18:271–7.
84. O-Keefe T, Patterson EJ. Evidence supporting routine polysomnography before bariatric surgery. Obes Surg 2004;14:23–6.
85. Salord N, Mayos M, Miralda R, et al. Respiratory sleep disturbances in patients undergoing gastric bypass surgery and their relation to metabolic syndrome. Obes Surg 2009;19(1):74–9.
86. Ramaswamy A, Gonzalez R, Smith CD. Extensive preoperative testing is not necessary in morbidly obese patients undergoing gastric bypass. J Gastrointest Surg 2004;8:159–65.
87. McCullough PA, Gallagher MJ, deJong AT, et al. Cardiorespiratory fitness and short-term complications after bariatric surgery. Chest 2006;13:517–25.
88. Collazo-clavell ML, Clark M, McAlpine DE, et al. Assessment and preparation of patients for bariatric surgery. Mayo Clin Proc 2006;81(10 Suppl):S11–7.
89. Sjostrom L, Narbo K, Sjostrom CD, et al. Effects of bariatric surgery on mortality in Swedish obese subjects. N Engl J Med 2007;357:741–52.
90. Kini S, Herron DM, Yanagisawa RT. Bariatric surgery for morbid obesity – a cure for metabolic syndrome? Med Clin North Am 2007;91:1255–71.
91. Chen SB, Lee YC, Ser KH, et al. Serum C-reactive protein and white blood cell count in morbidly obese surgical patients. Obes Surg 2009;19(4):461–6.
92. Batsis JA, Romero-Corral A, Collazo-Clavell ML, et al. Effect of bariatric surgery on the metabolic syndrome: a population-based, long-term controlled trial. Mayo Clin Proc 2008;83:897–907.
93. Klein S, Fontana L, Young VL, et al. Absence of an effect of liposuction on insulin action and risk factors for coronary heart disease. N Engl J Med 2004;350: 2549–57.
94. Giugliano G, Nicoletti G, Grella E, et al. Effect of liposuction on insulin resistance and vascular inflammatory markers in obese women. Br J Plast Surg 2004;57: 190–4.
95. Rizzo MR, Paolisso G, Grella R, et al. Is dermolipectomy effective in improving insulin action and lowering inflammatory markers in obese women? Clin Endocrinol (Oxf) 2005;63:253–8.
96. Tuttnauer A, Levin PD. Diabetes mellitus and anesthesia. Anesthesiol Clin 2006; 24:579–97.
97. Le Manach Y, Godet G, Coriat P, et al. The impact of postoperative discontinuation or continuation of chronic statin therapy on cardiac outcome after major vascular surgery. Anesth Analg 2007;104:1326–33 [table].

98. Pan W, Pintar T, Anton J, et al. Statins are associated with a reduced incidence of perioperative mortality after coronary artery bypass graft surgery. Circulation 2004;110:II45–9.
99. Le Manach Y, Coriat P, Collard CD, et al. Statin therapy within the perioperative period. Anesthesiology 2008;108:1141–6.
100. Poldermans D, Bax JJ, Kertai MD, et al. Statins are associated with a reduced incidence of perioperative mortality in patients undergoing major noncardiac vascular surgery. Circulation 2003;107:1848–51.
101. Lindenauer PK, Pekow P, Wang K, et al. Lipid-lowering therapy and in-hospital mortality following major noncardiac surgery. JAMA 2004;291:2092–9.
102. Hindler K, Shaw AD, Samuels J, et al. Improved postoperative outcomes associated with preoperative statin therapy. Anesthesiology 2006;105:1260–72.
103. Spencer FA, Allegrone J, Goldberg RJ, et al. Association of statin therapy with outcomes of acute coronary syndromes: the GRACE study. Ann Intern Med 2004;140:857–66.
104. Devereaux PJ, Yang H, Yusuf S, et al. Effects of extended-release metoprolol succinate in patients undergoing non-cardiac surgery (POISE trial): a randomised controlled trial. Lancet 2008;371:1839–47.
105. Sear JW, Giles JW, Howard-Alpe G, et al. Perioperative beta-blockade, 2008: what does POISE tell us, and was our earlier caution justified? Br J Anaesth 2008;101:135–8.

Surgery in the Patient with Liver Disease

Diego J. Muilenburg, MD[a], Amrik Singh, MD[b], Guido Torzilli, MD[c],
Vijay P. Khatri, MBChB, FACS[a,d],*

KEYWORDS

- Cirrhosis • Liver dysfunction • Ascites • Jaundice
- Hepatorenal syndrome • Hepatopulmonary syndrome
- Portal hypertension

Liver dysfunction is a prominent entity in Western medicine that has historically affected patients suffering from chronic viral or alcoholic hepatitis. The incidence of these conditions has not changed dramatically in recent years but the overall number of patients with liver dysfunction has increased considerably with the emergence of the obesity epidemic. Nonalcoholic fatty liver disease (NAFLD) has become increasingly recognized as the most common cause of chronic liver disease in the United States.[1] Although the rate of progression of NAFLD to overt cirrhosis is low, the high prevalence of this condition, combined with the moderate degree of liver dysfunction it engenders, has resulted in a significant increase in the number of patients with liver disease that can be encountered by a surgical practice.[2]

Any degree of clinically evident liver disease in a prospective surgical patient should raise concern for the entire surgical team. This particularly applies to intraabdominal surgery whereby the presence of hepatomegaly, portal hypertension, variceal bleeding, and ascites can turn even the most routine operation into a morbid and life-threatening procedure. Nonabdominal surgery avoids some of the technical challenges presented by liver disease but the anesthetic management of a cirrhotic patient still makes any operation potentially more dangerous. In this article, approaches to minimize the risk when surgery becomes necessary in the presence of liver disease are discussed.

[a] Department of Surgery, University of California-Davis, 2315 Stockton Boulevard, Sacramento, CA 95817, USA
[b] Department of Anesthesia and Pain Medicine, University of California Davis Medical Center, 4150 V Street, PSSB 1200, Sacramento, CA 95817, USA
[c] Third Department of Surgery, University of Milan, School of Medicine, IRCCS Istituto Clinico Humanitas, Via Manzoni 56, 20089, Rozzano, Milan, Italy
[d] Division of Surgical Oncology, University of California-Davis, School of Medicine, 4501 X Street, Sacramento, CA 95817, USA
* Corresponding author. Division of Surgical Oncology, University of California-Davis, School of Medicine, 4501 X Street, Sacramento, CA 95817.
E-mail address: vijay.khatri@ucdmc.ucdavis.edu (V.P. Khatri).

Med Clin N Am 93 (2009) 1065–1081
doi:10.1016/j.mcna.2009.05.008
0025-7125/09/$ – see front matter © 2009 Elsevier Inc. All rights reserved.

DEFINITION OF LIVER DYSFUNCTION

The spectrum of liver dysfunction ranges from mild diffuse inflammation seen in early hepatitis or infiltration of the liver with fat seen in hepatic steatosis to the development of the histologic changes associated with cirrhosis. These changes consist of regenerative nodules of hepatocytes surrounded by fibrous bands formed in response to prolonged and repeated liver injury. These fibrous bands eventually distort the hepatic vasculature and lead to portal hypertension and shunting of the portal and arterial blood directly into the hepatic outflow. The exposure of hepatocytes to hepatic blood flow is effectively diminished resulting in the impaired hepatocyte function that is one of the cardinal features of end-stage liver disease.[3] The varied metabolic derangements that develop over time in a patient as hepatocyte function declines manifest pathologic changes in every organ system and pose a formidable problem to the surgeon and anesthesiologist during surgery.

Classification of Liver Dysfunction

Two main classification systems have been developed to stratify patients with liver dysfunction. Both systems were developed initially to differentiate between patients belonging to specific populations but were then extended and extrapolated to all patients with liver disease.

The Child-Turcotte-Pugh (CTP) system, initially developed in 1964 as the Child-Turcott system, characterized the degree of liver disease in patients undergoing portosystemic shunting procedures.[4] Patient were assessed using serum albumin level, serum bilirubin level, ascites, encephalopathy, and nutritional status, and then assigned to a class: A (good, 4% 3-month mortality), B (intermediate, 14% 3-month mortality), or C (poor, 51% 3-month mortality). The category of nutritional status was replaced with prothrombin time by Pugh in 1970 to decrease the subjectivity of the score (**Table 1**). The system evolved into a widely accepted stratification method for all patients with liver dysfunction and became a common term in medical language when discussing a patient with liver disease. It was also a key component in the algorithm for liver transplant allocation until it was supplanted by the Model for End-Stage Liver Disease (MELD) in 2002. Surgeons have long used the CTP score to predict operative mortality for hepatic and nonhepatic surgery in patients with liver disease. The benefits of the CTP score lie in its ease of calculation, which can be performed mentally at the bedside, and its familiarity across fields of medicine. The system has withstood the test of time, with multiple studies showing independent prognostic value across varied clinical settings, medical and surgical.[5]

Table 1 Childs-Turcotte-Pugh score			
Characteristic	1 Point	2 Points	3 Points
Ascites	None	Controlled	Refractory
Encephalopathy	Absent	Controlled	Dense
Albumin (g/L)	>3.5	2.8–3.5	<2.8
Bilirubin (mg/dL)	<2	2–3	>3
INR	<1.7	1.7–2.3	>2.3

CTP class A: 5–6 total points. Low risk, 4% 3-month mortality.
CTP class B: 7–9 total points. Intermediate risk, 14% 3-month mortality.
CTP class C: 10–15 total points. High risk, 51% 3-month mortality.

The main weakness of the CTP score stems from the subjective measurements of ascites and encephalopathy that can skew the scoring system significantly between individuals. This issue came to a head for the United Network for Organ Sharing (UNOS) in the late 1990s when public pressure to make the allocation of liver transplants more objective caused them to abandon the CTP score in favor of the MELD score. This system was created at the Mayo Clinic to assess mortality risk in patients undergoing the transjugular intrahepatic portosystemic shunt (TIPS) procedure and has several benefits over the CTP score. The MELD score is calculated from the objective values of serum bilirubin level, serum creatinine level, and international normalized ratio (INR), which were determined by statistical analysis to be highly predictive of mortality in cirrhosis (**Box 1**). The values are weighted by logarithmic calculations to reflect their relative influence on mortality, giving the most weight to renal function as this has been shown to be a key component of predicting survival in cirrhosis. The MELD score has been evaluated in multiple studies[6] and has proved to be effective in predicting mortality in cirrhosis. It has also been compared with the CTP score in several articles to clarify for clinicians which system should be used with the following conclusions.[5,7]

1. Both scores are able to reliably predict mortality in cirrhotic patients, but the MELD is a more uniform system and more applicable to comparing multiple patients or groups of patients due to its lack of subjectivity.
2. The CTP score is well suited to evaluation of an individual patient because of its familiarity and ease of use. However, care should be taken when applying it to a patient with Childs class A or B with concomitant renal dysfunction, as this is not accounted for in the CTP system but has important prognostic significance in cirrhosis.

Befeler and colleagues performed a retrospective study of 53 patients with cirrhosis undergoing abdominal surgery, and concluded that the MELD provided a more accurate prediction of patient outcomes than the CTP score. The investigators proposed using a "cutoff" MELD score of 14 to distinguish between patients likely to have either a good or bad outcome following abdominal surgery, stating that the positive and negative predictive values of the MELD were more accurate than the three classes of the CTP score.[8] Although this is a small series, it directly addresses the need to assess perioperative mortality/morbidity in surgical patients. These investigators' strong endorsement of the MELD system perhaps warrants further attempts to implement the MELD score into routine preoperative assessment.

To summarize, at present there is no consensus on which score to use when assessing a patient with liver disease who requires surgery. The surgeon can use either the MELD or CTP scores to assess the patient's hepatic condition, but further laboratory and cardiopulmonary testing are advisable to assess the individual patient's overall condition.

Box 1

MELD score formula

MELD score = $(0.957 \times \log_e[\text{serum creatinine(mg/dL)}] + 0.378 \times \log_e[\text{total serum bilirubin (mg/dL)}] + 1.120 \times \log_e[\text{INR}]) \times 10$

- Minimum for all values is 1.
- Maximum value for creatinine is 4.
- Cause of cirrhosis recently removed from UNOS calculation

PREOPERATIVE PREPARATION

Complete blood count, coagulation studies, and a complete metabolic panel begins the workup for a patient with known or suspected liver disease undergoing surgery. These tests are necessary for calculation of the CTP and MELD scores and to detect anemia and renal dysfunction. There are multiple tests that evaluate hepatic reserve specifically by measuring clearance of labeled compounds with special imaging techniques.[9] The most widely used of these tests currently is the indocyanine green retention rate at 15 minutes (ICGR-15). This test indirectly measures the degree of hepatic sinusoidal capillarization by assessing hepatic perfusion and biliary anion excretion. Multiple investigators have reported that the ICGR-15 accurately predicts mortality following hepatectomy.[10–14] One notable example is the work of Imamura and colleagues,[15] who described a simple decision tree for hepatectomy, incorporating the presence of ascites, bilirubin level, and ICGR-15, that resulted in 1 mortality in 1429 consecutive hepatectomies.

Whereas ICGR-15 and similar tests are an important part of the preoperative evaluation for hepatectomy, they are rarely employed in the workup for nonhepatic surgery. For nonhepatic surgery, the approach focuses on addressing the wide range of physiologic derangements caused by declining liver function. Each of these is discussed systematically in the following paragraphs.

Malnutrition

Nutritional status is frequently poor in patients with cirrhosis. Serum albumin, prealbumin, and triglyceride levels are helpful to objectively quantify the patient's nutritional status, in addition to observing physical signs of cachexia and wasting. If the patient is undergoing elective surgery, every effort should be made to improve their nutritional status before surgery. Hospitalized patients should be evaluated for supplemental naso-enteric tube feeding if their oral intake is inadequate. Nonhospitalized patients may need to consume higher calorie foods to limit their volume intake if they have significant ascites. Patients with encephalopathy may be limited by enteral protein restriction, particularly if they have had a portosystemic shunt procedure, as hyperammonemia has been demonstrated following enteral glutamine administration in this population. This specific group of patients may benefit from parenteral nutrition preoperatively if their malnutrition is severe.[16,17]

Encephalopathy

As the liver's metabolic capacity diminishes with advancing disease, its ability to clear the portal blood of nitrogenous compounds generated by intestinal bacteria fails. Several such compounds have been implicated in hepatic encephalopathy, but ammonia has the most supporting evidence for a causative role. High serum ammonia levels are associated with increased risk of cerebral herniation, but no clear causative relationship has been established. Nevertheless, ammonia levels are followed by hepatologists and all treatments of hepatic encephalopathy are aimed at reducing the production of nitrogenous compounds by intestinal flora. It should be emphasized that hepatic encephalopathy is a diagnosis of exclusion and all other possible causes for a patient's confusion should be examined. The mainstay of treatment of hepatic encephalopathy is to rule out other causes of delirium, optimize the patient's care for any other comorbidities or cirrhosis complications, and administer lactulose enterally, titrating for three soft bowel movements per day. With the onset of acute encephalopathy, protein intake may be held for 24 hours, but should be reinstated thereafter with a goal of 1 to 1.5 g/kg/d. Patients with zinc deficiency should receive supplementation. Other less frequently used therapies include other laxatives as well as neomycin or metronidazole to decrease intestinal bacterial load. Close communication with the patient's hepatologist preoperatively is crucial to optimize the patient's medical care before surgery if they show signs of encephalopathy. Postoperatively, special care should be directed to limiting medications that may affect mental status as patients with preoperative encephalopathy are likely to manifest severe delirium postoperatively due to the stresses of surgery.[18]

Coagulopathy

A cardinal feature of cirrhosis is the development of coagulopathy secondary to the declining synthetic function of the liver, leading to prolongation of the prothrombin time (PT) and easy bruising or excessive bleeding. Although coagulopathy is usually due to poor hepatic function, concomitant poor nutrition or malabsorption can lead to vitamin K deficiency, which can exacerbate the problem. As it is difficult to distinguish the two causes, a single 10-mg dose of intramuscular vitamin K should be administered before surgery. Coagulopathy due to poor liver synthetic function is correctable with fresh frozen plasma (FFP), which contains all the necessary clotting factors. The short serum half-life of factor VII (3–5 hours) necessitates administration of the FFP immediately before surgery and frequently throughout the case, with intraoperative monitoring of coagulation parameters.[19] Finally, recombinant factor VII is highly effective at rapidly providing temporary correction of cirrhotic coagulopathy, but due to exorbitant cost and limited availability it should be reserved for emergency surgery in patients with severe coagulopathy or concomitant intracranial bleeding.[20]

Platelet counts are often low in patients with cirrhosis secondary to sequestration due to portal hypertension and splenomegaly. Significant thrombocytopenia (<20,000) should prompt platelet transfusion preoperatively, but not with more moderate levels of thrombocytopenia as the platelets function normally. The presence of coexisting renal failure and uremia may alter this decision as intrinsic platelet function may be compromised. Administration of 1-deamino-8-D-arginine vasopressin, which causes a transient increase in expression of the von Willebrand factor, can improve clotting temporarily.

Ascites and Hyponatremia

Ascites is the most common complication of cirrhosis and is associated with increased infections, increased incidence of renal failure, increased complication rate, poor quality of life, and worse long-term outcome. Ascites develops as hepatic resistance to portal blood flow increases, causing the gradual development of portal hypertension, collateral vein formation, and shunting of blood to the systemic circulation. Increased local production of vasodilators like nitric oxide leads to splanchnic arterial vasodilation, which, combined with portal hypertension, results in abdominal lymph production exceeding lymph resorption and accumulation of intraabdominal fluid. In the later stages of cirrhosis, the splanchnic vasodilation becomes so profound that it overcomes the compensatory cardiovascular and renal responses, decreasing effective circulating volume and ultimately leading to the hepatorenal syndrome.[21]

The presence of symptomatic ascites presents a significant problem for intraabdominal surgery. The sudden release of many liters of ascites at laparotomy can result in paracentesis-induced circulatory dysfunction (PICD), which involves activation of the renin-angiotensin-aldosterone system (RAAS) by an acute increase in splanchnic vasodilation, although the exact mechanism is not known. The incidence of PICD is reduced by preemptive administration of volume expanders, namely intravenous albumin at 8 g/L of ascites removed.[22,23] Most patients with symptomatic, large-volume ascites will benefit from preoperative paracentesis, diuretic therapy, and stringent limitation of salt intake to 1.5 to 2 g/d to minimize reaccumulation of the ascitic fluid. This regimen prevents PICD from appearing in the intra- and postoperative period, compounding the already complex care of a cirrhotic patient. In the case of emergent surgery when preoperative paracentesis is not possible, intravenous volume expansion before and during laparotomy should help to alleviate the effect of the rapid ascites removal. An alternative to large-volume paracentesis in patients with severe, refractory ascites is the TIPS procedure, which is effective in decreasing portal hypertension and splanchnic vasodilation, thereby reducing ascites formation.

TIPS is well accepted as a bridging therapy to transplantation but more recently has been evaluated by two large meta-analyses, including a Cochrane review,[24] as a primary treatment of refractory ascites. These analyses showed that TIPS effectively decreases ascitic fluid build up to manageable levels with no increase in mortality over paracentesis. However, there is a significant increase in the incidence of encephalopathy noted with TIPS, particularly in patients with prior encephalopathy, greater than 60 years old, or renal insufficiency.[25] Patients with these risk factors should not undergo TIPS, but in patients who are considered good candidates for TIPS, consideration should be given to performing the procedure before attempting nonurgent abdominal surgery. To date, this has not been evaluated in a large trial, but two small series have reported successful preoperative TIPS placement in patients with severe portal hypertension, for whom abdominal surgery was contraindicated, with enough improvement in their portal hypertension to allow the abdominal surgery to proceed.[26,27]

Hyponatremia can complicate the treatment of ascites significantly, as the patient may have low total body sodium secondary to hypersecretion of antidiuretic hormone (ADH), which is in response to activation of the RAAS by a low effective circulating volume. The initial treatment of hyponatremia is fluid restriction but this can be difficult to accomplish because the inciting cause in this case is an effective low-volume state, prompting RAAS activation and leading ultimately to development of the hepatorenal syndrome. Thus, in this setting volume restriction may hasten the development of renal impairment.[21]

A new class of drugs, known as vaptams or aquaretics, selectively inhibits V2 receptors in the renal collecting tubules, increasing free water clearance and showing some promise in treating hyponatremia of cirrhosis in preliminary clinical studies.[28] Further studies are needed before these agents will be available for routine treatment in clinical practice, however; meanwhile management is limited to negotiating a tenuous balance between diuretic therapy, salt limitation, and volume restriction, all while preserving the patient's often marginal renal function.[23,28]

Cardiovascular Issues and Cardiac Evaluation

Although the sequelae of portal hypertension cause most of the morbidity in cirrhosis, the systemic cardiovascular derangements associated with cirrhosis are pronounced and can impact significantly on morbidity and mortality. The predominant feature of a cirrhotic patient's cardiovascular system is a generalized hyperdynamic state, consisting of increased heart rate, cardiac output, and plasma volume, with reduced systemic vascular resistance and blood pressure. Early in cirrhosis these changes are subtle but they increase with disease progression, aided by the development of arteriovenous communications and autonomic dysfunction. Research indicates that the inciting cause of this condition may be increased production of nitric oxide in response to portal hypertension, which results in splanchnic vasodilation. A hyperdynamic circulatory response ensues to compensate for the perceived central hypovolemia due to pooled blood in the splanchnic vasculature. As the splanchnic vasodilation becomes severe in advanced cirrhosis, the hyperdynamic circulatory compensation is exhausted and systemic blood pressure is maintained mainly by vasoconstriction in the renal, cerebral, and hepatic vascular beds mediated by norepinephrine, vasopressin, and angiotensin II. The systemic nature of these metabolic and cardiac events leads to the overall poor functional status of a patient with end-stage cirrhosis and their inability to withstand the typical burdens of surgery.[22,29]

From a practical standpoint, the hemodynamic changes described earlier cause patients with cirrhosis to have increased total blood volume but decreased central and effective arterial volume, and are therefore functionally hypovolemic. Their peripheral circulation is increased, however, which can be deceptive on physical examination. Their hemodynamic compensatory systems are maximized, and their renal perfusion is already decreased at baseline, so acute volume depletion or hemorrhage is not well tolerated. It is advisable to obtain central venous access before commencing any intraabdominal surgery to reliably monitor the volume status of the central vasculature.

The heart is not spared the ravages of cirrhosis. Cirrhotic cardiomyopathy was for years confused with alcoholic cardiomyopathy but has recently been recognized and classified as a separate entity.[22] Systolic dysfunction, consisting of a blunted contractility response, and diastolic dysfunction are present, as well as electromechanical abnormalities. Although the penetrance of cardiac dysfunction in cirrhosis is variable, routine preoperative cardiac testing is advisable to identify patients with limited cardiac reserve. Electrocardiography can identify a characteristic increase in the Q-T interval, reflecting a prolonged repolarization time, which has been shown to significantly correlate with severity of liver disease, elevated brain natriuretic peptide (BNP) level, and decreased survival.[30] A preoperative stress echocardiogram can identify systolic dysfunction, as the expected increases in stroke volume and ejection fraction will be diminished or absent, reflecting an inadequate contractility response to increased ventricular filling pressure.[31] Diastolic dysfunction can be detected on Doppler echocardiogram as an abnormally low ratio of early to late (atrial) left ventricular filling, representing impaired left ventricular relaxation.

Pulmonary Issues and Pulmonary Evaluation

Patients with cirrhosis should also undergo pulmonary evaluation before surgery as the incidence of hepatopulmonary syndrome (HPS) approaches 30% in patients with end-stage liver disease and is associated with increased complications and mortality. This syndrome is defined as an arterial oxygenation defect induced by intrapulmonary vascular dilatations associated with hepatic disease. Increased pulmonary nitric oxide production is implicated in the pathogenesis of this condition, similar to that of splanchnic vasodilatation. This produces an increase in the shunt fraction, resulting in a ventilation-perfusion mismatch. Typical clinical findings in HPS include platypnea and orthodeoxia, consisting of dyspnea and measurable hypoxia, respectively, on moving from a supine to an upright position. Physical examination findings indicating chronic hypoxia, such as digital clubbing, spider nevi, and cyanotic lips and nail beds, are seen in advanced HPS although they are not specific to this condition.[32,33]

The recommended algorithm to screen for HPS in a patient with liver disease and hypoxia consists first of measurement of arterial blood gasses. A PaO_2 of less than 80 mmHg, or an alveolar-arterial oxygen tension difference greater than 15 mmHg, indicating significant shunting, is a concern for HPS, and should prompt further testing with contrast echocardiography. Contrast echocardiography is considered the gold standard test for HPS and consists of injecting a normal saline solution of microbubbles in a peripheral vein while performing transthoracic or transesophageal echocardiography. The bubbles are trapped and absorbed by normal alveoli so the appearance of any bubbles in the left atrium constitutes a positive test.[32]

There are no effective perioperative therapies to improve the pulmonary vascular abnormalities, hypoxemia, and ventilation-perfusion mismatches associated with HPS. Liver transplant is the only treatment shown to be effective in improving this condition. Patients with significant hypoxemia require long-term supplemental oxygen therapy. The prognosis with HPS is poor. In a prospective trial of 111 patients with cirrhosis, Schenk and colleagues[34] demonstrated that the presence of HPS in Child class C patients imparted a 5 times greater mortality rate.

Gastric and Esophageal Varices

Depending on the type of surgery anticipated, a preoperative esophagogastroduodenoscopy may be useful to evaluate the extent of the varices present in a cirrhotic patient's esophagus and stomach. This especially applies if the patient is to undergo foregut surgery, as this will better delineate the anatomy of interest preoperatively. If the patient has a history of prior upper gastrointestinal bleeding, it is prudent to perform endoscopy before surgery if not recently done already.

INTRAOPERATIVE MANAGEMENT

The presence of ascites, higher Child-Pugh class dysfunction, renal impairment, coexisting respiratory disease, higher American Society of Anesthesiologists (ASA) physical classification status, higher surgical score, and intraoperative hypotension have been shown to correlate with increased perioperative morbidity and mortality.[35,36] Preoperative risk reduction strategies such as paracentesis, treatment of coagulopathy, hypovolemia and respiratory dysfunction, and improving nutritional status should be employed to improve perioperative outcome.

Emergent Versus Elective Surgery

Numerous studies have shown increased mortality in cirrhotic patients undergoing emergent surgery. Wahlstrom and colleagues[37] demonstrated that cirrhotic trauma patients who underwent emergent laparotomy had 44% mortality and 71% morbidity. In a retrospective review of 40 patients with cirrhosis who underwent various surgical procedures, Franzetta and colleagues[38] concluded that the emergency nature of the procedure, in combination with Child class, was a significant factor in predicting perioperative mortality. Friedman proposed the following list of contraindications to elective surgery in patients with liver disease:[39]

- Acute viral hepatitis
- Acute alcoholic hepatitis
- Fulminant hepatic failure
- Severe chronic hepatitis
- Child class C cirrhosis
- Severe coagulopathy (prolongation of the PT of >3 s despite vitamin K administration; platelet count <50,000/mm^3)
- Severe extrahepatic complications (hypoxemia, cardiomyopathy, heart failure, acute renal failure)

On the other hand, patients with abnormal preoperative liver enzymes but mild or no clinical symptoms of liver failure can undergo surgery with minimal or no increase in perioperative morbidity and mortality.[40]

Anesthetic Management

The ultimate goal of intraoperative management is to minimize perturbations of the hepatic oxygen supply and demand ratio. In normal, healthy individuals hepatic blood flow is provided by the hepatic artery (30%) and the portal vein (70%), with 50% oxygen supply from each. If portal vein blood flow is reduced, hepatic artery flow increases to maintain adequate oxygen supply. This autoregulation is disrupted by hepatic disease and volatile anesthetic agents. In an animal model of inhaled anesthetics, isoflurane increased hepatic artery flow but decreased portal vein flow.[41] Desflurane and sevoflurane affect hepatic circulation in a manner similar to isoflurane. Halothane decreases the portal vein flow but causes no increase in hepatic artery flow (**Fig. 1**).

As discussed earlier, patients with liver failure often exhibit a hyperdynamic vascular state with vasodilation and low systemic vascular resistance. Further myocardial depression and systemic vasodilation by anesthetic agents can lead to hypotension that is unresponsive to catecholamines. The normal compensatory baroreceptor mechanism and the regulatory systems of cardiovascular homoeostasis are impaired.[42] Mechanical ventilation can further reduce the venous return, causing hepatic congestion and lower cardiac output. Preoperative paracentesis can lead to hypovolemia, further contributing to intraoperative hypotension.

Other intraoperative events that can compromise liver blood flow and oxygen supply include acute hypotension, sympathomimetic drugs, and increased splanchnic vascular resistance from surgical manipulation. These periods of hepatic hypoxemia are the most common cause of postoperative liver dysfunction in all patients, and this effect is more pronounced in patients with preexisting liver disease.[43] Anesthetic management of patients with cirrhosis is therefore focused on minimizing the periods of time when the liver is subjected to suboptimal perfusion and oxygenation.

Not surprisingly, postoperative liver dysfunction is even more pronounced in cirrhotic patients anesthetized with halothane, and it is not indicated for use in these patients. In addition to its untoward effects on liver blood flow, halothane is also

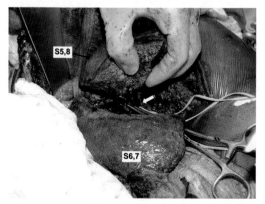

Fig. 1. Intraoperative view of a cirrhotic liver during resection of a right anterior sector (*black arrow*, segment 5,8) hepatocellular carcinoma. *White arrow* points to the clamped portal pedicle for the right anterior sector before transection with a stapler.

associated with rare but severe hepatitis, which is believed to be immune mediated.[44] Other inhaled anesthetics are also associated with severe postoperative liver failure, but with much lower incidence.

Patients with liver disease have altered pharmokinetics of systemically administered drugs due to increased volume of distribution, decreased cytochrome P450 enzyme metabolism, decreased serum drug binding secondary to low protein/albumin levels, and sometimes decreased biliary drug excretion. Drug elimination is largely unchanged after a single induction dose of intravenous anesthetics such as sodium thiopental or propofol, but multiple doses or a continuous infusion can lead to prolonged clinical effects.[45] Opioids such as morphine, meperidine, and oxycodone have a prolonged half-life and increased bioavailability, whereas fentanyl and remifentanil clearance is unaffected.[46] If the use of longer acting opioids is desired, lower doses at less frequent intervals should be administered. Slower metabolism of benzodiazepines such as diazepam and midazolam can lead to accumulation and prolonged clinical effects. The neuromuscular blocking agents vecuronium and rocuronium are degraded by the hepatic system exclusively.[47] Atracurium and cisatracurium are metabolized independent of the liver and are therefore preferred in patients with liver disease. Plasma cholinesterase levels are decreased in severe liver disease, possibly resulting in the observed prolonged duration of mivacurium.[48]

There is no difference in clinical outcomes related to the anesthetic technique. Because most patients with significant liver disease have coagulation defects, most surgeries are performed under general anesthesia. Regional anesthesia with spinal, epidural, or peripheral nerve block can be considered in the presence of normal coagulation status. Airway management is dictated by physical evaluation, gastric aspiration risk, and nature of surgery. In general, nasal intubation is avoided in the presence of coagulopathy. Esophageal and gastric instrumentation should be minimized due to the risk of bleeding.

Hemodynamic monitoring is dependent on the physiologic state of the patient and magnitude of the proposed surgery. Preoperative fasting can lead to hypoglycemia necessitating periodic plasma glucose monitoring and infusion of glucose-containing fluids. An arterial catheter is usually indicated to continuously monitor blood pressure, allow rapid blood sampling, and, with newer devices, monitor cardiac output using the peripheral arterial waveform. A central venous pressure (CVP) catheter is usually necessary to monitor intravascular volume status and to administer vasoactive drugs if necessary. For larger procedures, a pulmonary artery catheter should be placed or at least a central catheter capable of accommodating intraoperative pulmonary artery catheter placement. Ongoing coagulation defects should be corrected with FFP before inserting invasive lines, except under emergent conditions. Blood gas analysis should be performed as needed to monitor acid base status, as alkalosis can further exacerbate ammonia diffusion across the blood-brain barrier. Patients should at least be typed and screened for blood transfusion as possible previous transfusions could induce plasma antibodies requiring longer type and cross-matching time. Patients with liver disease have slow citrate clearance, so blood is transfused slowly if possible.

Overall, a restrictive transfusion policy is preferable to avoid postoperative hyperbilirubinemia, and primary volume replacement for blood loss should be with FFP and secondarily lactated Ringer solution.[49] Intraoperative fluid management can be difficult, as many patients are already functionally hypovolemic and the anesthetics cause hypotension, yet the blood pressure must be kept adequate to perfuse the liver and sympathomimetics are often counterproductive. Thus, there is often a need to administer significant volume, but this must be minimized as much as possible to limit total body volume overload. In these settings a pulmonary artery catheter can provide useful information regarding central volume status and cardiac performance and should direct resuscitative efforts. Diligent reassessment of these parameters and aggressive tapering of the rate of fluid infusion should reduce overall volume administration. Overall the amount of fluid administered should be restricted during surgery (rather than the usual 10 mL/kg/h to the 4.5 to 5 mL/kg/h) in addition to maintaining a low CVP.

Care of the Acutely Alcohol Intoxicated Patient

Patients with alcohol-related chronic liver disease have a significant increase in perioperative morbidity[50] and can present for emergent surgery in an acutely intoxicated condition. In addition to chronic alcohol abuse-related complications such as malnutrition, suboptimal immune response, fluid and electrolyte disturbances, and cardiomyopathy, acute intoxication causes central nervous system depression and lower anesthetic requirements, higher risk of gastric content aspiration, and higher risk of intraoperative hypotension secondary to dehydration and hypovolemia. In addition, all alcoholic patients should be observed postoperatively for development of alcohol withdrawal symptoms.

Summary of Intraoperative Management

Although every patient is evaluated and treated individually, the following general recommendations can be made for the intraoperative care of patients with liver disease:

- Postpone elective surgery until acute hepatitis resolves.
- Maintain hepatic blood flow and oxygenation by sustaining a normal blood pressure and cardiac output, avoiding sympathomimetic drugs, and minimizing surgical manipulation of the porta hepatis.
- Isoflurane is the preferred volatile anesthetic agent. Preferentially use drugs with minimal or no hepatic degradation. Titrate drugs to achieve the desired clinical effect. Use a twitch monitor to guide muscle relaxation.
- Avoid nasal and esophageal/gastric instrumentation to prevent bleeding. Employ gastric aspiration prophylaxis. Correct coagulation defects before inserting invasive vascular lines.

POSTOPERATIVE CARE

Postoperative care is arguably the most difficult aspect of performing surgery on a patient with cirrhosis, as they tend to have a high rate of complications, particularly following abdominal surgery. The complications are influenced by the degree of liver disease the patient had preoperatively and the complexity of the operation performed. As discussed earlier, Child class C and elevated MELD scores of greater than 14 portend postoperative complications. Hernia repairs and laparoscopic cholecystectomy impart a low mortality, whereas that of open alimentary tract surgery is significantly higher.[51]

To minimize the development of postoperative complications, the surgeon should adopt a proactive and preemptive role to optimize the patient's physiology and employ sensitive monitoring systems to detect the earliest signs of development of complications. The first step should be to place all postoperative patients with Child B or C cirrhosis in a monitored unit, preferably an intensive care unit, even if they have been successfully extubated and seem stable. The decreased metabolic capacity of patents with cirrhosis makes them ill-equipped to clear anesthetic agents and pain medications, resulting in an increased risk of somnolence and hypoventilation. Furthermore, the inevitable postoperative fluid shifts resulting in impaired hepatic perfusion could make a single night in an unmonitored setting catastrophic. Continuous cardiac monitoring and hourly vital signs are prudent for all patients with cirrhosis for the first night postoperatively.

Patients who undergo open abdominal surgery should have central venous access and an arterial catheter in place. These should be maintained for at least 24 hours and longer if the patient is not showing clear signs of recovery, such as adequate urine output, clear mental status, and reassuring cardiac and pulmonary parameters. Continuous or hourly monitoring of CVP for the first 24 hours will help the team maintain adequate volume status (CVP 8–12 in the extubated patient) without reaching fluid overload. This is of critical importance to maximize cardiac output and maintain good perfusion to the liver, which will usually have suffered some degree of ischemic insult from intraoperative anesthetics, surgical manipulation, or hemorrhage. Depending on how much hepatic reserve the patient has, this could make the difference between recovery and slipping into acute liver failure. In addition, all potentially hepatotoxic agents should be minimized or avoided. Preference should be given to medications that are cleared by the kidneys. Acetaminophen should not be given in excess of 2 g/d.[52]

Enteral nutrition is more conducive to hepatic recovery than parenteral nutrition, and oral intake or tube feedings should be started as soon as possible. Oral feeding also reduces the risk of spontaneous bacterial peritonitis in the postoperative period. Even trophic feedings with supplemental parenteral nutrition may be beneficial to the intestinal mucosa.[16]

Laboratory studies, including blood count, electrolytes with ionized calcium, and coagulation parameters should be sent immediately on the patient's return from surgery. Serum potassium, magnesium, and calcium levels should be aggressively replaced, which provides another practical reason for central venous access postoperatively. The patient's INR should be less than 1.5 (and preferably lower), which will frequently require additional FFP. Platelets should be transfused to maintain levels more than 50,000 for the first 12 to 24 hours.

Pain management can be particularly difficult in the postoperative patient with cirrhosis for reasons alluded to earlier. It is difficult to estimate how the cirrhotic liver will clear medications metabolized by the cytochrome P450 enzyme system, and thus the doses of most opiates must be significantly reduced. Fentanyl is minimally affected but has such a short duration of action that it is poorly suited to managing postoperative pain, except in a patient with pre- or postoperative encephalopathy for whom a short-acting agent could be beneficial. Intermediate duration agents such as morphine are commonly used but initial dosing should be started at half the usual dose, calculated based on the patient's ideal body weight.

Two postoperative problems that apply particularly to the patient with liver disease are postoperative ascites leak and postoperative jaundice.

Postoperative Ascites Leak

Although attempts are presumably made intraoperatively to minimize the amount of parenteral fluid administered, patients almost always have an increased total body fluid volume. Combined with the inevitable intraabdominal inflammation and preexisting portal hypertension, this leads to third-spacing of fluid and a rapid reaccumulation of ascites. Whether this fluid leaks through the laparotomy incision depends on the size of the incision, the nutritional status of the patient, and the rapidity with which the intraabdominal pressure reaccumulates. If the peritoneum and skin can bridge the gap of the incision before the pressure builds up, the ascites may be contained.

Ensuring adequate postoperative nutrition is important for early wound closure and the patient should be fed enterally as soon as possible.

Once ascites begins leaking from the patient's wound, treatment is mostly supportive. Frequent dressing changes are required to minimize skin maceration. The skin incision should only be reopened if there is clinical evidence of a wound infection. A vacuum-assisted closure device may then facilitate wound closure, although this must be balanced with the risk of increased ascitic fluid (and therefore protein) loss. Stawicki and colleagues[53] recently reported that a small series of four patients with severe postoperative ascites leaks were effectively managed with these devices.

With continued ascitic fluid leak, the risk of contamination of the abdomen and subsequent bacterial peritonitis increases. If the patient does develop clinical evidence of systemic infection and no other source is identified, cultures of the ascitic fluid should be obtained to analyze the type of organism, to determine antibiotic therapy and define the source of the infection. If staphylococcal and streptococcal species are cultured, the infection can be assumed to have originated from the wound. However, if enteric bacteria are encountered, the source may be either from intraoperative contamination or postoperative bowel perforation, anastomotic leakage, or spontaneous bacterial peritonitis, which carry grave prognoses.[54,55] The nature of the operation will also guide this line of investigation.

Postoperative Jaundice

The overall incidence of postoperative jaundice is reported to be less than 1% in minor abdominal surgeries and up to 17% following major abdominal surgery. In patients with preexisting liver dysfunction, up to 45% will become icteric following surgery.[56] The causes of postoperative jaundice can be categorized by three main pathologic mechanisms: (1) increased pigment load; (2) impaired hepatocellular function; (3) posthepatic obstruction.

Increased pigment load in the postoperative setting is most commonly due to hemolysis of transfused erythrocytes, particularly if a minor transfusion reaction occurred. Other causes include drug-induced hemolysis, resorption of hematoma, or gastrointestinal hemorrhage from an esophageal varix disrupted by nasogatric tube trauma or intraoperative manipulation. Intraluminal bleeding from a recent intestinal anastamosis must also be considered, although these last two reasons should manifest more apparent clinical signs of blood loss before the onset of jaundice.

Impaired hepatocyte function is the most likely cause of postoperative jaundice in a patient with preexisting liver dysfunction. As discussed earlier, certain anesthetic agents can diminish hepatic blood flow, as can episodes of intraoperative hypotension, use of sympathomimetic agents, and surgical manipulation. Postoperative sepsis or hypovolemia will contribute to the damage. These insults are poorly tolerated by the cirrhotic liver and irreversible hepatocyte injury can result, causing a spectrum of liver dysfunction from mild jaundice to fulminant hepatic failure.

Posthepatic obstruction can result from iatrogenic intraoperative causes or passage of a gallstone. A rare but important cause is acalculous cholecystitis.[57] This condition typically occurs in elderly patients or those with significant comorbidities, and is usually seen in the setting of sepsis or some other critical illness. Patients usually have the classic symptoms of calculous cholecystitis, including upper abdominal pain, fever, nausea, and leukocytosis. However, in the critically ill, postoperative, cirrhotic patient few or none of these symptoms will stand out and the diagnosis is made by ultrasound prompted by a high index of suspicion. Treatment is, ideally, cholecystectomy. However, if the patient is too ill to return to the operating room, a percutaneous cholecystostomy tube placed at the bedside will drain the gallbladder and temporize the situation until the patient can undergo a definitive operation.[56]

SUMMARY

The surgical management of the patient with cirrhosis is challenging. The ravages of cirrhosis are broad, affecting all major organ systems and causing a wide range of clinical symptoms, which can be dramatic and obvious like ascites, or subtle but deadly like hepatopulmonary syndrome. Those caring for patients with cirrhosis should carry a healthy respect for the disease and have a high index of suspicion for possible complications. Surgeons who treat patients with cirrhosis infrequently should enlist the support of a hepatologist preoperatively to assist in optimizing the patient's condition before attempting any elective procedures. The following general guidelines are proposed for managing surgical patients with Child Class B or C cirrhosis:

- Operate only on patients with a compelling need for surgery.
- Assess the patient's cardiovascular and pulmonary status objectively, as the presence of a severely hyperdynamic state or the hepatopulmonary syndrome alter the risk-benefit consideration significantly.
- Transfuse FFP for coagulopathy immediately before arrival in the operating room, as the short half-life of factor VII limits its duration of action.
- Address symptomatic ascites preoperatively with large-volume paracentesis and volume expansion with albumin.
- Minimize operative time and avoid hypothermia.
- Strongly consider intensive care unit observation for the first night following surgery, even if the patient seems to be recovering well.

REFERENCES

1. Abdelmalek MF, Diehl AM. Nonalcoholic fatty liver disease as a complication of insulin resistance. Med Clin North Am 2007;91(6):1125–49, ix.
2. Adams LA, Angulo P, Lindor KD. Nonalcoholic fatty liver disease. CMAJ 2005; 172(7):899–905.
3. Schuppan D, Afdhal NH. Liver cirrhosis. Lancet 2008;371(9615):838–51.
4. Child CG, Turcotte JG. Surgery and portal hypertension. Major Probl Clin Surg 1964;1:1–85.
5. Durand F, Valla D. Assessment of the prognosis of cirrhosis: Child-Pugh versus MELD. J Hepatol 2005;42(Suppl 1):S100–7.
6. Bingener J, Cox D, Michalek J, et al. Can the MELD score predict perioperative morbidity for patients with liver cirrhosis undergoing laparoscopic cholecystectomy? Am Surg 2008;74(2):156–9.
7. Farnsworth N, Fagan SP, Berger DH, et al. Child-Turcotte-Pugh versus MELD score as a predictor of outcome after elective and emergent surgery in cirrhotic patients. Am J Surg 2004;188(5):580–3.
8. Befeler AS, Palmer DE, Hoffman M, et al. The safety of intra-abdominal surgery in patients with cirrhosis: model for end-stage liver disease score is superior to Child-Turcotte-Pugh classification in predicting outcome. Arch Surg 2005; 140(7):650–4 [discussion: 655].
9. Schneider PD. Preoperative assessment of liver function. Surg Clin North Am 2004;84(2):355–73.

10. Lau H, Man K, Fan ST, et al. Evaluation of preoperative hepatic function in patients with hepatocellular carcinoma undergoing hepatectomy. Br J Surg 1997;84(9):1255–9.

11. Hemming AW, Scudamore CH, Shackleton CR, et al. Indocyanine green clearance as a predictor of successful hepatic resection in cirrhotic patients. Am J Surg 1992;163(5):515–8.

12. Hsia CY, Lui WY, Chau GY, et al. Perioperative safety and prognosis in hepatocellular carcinoma patients with impaired liver function. J Am Coll Surg 2000;190(5):574–9.

13. Poon RT, Fan ST. Assessment of hepatic reserve for indication of hepatic resection: how I do it. J Hepatobiliary Pancreat Surg 2005;12(1):31–7.

14. Lee SG, Hwang S. How I do it: assessment of hepatic functional reserve for indication of hepatic resection. J Hepatobiliary Pancreat Surg 2005;12(1):38–43.

15. Imamura H, Sano K, Sugawara Y, et al. Assessment of hepatic reserve for indication of hepatic resection: decision tree incorporating indocyanine green test. J Hepatobiliary Pancreat Surg 2005;12(1):16–22.

16. Cabre E, Gassull MA. Nutritional aspects of liver disease and transplantation. Curr Opin Clin Nutr Metab Care 2001;4(6):581–9.

17. Plauth M, Roske AE, Romaniuk P, et al. Post-feeding hyperammonaemia in patients with transjugular intrahepatic portosystemic shunt and liver cirrhosis: role of small intestinal ammonia release and route of nutrient administration. Gut 2000;46(6):849–55.

18. Blei AT, Cordoba J. Hepatic encephalopathy. Am J Gastroenterol 2001;96(7): 1968–76.

19. Bell CL, Jeyarajah DR. Management of the cirrhotic patient that needs surgery. Curr Treat Options Gastroenterol 2005;8(6):473–80.

20. Shami VM, Caldwell SH, Hespenheide EE, et al. Recombinant activated factor VII for coagulopathy in fulminant hepatic failure compared with conventional therapy. Liver Transpl 2003;9(2):138–43.

21. Gines P, Cardenas A, Arroyo V, et al. Management of cirrhosis and ascites. N Engl J Med 2004;350(16):1646–54.

22. Moller S, Henriksen JH. Cardiovascular complications of cirrhosis. Gut 2008; 57(2):268–78.

23. Kuiper JJ, van Buuren HR, de Man RA. Ascites in cirrhosis: a review of management and complications. Neth J Med 2007;65(8):283–8.

24. Saab S, Nieto JM, Lewis SK, et al. TIPS versus paracentesis for cirrhotic patients with refractory ascites. Cochrane Database Syst Rev 2006;(4):CD004889.

25. Russo MW, Sood A, Jacobson IM, et al. Transjugular intrahepatic portosystemic shunt for refractory ascites: an analysis of the literature on efficacy, morbidity, and mortality. Am J Gastroenterol 2003;98(11):2521–7.

26. Azoulay D, Buabse F, Damiano I, et al. Neoadjuvant transjugular intrahepatic portosystemic shunt: a solution for extrahepatic abdominal operation in cirrhotic patients with severe portal hypertension. J Am Coll Surg 2001;193(1):46–51.

27. Gil A, Martinez-Regueira F, Hernandez-Lizoain JL, et al. The role of transjugular intrahepatic portosystemic shunt prior to abdominal tumoral surgery in cirrhotic patients with portal hypertension. Eur J Surg Oncol 2004;30(1):46–52.

28. Dong MH, Saab S. Complications of cirrhosis. Dis Mon 2008;54(7):445–56.

29. Blei AT, Mazhar S, Davidson CJ, et al. Hemodynamic evaluation before liver transplantation: insights into the portal hypertensive syndrome. J Clin Gastroenterol 2007;41(Suppl 3):S323–9.

30. Zambruni A, Trevisani F, Caraceni P, et al. Cardiac electrophysiological abnormalities in patients with cirrhosis. J Hepatol 2006;44(5):994–1002.

31. Wong F, Girgrah N, Graba J, et al. The cardiac response to exercise in cirrhosis. Gut 2001;49(2):268–75.
32. Rodriguez-Roisin R, Krowka MJ, Herve P, et al. Pulmonary-hepatic vascular disorders (PHD). Eur Respir J 2004;24(5):861–80.
33. Hanje AJ, Patel T. Preoperative evaluation of patients with liver disease. Nat Clin Pract Gastroenterol Hepatol 2007;4(5):266–76.
34. Schenk P, Schoniger-Hekele M, Fuhrmann V, et al. Prognostic significance of the hepatopulmonary syndrome in patients with cirrhosis. Gastroenterology 2003; 125(4):1042–52.
35. Ziser A, Plevak DJ, Wiesner RH, et al. Morbidity and mortality in cirrhotic patients undergoing anesthesia and surgery. Anesthesiology 1999;90(1): 42–53.
36. Teh SH, Nagorney DM, Stevens SR, et al. Risk factors for mortality after surgery in patients with cirrhosis. Gastroenterology 2007;132(4):1261–9.
37. Wahlstrom K, Ney AL, Jacobson S, et al. Trauma in cirrhotics: survival and hospital sequelae in patients requiring abdominal exploration. Am Surg 2000; 66(11):1071–6.
38. Franzetta M, Raimondo D, Giammanco M, et al. Prognostic factors of cirrhotic patients in extra-hepatic surgery. Minerva Chir 2003;58(4):541–4.
39. Friedman LS. The risk of surgery in patients with liver disease. Hepatology 1999; 29(6):1617–23.
40. Sahin H, Pirat A, Arslan G. Anaesthesia and surgery in patients with abnormal preoperative liver enzymes. Eur J Anaesthesiol 2007;24(5):465–7.
41. Gelman S, Fowler KC, Smith LR. Liver circulation and function during isoflurane and halothane anesthesia. Anesthesiology 1984;61(6):726–30.
42. Moller S, Henriksen JH. Cardiopulmonary complications in chronic liver disease. World J Gastroenterol 2006;12(4):526–38.
43. Baden JM, Serra M, Fujinaga M, et al. Halothane metabolism in cirrhotic rats. Anesthesiology 1987;67(5):660–4.
44. Gut J, Christen U, Huwyler J. Mechanisms of halothane toxicity: novel insights. Pharmacol Ther 1993;58(2):133–55.
45. Servin F, Cockshott ID, Farinotti R, et al. Pharmacokinetics of propofol infusions in patients with cirrhosis. Br J Anaesth 1990;65(2):177–83.
46. Tegeder I, Lotsch J, Geisslinger G. Pharmacokinetics of opioids in liver disease. Clin Pharmacokinet 1999;37(1):17–40.
47. Lebrault C, Berger JL, D'Hollander AA, et al. Pharmacokinetics and pharmacodynamics of vecuronium (ORG NC 45) in patients with cirrhosis. Anesthesiology 1985;62(5):601–5.
48. Cook DR, Freeman JA, Lai AA, et al. Pharmacokinetics of mivacurium in normal patients and in those with hepatic or renal failure. Br J Anaesth 1992;69(6): 580–5.
49. Torzilli G, Makuuchi M, Inoue K, et al. No-mortality liver resection for hepatocellular carcinoma in cirrhotic and noncirrhotic patients: is there a way? A prospective analysis of our approach. Arch Surg 1999;134(9):984–92.
50. Tonnesen H, Kehlet H. Preoperative alcoholism and postoperative morbidity. Br J Surg 1999;86(7):869–74.
51. Mansour A, Watson W, Shayani V, et al. Abdominal operations in patients with cirrhosis: still a major surgical challenge. Surgery 1997;122(4):730–5 [discussion: 735–6].
52. Redai I, Emond J, Brentjens T. Anesthetic considerations during liver surgery. Surg Clin North Am 2004;84(2):401–11.

53. Stawicki SP, Schwarz NS, Schrag SP, et al. Application of vacuum-assisted therapy in postoperative ascitic fluid leaks: an integral part of multimodality wound management in cirrhotic patients. J Burns Wounds 2007;6:e7.
54. Mihas AA, Toussaint J, Hsu HS, et al. Spontaneous bacterial peritonitis in cirrhosis: clinical and laboratory features, survival and prognostic indicators. Hepatogastroenterology 1992;39(6):520–2.
55. Fernandez J, Navasa M, Planas R, et al. Primary prophylaxis of spontaneous bacterial peritonitis delays hepatorenal syndrome and improves survival in cirrhosis. Gastroenterology 2007;133(3):818–24.
56. Faust TW, Reddy KR. Postoperative jaundice. Clin Liver Dis 2004;8(1):151–66.
57. Rizvon MK, Chou CL. Surgery in the patient with liver disease. Med Clin North Am 2003;87(1):211–27.

Surgery in the Patient with Renal Dysfunction

Dean R. Jones, MD, FRCPC[a], H.T. Lee, MD, PhD[b],*

KEYWORDS

- Chronic kidney disease • Acute kidney injury • Renal failure
- Renal protection • Preoperative evaluation

Millions of patients with renal dysfunction have surgery each year. The social and financial impact on the health care system is enormous.[1] Preoperative evaluation should attempt to reduce morbidity and mortality and improve quality in this complex patient population.

Renal dysfunction represents a spectrum of disease with potentially far-ranging consequences on surgical and anesthetic management due to not only the underlying disease processes but also from the intervening medical and surgical therapies. Furthermore, optimization of the patient with renal dysfunction needs to not only consider the preexisting renal function but also the potential risk of acute kidney injury (AKI) in the perioperative setting.

In this context, the goal of this review is to focus on perioperative evaluation and optimization of care in surgical patients who have renal dysfunction. Two different sections are presented. The first section focuses on definitions and the epidemiology of chronic kidney disease (CKD), end-stage renal disease (ESRD), and AKI. The surgical risk factors for AKI are also reviewed. The second section focuses on an approach to preoperative evaluation, with particular emphasis on potential areas of conflict between the primary care physician or nephrologist, surgeon, and anesthesiologist. Recent research findings on perioperative renal protection strategies are also reviewed.

RENAL DYSFUNCTION
Chronic Kidney Disease

CKD as defined in 2002 by the Kidney Disease Outcomes Quality Initiative (K/DOQI) of the National Kidney Foundation is either kidney damage or decreased kidney function

---

This work was supported solely by the Intramural Research Fund of the Department of Anesthesiology at Columbia University.

[a] Department of Anesthesiology, Columbia University, PH 5-133, 622 West 168th Street, New York, NY 10032, USA
[b] Department of Anesthesiology, Anesthesiology Research Laboratories, Columbia University, P&S Box 46 (PH-5), 630 West 168th Street, New York, NY 10032-3784, USA
* Corresponding author.
E-mail address: tl128@columbia.edu (H.T. Lee).

for 3 or more months.[2] Proteinuria or abnormalities in imaging tests are markers for kidney damage and a reduction in glomerular filtration rate (GFR) is a marker for decreased kidney function.[3] ESRD is a government-derived administrative term that only indicates chronic treatment by dialysis or transplantation. It does not refer to a specific degree of kidney function.[3]

The National Kidney Foundation classifies CKD based on pathology:

- Diabetic glomerulosclerosis
- Glomerular diseases (primary or secondary)
- Vascular diseases (including hypertension and microangiopathy)
- Tubulointerstitial diseases (including obstructive or reflux nephropathy)
- Cystic diseases
- Diseases in renal transplant recipients (rejection, drug toxicity, recurrence of disease)

A GFR of less than 60 mL/min/1.73 m^2 is considered the threshold for CKD.[4] GFR varies with sex, age, and body size, and is typically estimated with calculations based on serum creatinine (SCr) level.[4] Stevens and colleagues[4] review the limitations of the SCr-based Cockcroft-Gault formula and the Modification of Diet in Renal Disease (MDRD) equation. Proximal tubular cells in the kidney secrete creatinine and therefore creatinine clearance surpasses GFR. However, in the steady state SCr is related to the reciprocal of GFR.[4]

As shown in **Table 1**, there are 5 different stages of CKD.[2] Kidney failure is defined as either GFR less than 15 mL/min/1.73 m^2 or a need for dialysis or renal transplantation.

Acute Kidney Injury

There are many different definitions for an acute change in renal function. The term acute renal failure (ARF) has been supplanted by the term AKI.[5] AKI encompasses the entire range of ARF from small changes in SCr to loss of function requiring dialysis. In an effort to standardize the classification of AKI, in 2004 the Acute Dialysis Quality Initiative (ADQI) Group proposed the RIFLE criteria.[6] As shown in **Fig. 1**, RIFLE stands for Risk of renal dysfunction; Injury to the kidney; Failure of kidney function; Loss of kidney function; and End-stage kidney disease. It relies on measurement of GFR or SCr and urine output (UO) to classify the severity of ARF. Since their initial publication, the RIFLE criteria have been validated in numerous studies of intensive care unit (ICU), postsurgical, and hospital patients as independent predictors of mortality.[7-9] In 2007 the Acute Kidney Injury Network (AKIN) proposed a modification to the RIFLE criteria.[5] As shown in **Table 2**, the AKIN definition considers 3 different stages of AKI, adds a 48-hour time frame for the diagnosis of AKI, and changes the criteria for "Risk,"

Table 1		
Stages of chronic kidney disease		
Stage	**Description**	**GFR (mL/min/1.73 m^2)**
1	Kidney damage with normal or increased GFR	≥90
2	Kidney damage with mild decrease in GFR	60–89
3	Moderate decrease in GFR	30–59
4	Severe decrease in GFR	15–29
5	Kidney failure	<15 (or dialysis)

GFR Criteria*   Urine Output Criteria

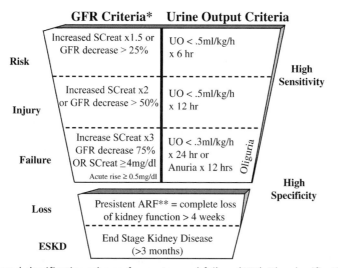

Fig. 1. Proposed classification scheme for acute renal failure (ARF). The classification system includes separate criteria for creatinine and output (UO). A patient can fulfill the criteria through changes in serum creatinine (SCreat) or changes in UO, or both. ARF, acute renal failure; GFR, glomerular filtration rate. (*From* Bellomo R, Ronco C, Kellum JA, et al. Acute renal failure – definition, outcome measures, animal models, fluid therapy and information technology needs: the Second International Consensus Conference of the Acute Dialysis Quality Initiative (ADQI) Group. Crit Care 2004;8(4):R204–12; with permission.)

or Stage 1 AKI, to include patients with increases in SCr level of greater than or equal to 0.3 mg/dL ($\geq$26.4 μmol/L). In a 5-year analysis of more than 120,000 ICU admissions in Australia, investigators found no significant differences in the predictive ability of the RIFLE criteria compared with the AKIN definition.[10]

Despite their use in current definitions of AKI, SCr and UO are not the ideal markers for AKI and significant research efforts are underway to identify biomarkers of AKI.[11] Potential biomarkers of AKI include neutrophil gelatinase-associated lipocalin (NGAL), cystatin C, and interleukin-18.[11]

AKI can be classified according to prerenal, renal, and postrenal causes.[12] Perioperatively the most common cause of AKI is secondary to acute tubular necrosis (ATN).[12] A study in ICU patients found the most common causes of AKI were septic shock, major surgery, cardiogenic shock, hypovolemia, and drug-induced AKI.[13]

Surgical Risk Factors for AKI

Patients with kidney disease may present for a wide variety of surgical procedures. Access for dialysis is the most common procedure followed by procedures for peripheral vascular disease, coronary artery disease, and kidney transplantation.[14]

Overall, the risk of AKI in surgical patients has been estimated to be approximately 1%.[15] However, certain patient populations are at much higher risk. Factors identified as increasing the risk of AKI include age, past history of kidney disease, left ventricular ejection fraction less than 35%, cardiac index less than 1.7 L/min/m^2, hypertension, peripheral vascular disease, diabetes mellitus, emergency surgery, and type of surgery.[15] The highest risk surgeries include coronary artery surgery, cardiac valve surgery, aortic aneurysm surgery, and liver transplant surgery.[16–18] The literature is difficult to evaluate given the many different definitions of AKI, but rates of AKI or

Table 2 Classification/staging system for AKI[a]		
Stage	**Serum Creatinine Criteria**	**Urine Output Criteria**
1	Increase in serum creatinine of more than or equal to 0.3 mg/dL ($\geq$ 26.4 μmol/l) or increase to more than or equal to 150% to 200% (1.5- to 2-fold) from baseline	Less than 0.5 mL/kg/h for more than 6 h
2[b]	Increase in serum creatinine to more than 200% to 300% (>2- to 3-fold) from baseline	Less than 0.5 mL/kg/h for more than 12 h
3[c]	Increase in serum creatinine to more than 300% (>3-fold) from baseline (or serum creatinine of more than or equal to 4.0 mg/dL [$\geq$ 354 μmol/l] with an acute increase of at least 0.5 mg/dL [44 μmol/l])	Less than 0.3 mL/kg/h for 24 h or anuria for 12 h

[a] Modified from the RIFLE (Risk, Injury, Failure, Loss, and End-stage kidney disease) criteria. The staging system proposed is a highly sensitive, interim, staging system and is based on recent data indicating that a small change in serum creatinine level influences outcome. Only 1 criterion (creatinine level or urine output) has to be fulfilled to qualify for a stage.
[b] 200% to 300% increase = 2- to 3-fold increase.
[c] Given wide variation in indication and timing of initiation of renal replacement therapy (RRT). Individuals who receive RRT are considered to have met the criteria for stage 3 irrespective of the stage they are in at the time of RRT.
Adapted from Mehta RL, Kellum JA, Shah SV et al Acute Kidney Injury Network: report of an initiative to improve outcomes in acute kidney injury. Crit Care 2007;11(2):R31; with permission.

need for dialysis range from 3% to 5% for cardiac surgery with cardiopulmonary bypass to more than 50% for emergency abdominal aortic aneurysm repair.[15]

Perioperative Morbidity of Kidney Disease

The United Stated Renal Data System (USRDS) collects data on the ESRD population in the United States.[1] The 2007 USRDS report estimates that approximately 15% of the general population has CKD.[1] They also estimate that all-cause hospitalization rates are 3 times higher for patients with CKD and that rates of hospitalization due to AKI are approximately 6 times higher for patients with CKD.

The presence of CKD increases the rates of morbidity and mortality for several different surgical procedures. Investigators found estimated GFR (eGFR) calculated by the MDRD equation to be an independent predictor of mortality after coronary artery bypass graft surgery (CABG).[19] The mean eGFR was 64.7 mL/min/1.73 m[2] for survivors compared with 57.9 mL/min/1.73 m[2] in the patients who died.[19] Similar findings correlating eGFR with increased morbidity and mortality have also been published for elective major vascular surgery, hip fracture and repair, and endovascular aortic aneurysm surgery.[20–23]

A review found the overall mortality rate from AKI between 1956 and 2003 was comparatively unchanged at approximately 50%.[24] AKI during the perioperative period had an even poorer prognosis with mortality rates of 64% to 83% depending on the surgical population.[24,25] Even small changes in SCr correlate with a significant increase in the risk of death. In 1 study, patients with SCr increases of 0.3 to 0.4 mg/dL had a 70% increase in the risk for death compared with patients with little or no change in SCr.[25]

An important point is that surgery presents significant risks to patients with CKD or to those with, or at risk of, AKI. These risks need to be effectively communicated to patient and family so they can make informed decisions about their medical therapy. Furthermore, when evaluating the health care systems for patients with CKD, systems need to be in place to manage a potential deterioration in renal function in the perioperative period.

PREOPERATIVE EVALUATION AND PERIOPERATIVE RENAL PROTECTION

Given the array of diseases that can affect kidney function, a patient with kidney dysfunction who presents for surgery requires a comprehensive evaluation. The National Kidney Foundation recommends the following assessments for patients with CKD:[2]

- Diagnosis (type of kidney disease)
- Comorbid conditions
- Severity, assessed by level of kidney function
- Complications, related to level of kidney function
- Risk for loss of kidney function
- Risk for cardiovascular disease

These assessments hold true for the preoperative evaluation but they must be put into context of the requirement for the underlying surgery and the inherent surgical risk. As should be apparent, patients with CKD may have complex and overlapping medical problems: diabetes, cardiovascular disease, hypertension, anemia, dyslipidemia, poor nutritional status, bone disease, neuropathy, and an overall decreased quality of life.[2] Optimization of modifiable risk factors is the main goal of the preoperative assessment. Depending on the patient's status and the surgical procedure, the preoperative evaluation may require close communication between the primary care physician, nephrologist, surgeon, and anesthesiologist to determine if a patient is optimized for surgery. It cannot be stressed enough that a patient with kidney dysfunction is not cleared for surgery. The dictum "avoid hypoxia, avoid hypotension, avoid succinylcholine" is similarly ineffective. Areas that require close coordination to avoid conflict include the following:

- Preoperative goals: blood pressure, timing of dialysis
- Medications in the perioperative period
- Preoperative laboratory studies
- Preoperative tests

Preoperative Goals

Intraoperative hypotension and decreased renal perfusion is often considered a risk factor for the development of perioperative AKI.[11] Patients with hypertension and diabetes undergoing noncardiac surgery with a mean arterial pressure greater than 110 mmHg are at increased risk of intraoperative hypotension, and hypotension and hypertension are associated with higher rates of cardiovascular and renal complications.[26] Hence, adequate control of blood pressure before a patient undergoes surgery is paramount. The seventh report of the Joint National Committee on prevention, detection, evaluation, and treatment of high blood pressure (JNC VII) recommends patients with CKD or diabetes have a blood pressure less than 130/80 mmHg.[27] To minimize the risks of volume overload, electrolyte imbalances, and uremic bleeding, arrangements should be made for patients requiring dialysis to receive it within 24 hours of surgery.[28]

Medications in Perioperative Period

Angiotensin-converting enzyme inhibitors (ACEI) and angiotensin II antagonists (ARA) are commonly used to treat hypertension in patients with CKD, and they are also commonly associated with intraoperative hypotension, particularly with induction of general anesthesia.[29,30] Discontinuation of ACEI or ARA therapy for at least 10 hours before general anesthesia is recommended to reduce the risk of postinduction hypotension.[30] Given the risk of cardiovascular disease, ischemic stroke, and peripheral arterial disease, clopidogrel bisulfate (Plavix) is another medication commonly used in the CKD patient population. The decision to continue or hold clopidogrel in the perioperative period relates to the risk of the underlying condition indicated for its use, particularly in the setting of coronary stents, versus the risk of bleeding during surgery. For example, studies in the cardiac surgery literature recommend stopping clopidogrel for 5 to 7 days before cardiac surgery.[31] Anesthesiologists will not generally perform neuraxial techniques (epidural or spinal anesthesia) on patients who have taken clopidogrel within 7 days of surgery.[32] Ultimately the decision to continue or hold clopidogrel will depend on a risk assessment of the underlying condition, the bleeding risk during surgery, and the choice of anesthetic technique.

Preoperative Laboratory Studies

Several preoperative laboratory studies are recommended for patients with CKD but the more important question is what to do with the results. An eGFR should be calculated to not only ensure that correct dosage adjustments are made for renally excreted medications but also to help quantify perioperative risk. AKI in the setting of CKD should prompt an evaluation to identify precipitating factors and elective procedures should be postponed until resolution. Urgent surgical procedures, such as those related to underlying cancer or certain orthopedic injuries, in patients with AKI require an evaluation to determine if the precipitating cause(s) of AKI can be managed before the surgical issue deteriorates further.

Anemia may necessitate preoperative transfusion or supplementation with iron or erythropoietin. Typing and screening for blood should be done before operations with potential for significant blood loss. Patients with CKD may have received multiple transfusions and they can develop antibodies that can significantly delay processing for packed red blood cells. Electrolyte disturbances are common and hyperkalemia is a frequent concern. It is typically recommended that potassium levels be no more than 5 to 5.5 mmol/L. However, there are studies that show hyperkalemia is not associated with increased morbidity in vascular access surgery patients or when succinylcholine is used as a muscle relaxant.[33,34] These studies underscore that the management of patients with CKD needs to be individualized, as mild to moderate hyperkalemia is common in patients with CKD. Some studies suggest that more than 50% of patients with CKD have hyperkalemia and that acute intervention should be reserved for potassium levels greater than 6.5 mmol/L.[35] Overall, the preoperative potassium level needs to be evaluated in the context of its rate of change from previous levels, the potential blood transfusion requirements during surgery, and the potential for alterations in acid/base status perioperatively.

Preoperative Tests

The extent of preoperative testing is dependent on a patient's comorbid diseases and often includes an electrocardiogram and chest radiograph. Cardiovascular disease is the number 1 cause of mortality in patients with kidney failure.[2] To stratify cardiovascular risk the American College of Cardiology/American Heart Association 2007 guidelines on perioperative cardiovascular evaluation for noncardiac surgery are recommended.[36]

Surgical Risk

Surgical risk as related to CKD can be divided into the following areas: need for surgery, specific surgical techniques, fluid shifts and blood loss, analgesic requirements, intravenous access, anesthetic techniques, and expected disposition.

The need for surgery can be stratified as elective, urgent, or emergent. As discussed previously, emergent surgery is associated with increased morbidity and mortality for patients with CKD. Urgent and elective surgery can be deferred until the patient's status is optimized, particularly if they have concomitant AKI. Surgery can help to expedite the resolution of AKI if it is treating the underlying precipitating event. Again, communication between primary care and perioperative physicians is crucial to make this determination and to plan an appropriate course of action.

Surgical techniques include the use of nonionic contrast agents or the use of intra-abdominal laparoscopy and they may need to be modified for patients with CKD or AKI. Earlier studies on endovascular patients with CKD suggested that nonionic contrast agents might increase the risk of death in patients with CKD.[37] Other studies show clinically insignificant changes, particularly when preoperative prevention strategies are employed.[38] The ideal strategy to prevent contrast-induced nephropathy (CIN) is unknown but current recommendations include hydration, avoidance of other nephrotoxic medications, prevention of hypotension, and possibly use of adjuvants such as sodium bicarbonate or N-acetylcysteine.[39,40] Laparoscopic surgery with abdominal pneumoperitoneum is a common technique favored for its noninvasive nature, faster wound healing, and reduction in postoperative pain. However, laparoscopy is also associated with a reduction in renal perfusion.[41] To preserve renal blood flow, abdominal insufflation pressures more than 15 mmHg are not recommended. Laparoscopy can also cause hypotension, which will further aggravate reductions in renal perfusion. To mitigate these changes, adequate fluid replacement is recommended.[41,42]

Maintenance of euvolemia and renal perfusion seem like obvious goals for patients with CKD or AKI. However, assessing their adequacy in the perioperative period is not a simple task. Features of hypovolemia can be masked by anesthesia and surgery. Invasive monitoring may improve assessment but disease states, such as sepsis, can cause maldistribution of intravascular volume due to vasodilatation and altered capillary permeability.[11] Intraoperative blood loss and fluid shifts during surgery can compound these problems. Typically the anesthesia team will aim for a mean arterial pressure greater than 65 to 70 mmHg, or higher for the uncontrolled hypertensive patient, UO >0.5 ml/kg/h as applicable, central venous pressure 10 to 15 mmHg, and pulmonary artery wedge pressure of 10 to 15 mmHg. Intraoperative transesophageal echocardiography and newer monitors of stroke volume may also be used to assess adequacy of cardiac preload.[11,42] Fluid resuscitation is typically with either crystalloids or colloids or blood products as indicated. The ideal crystalloid is debatable and many texts continue to recommend normal saline as the choice of intravenous fluid for patients with kidney dysfunction.[43] Normal saline is hypertonic and hyperchloremic compared with plasma and volumes of greater than 30 ml/kg can lead to hyperchloremic metabolic acidosis and exacerbation of hyperkalemia. A study of kidney transplant recipients found that normal saline for fluid management was associated with a higher incidence of hyperkalemia and acidosis than patients managed with lactated Ringer solution.[43] Over hydration and goal-directed therapy to supranormal values can have a negative effect on patient outcome such as ileus, pulmonary edema, and prolonged hospital admission.[42]

Analgesic requirement in the perioperative period is an important area to consider given that opioids may accumulate in patients with CKD, placing them at higher risk of respiratory depression.[44] Nonsteroidal antiinflammatory drugs are not recommended for patients with CKD or AKI. Other options for moderate to severe postoperative pain include indwelling peripheral nerve catheters, long-lasting peripheral nerve blocks, or epidural catheters, as applicable. Managing postoperative pain in patients with CKD may require inpatient admission or coordination of outpatient nursing services.

Intravenous access is not a trivial matter for patients with CKD. Hemodialysis fistulas, previous blood draws, and previous surgeries all contribute to making intravenous access more difficult in this patient population. Central line placement may be required or a peripherally inserted central catheter (PICC) can be placed preoperatively for cases not associated with significant fluid losses or for cases requiring ongoing postoperative intravenous medical therapies.

Anesthetic techniques for surgery can be grouped into general anesthesia, neuraxial anesthesia, peripheral nerve blockade, or sedation. The ideal anesthetic technique for a patient with CKD or AKI having a particular procedure is unknown. Studies comparing general anesthesia versus regional anesthesia often look at outcomes such as functional recovery, bleeding risks, coagulation risks, or neurologic outcome. Ultimately the selected anesthetic technique will be determined by the patient's coexisting disease, surgical approach, and desired anesthetic goals.

After surgery, patients will generally be discharged from the postanesthesia care unit to home (outpatient surgery), hospital admission, or the ICU. Patients with CKD are at higher risk of complications and prolonged hospital or ICU stay.[14]

Perioperative Renal Protection

Beyond the standard goals of maintaining euvolemia, maintaining renal perfusion, and avoiding nephrotoxins, there is a great deal of research underway to identify methods of perioperative renal protection. Unfortunately, often promising results in animal models of AKI have not translated into successful clinical trials in humans.[45] Recent research suggests that fenoldopam may hold promise in this area.

Fenoldopam mesylate is a dopamine-1 receptor agonist that was initially approved for treatment of hypertensive emergencies. It has been studied in a variety of surgical and intensive care populations and been shown to reduce the risk of AKI.[46,47] A meta-analysis of 16 randomized studies found that fenoldopam reduced the risk of AKI and in-hospital death.[48] Doses of fenoldopam vary, but many of the positive trials used approximately 0.1 μg/kg/min and initiated treatment with the induction of surgery. These findings if replicated in a multicentered randomized controlled trial would represent a breakthrough in the treatment of AKI.

SUMMARY

Patients with CKD or AKI who present for surgery often have complex medical problems. Preoperative evaluation should strive to identify and correct any modifiable risks. Communication between the primary care team, nephrologist, surgeon, and anesthesiologist should ensure timely and appropriate investigation. Despite optimization, patients with CKD or AKI are at significantly higher risk of morbidity and mortality during the perioperative period. These risks need to be communicated to the patient or caregivers so that informed medical decisions can be made. Perioperative goals for euvolemia, maintenance of renal perfusion, and avoidance of nephrotoxins may require modifications in the usual surgical or anesthetic care. Despite intense research into perioperative renal protection, many successful therapies in animal models have not achieved success in human populations. Fenoldopam, as a prophylactic therapy in patients with CKD undergoing high risk surgery or for those patients at high risk of AKI, may be beneficial. Ultimately more research is required for a definitive answer to this elusive goal.

REFERENCES

1. US Renal Data System. USRDS 2007 Annual Data Report: atlas of chronic kidney disease and end-stage renal disease in the United States. Bethesda (MD): National Institutes of Health, National Institute of Diabetes and Digestive and Kidney Diseases; 2007.
2. National Kidney Foundation. K/DOQI clinical practice guidelines for chronic kidney disease: evaluation, classification, and stratification. Am J Kidney Dis 2002;39(2 Suppl 1):S1–266.
3. Levey AS, Coresh J, Balk E, et al. National Kidney Foundation practice guidelines for chronic kidney disease: evaluation, classification, and stratification. Ann Intern Med 2003;139(2):137–47.
4. Stevens LA, Coresh J, Greene T, et al. Assessing kidney function – measured and estimated glomerular filtration rate. N Engl J Med 2006;354(23):2473–83.
5. Mehta RL, Kellum JA, Shah SV, et al. Acute Kidney Injury Network: report of an initiative to improve outcomes in acute kidney injury. Crit Care 2007; 11(2):R31.
6. Bellomo R, Ronco C, Kellum JA, et al. Acute renal failure – definition, outcome measures, animal models, fluid therapy and information technology needs: the Second International Consensus Conference of the Acute Dialysis Quality Initiative (ADQI) Group. Crit Care 2004;8(4):R204–12.
7. Kuitunen A, Vento A, Suojaranta-Ylinen R, et al. Acute renal failure after cardiac surgery: evaluation of the RIFLE classification. Ann Thorac Surg 2006;81(2): 542–6.
8. Abosaif NY, Tolba YA, Heap M, et al. The outcome of acute renal failure in the intensive care unit according to RIFLE: model application, sensitivity, and predictability. Am J Kidney Dis 2005;46(6):1038–48.
9. Uchino S, Bellomo R, Goldsmith D, et al. An assessment of the RIFLE criteria for acute renal failure in hospitalized patients. Crit Care Med 2006;34(7):1913–7.
10. Bagshaw SM, George C, Bellomo R. A comparison of the RIFLE and AKIN criteria for acute kidney injury in critically ill patients. Nephrol Dial Transplant 2008;23(5): 1569–74.
11. Jones DR, Lee HT. Perioperative renal protection. Best Pract Res Clin Anaesthesiol 2008;22(1):193–208.
12. Lameire N, Van Biesen W, Vanholder R. Acute renal failure. Lancet 2005; 365(9457):417–30.
13. Uchino S, Kellum JA, Bellomo R, et al. Acute renal failure in critically ill patients: a multinational, multicenter study. JAMA 2005;294(7):813–8.
14. Krishnan M. Preoperative care of patients with kidney disease. Am Fam Physician 2002;66(8):1471–6.
15. Carmichael P, Carmichael AR. Acute renal failure in the surgical setting. ANZ J Surg 2003;73(3):144–53.
16. Bove T, Calabro MG, Landoni G, et al. The incidence and risk of acute renal failure after cardiac surgery. J Cardiothorac Vasc Anesth 2004;18(4):442–5.
17. Kashyap VS, Cambria RP, Davison JK, et al. Renal failure after thoracoabdominal aortic surgery. J Vasc Surg 1997;26(6):949–55.
18. Cabezuelo JB, Ramirez P, Rios A, et al. Risk factors of acute renal failure after liver transplantation. Kidney Int 2006;69(6):1073–80.
19. Hillis GS, Croal BL, Buchan KG, et al. Renal function and outcome from coronary artery bypass grafting: impact on mortality after a 2.3-year follow-up. Circulation 2006;113(8):1056–62.

20. Kertai MD, Boersma E, Bax JJ, et al. Comparison between serum creatinine and creatinine clearance for the prediction of postoperative mortality in patients undergoing major vascular surgery. Clin Nephrol 2003;59(1):17–23.
21. Ensrud KE, Lui LY, Taylor BC, et al. Renal function and risk of hip and vertebral fractures in older women. Arch Intern Med 2007;167(2):133–9.
22. Singh Mangat K, Mehra A, Yunas I, et al. Is estimated peri-operative glomerular filtration rate associated with post-operative mortality in fractured neck of femur patients? Injury 2008;39:1141–6.
23. Azizzadeh A, Sanchez LA, Miller CC 3rd, et al. Glomerular filtration rate is a predictor of mortality after endovascular abdominal aortic aneurysm repair. J Vasc Surg 2006;43(1):14–8.
24. Ympa YP, Sakr Y, Reinhart K, et al. Has mortality from acute renal failure decreased? A systematic review of the literature. Am J Med 2005;118(8):827–32.
25. Chertow GM, Burdick E, Honour M, et al. Acute kidney injury, mortality, length of stay, and costs in hospitalized patients. J Am Soc Nephrol 2005;16(11):3365–70.
26. Charlson ME, MacKenzie CR, Gold JP, et al. Preoperative characteristics predicting intraoperative hypotension and hypertension among hypertensives and diabetics undergoing noncardiac surgery. Ann Surg 1990;212(1):66–81.
27. Chobanian AV, Bakris GL, Black HR, et al. Seventh report of the Joint National Committee on prevention, detection, evaluation, and treatment of high blood pressure. Hypertension 2003;42(6):1206–52.
28. Stoelting RK, Dierdorf SF. Anesthesia and co-existing disease. Philadelphia: Churchill Livingstone; 2002.
29. Bertrand M, Godet G, Meersschaert K, et al. Should the angiotensin II antagonists be discontinued before surgery? Anesth Analg 2001;92(1):26–30.
30. Comfere T, Sprung J, Kumar MM, et al. Angiotensin system inhibitors in a general surgical population. Anesth Analg 2005;100(3):636–44.
31. Dunning J, Versteegh M, Fabbri A, et al. Guideline on antiplatelet and anticoagulation management in cardiac surgery. Eur J Cardiothorac Surg 2008;34(1):73–92.
32. Horlocker TT, Wedel DJ, Benzon H, et al. Regional anesthesia in the anticoagulated patient: defining the risks (the second ASRA Consensus Conference on Neuraxial Anesthesia and Anticoagulation). Reg Anesth Pain Med 2003;28(3):172–97.
33. Schow AJ, Lubarsky DA, Olson RP, et al. Can succinylcholine be used safely in hyperkalemic patients? Anesth Analg 2002;95(1):119–22.
34. Olson RP, Schow AJ, McCann R, et al. Absence of adverse outcomes in hyperkalemic patients undergoing vascular access surgery. Can J Anaesth 2003;50(6):553–7.
35. Gennari FJ, Segal AS. Hyperkalemia: an adaptive response in chronic renal insufficiency. Kidney Int 2002;62(1):1–9.
36. Fleisher LA, Beckman JA, Brown KA, et al. ACC/AHA 2007 Guidelines on Perioperative Cardiovascular Evaluation and Care for Noncardiac Surgery: executive summary: a report of the American College of Cardiology/American Heart Association Task Force on Practice Guidelines (Writing Committee to Revise the 2002 Guidelines on perioperative cardiovascular evaluation for noncardiac surgery) developed in collaboration with the American Society of Echocardiography, American Society of Nuclear Cardiology, Heart Rhythm Society, Society of Cardiovascular Anesthesiologists, Society for Cardiovascular Angiography and Interventions, Society for Vascular Medicine and Biology, and Society for Vascular Surgery. J Am Coll Cardiol 2007;50(17):1707–32.

37. Walker SR, Yusuf SW, Wenham PW, et al. Renal complications following endovascular repair of abdominal aortic aneurysms. J Endovasc Surg 1998;5(4):318–22.
38. Mehta M, Veith FJ, Lipsitz EC, et al. Is elevated creatinine level a contraindication to endovascular aneurysm repair? J Vasc Surg 2004;39(1):118–23.
39. Wong GT, Irwin MG. Contrast-induced nephropathy. Br J Anaesth 2007;99(4): 474–83.
40. Lameier NH. Contrast-induced nephropathy – prevention and risk reduction. Nephrol Dial Transplant 2006;21(6):i11–23.
41. Demyttenaere S, Feldman LS, Fried GM. Effect of pneumoperitoneum on renal perfusion and function: a systematic review. Surg Endosc 2007;21(2):152–60.
42. Demyttenaere SV, Taqi A, Polyhronopoulos GN, et al. Targeting individual hemodynamics to maintain renal perfusion during pneumoperitoneum in a porcine model. Surgery 2007;142(3):350–6.
43. O'Malley CM, Frumento RJ, Hardy MA, et al. A randomized, double-blind comparison of lactated Ringer's solution and 0.9% NaCl during renal transplantation. Anesth Analg 2005;100(5):1518–24.
44. Kurella M, Bennett WM, Chertow GM. Analgesia in patients with ESRD: a review of available evidence. Am J Kidney Dis 2003;42(2):217–28.
45. Jones DR, Lee HT. Protecting the kidney during critical illness. Curr Opin Anaesthesiol 2007;20(2):106–12.
46. Cogliati AA, Vellutini R, Nardini A, et al. Fenoldopam infusion for renal protection in high-risk cardiac surgery patients: a randomized clinical study. J Cardiothorac Vasc Anesth 2007;21(6):847–50.
47. Morelli A, Ricci Z, Bellomo R, et al. Prophylactic fenoldopam for renal protection in sepsis: a randomized, double-blind, placebo-controlled pilot trial. Crit Care Med 2005;33(11):2451–6.
48. Landoni G, Biondi-Zoccai GG, Tumlin JA, et al. Beneficial impact of fenoldopam in critically ill patients with or at risk for acute renal failure: a meta-analysis of randomized clinical trials. Am J Kidney Dis 2007;49(1):56–68.

Anemia in the Preoperative Patient

Manish S. Patel, MD[a],*, Jeffrey L. Carson, MD[a]

KEYWORDS

- Anemia • Erythrocyte transfusion • Surgery
- Preoperative care • Anesthesia

ANEMIA

Anemia is the most common hematologic problem in the preoperative patient. Often, it is a sign of an underlying disease or condition that could affect the surgical outcome. Consequently, blood transfusions are commonly given perioperatively to anemic patients. In 2006, the supply of allogenic whole blood/red blood cells in the United States was estimated to be more than 15.7 million units, and an estimated 14.6 million units were transfused.[1] It has been shown that 40% to 70% of all red cell units are transfused in the surgical setting.[2–5] Therefore, an understanding of the causes and consequences of anemia and any potential treatments is crucial in the preoperative setting.

EVALUATION OF ANEMIA
History and Physical Examination

The evaluation of the anemic preoperative patient should always begin with a thorough history and physical examination. The history should first attempt to elicit symptoms of bleeding, such as menstrual blood loss, hematochezia, melena, hematemesis, hemoptysis, or hematuria. It is also important to ask about symptoms related to the anemia and the body's compensatory mechanisms, that is, anginal chest pain, dyspnea, fatigue, and palpitations. Any history of or symptoms of underlying illnesses, such as constitutional symptoms, malignancy, renal failure, endocrinopathies (eg, thyroid disorders), infections, or liver disease, should be targeted. Past history of anemia is also important, including previous hemoglobin values and therapies, onset, need for previous blood transfusions, splenectomy, and blood donations. The patient's family history may contain a history of anemia, bleeding, hematologic disorders, splenectomy, and early onset cholelithiasis, which may indicate congenital hemolytic

This work was supported by Grant No. U01 HL73958 from the National Heart, Lung and Blood Institute, National Institutes of Health.

[a] Department of Medicine, Division of General Internal Medicine, University of Medicine and Dentistry of New Jersey Robert Wood Johnson Medical School, 125 Paterson Street, New Brunswick, NJ 08903, USA
* Corresponding author.
E-mail address: patel168@umdnj.edu (M.S. Patel).

Med Clin N Am 93 (2009) 1095–1104
doi:10.1016/j.mcna.2009.05.007
0025-7125/09/$ – see front matter
medical.theclinics.com

disorders. The social history should take into account occupational hazards and exposures, dietary habits, alcohol and illicit drug use, and a detailed list of all prescription and nonprescription medications, including herbal and over-the-counter medications.

The physical examination should focus on manifestations and potential etiologies of the anemia, such as pallor of the skin and mucous membranes, jaundice, signs of bleeding, purpura, petechiae, hepatosplenomegaly, and lymphadenopathy. A heart murmur is sometimes heard, and this may be a flow murmur resulting from decreased blood viscosity and elevated cardiac output from the anemia, or it may indicate the presence of a prosthetic valve. A pelvic and rectal examination with stool guaiac may need to be performed to evaluate for possible sources of blood loss.

Diagnostic Evaluation

An approach to anemia is given in **Fig. 1**. Initial laboratory testing should include a complete blood count (CBC), peripheral blood smear, and a reticulocyte count. In addition, stool guaiac, radiologic, and endoscopic testing may be required in an effort to exclude blood loss. The reticulocyte count can be an indication of bone marrow production, but it usually needs to be corrected for differences in hematocrit and the effect of erythropoietin on the marrow. This is done by calculating a reticulocyte production index (RPI) (**Fig. 2**).

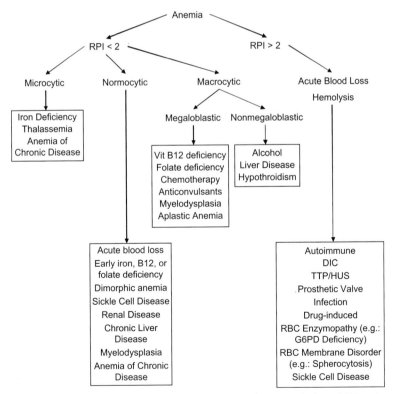

Fig. 1. Approach to anemia. DIC, disseminated intravascular coagulation; G6PD, glucose-6-phosphate dehydrogenase; RBC, red blood cell; RPI, reticulocyte production index; TTP/HUS, thrombotic thrombocytopenic purpura/hemolytic uremic syndrome.

$$\text{Reticulocyte Production Index} = \text{Retic Count} \times \frac{\text{Patient's Hematocrit}}{\text{Normal Hematocrit (45)}} \times \frac{1}{\text{Maturation Correction}}$$
$$\text{(RPI)}$$

Hematocrit (%)	Maturation Correction
36-45	1.0
26-35	1.5
16-25	2.0
≤ 15	2.5

RPI < 2 indicates an inappropriate/decreased marrow response to anemia
RPI > 2 indicates an appropriate marrow response to anemia, usually due to blood loss or hemolysis

Fig. 2. Calculating the reticulocyte production index.

An RPI of less than 2 usually indicates a hypoproliferative anemia or an inappropriate/decreased marrow response to the anemia. The next step would be to look at the mean corpuscular volume on the CBC to characterize the anemia as microcytic, normocytic, or macrocytic. Iron deficiency and thalassemia are the most common causes of microcytic anemia and, therefore, initial work-up includes obtaining serum ferritin, serum iron, and total iron-binding capacity. Further tests may consist of hemoglobin electrophoresis or a bone marrow biopsy. In normocytic anemia, acute blood loss must first be excluded. Additional causes of normocytic anemia may include underlying renal or liver disease; early iron, vitamin B12, or folate deficiency; dimorphic anemia, such as concurrent iron and vitamin B12 deficiency; myelodysplasia/aplastic anemia; or anemia of chronic disease resulting from an underlying inflammatory condition. The testing for normocytic anemia may entail many of the serologies discussed for microcytic anemia, assessment of renal and liver function, and bone marrow biopsy. Macrocytic anemia can be characterized as megaloblastic and nonmegalobloastic anemia. Megaloblastic anemia may be due to vitamin B12 or folate deficiency, drugs such as chemotherapeutic agents or anticonvulsants, and myelodysplasia. Nonmegaloblastic anemia includes alcohol ingestion, liver disease, or hypothyroidism. Initial work-up should comprise measurement of vitamin B12 and folate levels. Further tests may include thyroid or liver function tests and a bone marrow biopsy.

An RPI of greater than 2 demonstrates an appropriate marrow response to blood loss or may indicate hemolysis. Initial studies would include measuring direct and indirect bilirubin, lactate dehydrogenase, and haptoglobin levels, and direct and indirect Coombs test. The peripheral smear should also be reviewed for clues to the underlying process. Polychromasia, basophilic stippling, and nucleated red blood cells can all be seen in hemolytic anemia. In addition, several findings may point toward a specific cause. For example, schistocytes are generally associated with microangiopathic hemolytic anemias, such as those resulting from disseminated intravascular coagulation, thrombotic thrombocytopenic purpura/hemolytic uremic syndrome, and hemolysis from prosthetic valves. Spherocytes may be seen in hereditary spherocytosis, autoimmune hemolytic anemia, and microangiopathic hemolytic anemias.

RISK FOR ANEMIA IN SURGICAL PATIENTS

The risk for anemia in patients can be ascertained from studies involving those who decline blood transfusions. The largest such study was a retrospective cohort study performed on 1958 consecutive surgical patients who refused transfusions based on religious reasons. The overall 30-day risk of mortality increased with decreasing preoperative hemoglobin concentrations, especially in those patients with a hemoglobin level of less than 6 g/dL.[6] The risk for death was much greater, however, in patients with underlying cardiovascular disease and preoperative hemoglobin value of 10 g/dL or less. A subsequent study on the same population showed that none of the 99 patients with postoperative hemoglobin concentrations between 7 and 8 g/dL died, whereas there was a sharp increase in mortality in those patients with a hemoglobin concentration less than 5 to 6 g/dL.[7]

These results are consistent with a series of studies in which healthy subjects underwent acute isovolemic reduction to a hemoglobin level of 5 g/dL.[8–11] Two of these studies found evidence of asymptomatic and reversible ST-segment changes suggestive of myocardial ischemia in 5 of the 87 combined patients at hemoglobin concentrations between 5 and 7 g/dL.[8,11] Another study evaluated 8 healthy volunteers during isovolemic reduction and found increased self-assessed fatigue at a hemoglobin level of 7 g/dL, which then worsened further at hemoglobin levels of 6 g/dL and 5 g/dL.[9] Minor and reversible cognitive changes were seen in 9 healthy subjects, including decreased reaction times, at hemoglobin concentration of less than 6 g/dL and impaired immediate and delayed memory at hemoglobin levels less than 5 g/dL.[10] These studies show that even healthy subjects can exhibit clinical changes at hemoglobin concentrations between 5 and 7 g/dL.

Elderly patients, however, may respond to and tolerate preoperative anemia differently than younger patients. In a study of 20 patients older than 65 years and free from known cardiac disease, isovolemic anemia to a mean hemoglobin concentration of 8.8 g/dL was well tolerated.[12] Another study examined patients with known coronary artery disease and found that isovolemic anemia was well tolerated to hemoglobin value of 9.9 g/dL. In addition, the increase in cardiac index and oxygen extraction during hemodilution was found to be independent of age.[13] The results of these studies should be interpreted with caution because they involved small numbers of patients and very few were older than 80 years.[14]

A later study analyzed preoperative hematocrit levels in over 310,000 elderly veterans undergoing noncardiac surgery.[15] In contrast to the 2 previous studies, even mild anemia was associated with an increased risk of 30-day morbidity and mortality. There was a monotonic rise in mortality and cardiac events when the hematocrit level was less than 39%. These results, however, may not be able to be generalized to elderly females. Moreover, it is unclear whether the anemia is causal or associated with the increased morbidity and mortality and whether this risk may be corrected with transfusion.[16]

CURRENT EVIDENCE RELEVANT TO TRANSFUSION
Observational Studies

There have been many observational studies documenting the effect of anemia and red blood cell transfusions on clinical outcomes of patients undergoing surgery, of those with acute coronary syndromes, and of those admitted to intensive care units. A systematic review of the literature identified 45 cohort studies including 272,596 patients.[17] With the exception of 3 studies, the risks for transfusion appeared to outweigh the benefits. Transfusion was associated with an increased risk for death, infection, multiorgan dysfunction syndrome, and acute respiratory distress syndrome. However, this analysis has important limitations, including that the analysis did not take into account the hemoglobin concentration before transfusion and the very high likelihood of uncontrolled confounding.[18] Patients requiring blood transfusions are more severely ill than those who do not require them, and it is impossible to completely adjust for these differences between the patients who have received transfusions and those who have not. Therefore, the decision to transfuse a preoperative patient must rest on the strength of randomized clinical trials.

Randomized Clinical Trials

There are 10 randomized clinical trials in adults to date that distinguish the consequences of various transfusion thresholds.[19–26] The clinical settings of the studies were diverse, but each of the studies did randomize patients to receive transfusions based on a "restrictive" versus a "liberal" strategy. Of the 10 clinical trials, 5 took place within a surgical setting. One study evaluated 39 patients after myocardial revascularization and found no difference in morbidity between the conservative and liberal group, but mortality was not evaluated.[24] Another study involved 428 patients undergoing coronary artery bypass grafting who were randomized to receive transfusion for a hemoglobin threshold less than 9 g/dL and less than 8 g/dL.[20] There was no difference in mortality, morbidity, and clinical outcomes between the 2 groups. A third study included 127 patients undergoing knee arthroplasty who were assigned to receive either 2 units of autologous red blood cells immediately postoperatively or to be transfused only if the hemoglobin fell below 9 g/dL.[25] The mean postoperative hemoglobin values between both groups only differed by 0.7 g/dL. There were more nonsurgical complications in the conservative transfusion group. In another study, 84 hip fracture patients were randomized to receive blood transfusion either when the hemoglobin fell below 10 g/dL or if they became symptomatic (this also included transfusion if the hemoglobin level was less than 8 g/dL).[26] There were no statistical differences in morbidity, mortality, or functional recovery between the 2 groups, although a trend of increased 60-day mortality was seen in the liberal transfusion group (11.9% vs 4.8% in the restrictive group).

The largest randomized clinical trial, the only one with adequate power to assess clinical outcomes related to transfusion triggers, is the Transfusion Requirements in Critical Care (TRICC) trial.[23] About 838 normovolemic, critically ill patients were randomized to a restrictive transfusion strategy or a liberal strategy. In the restrictive transfusion group, patients were transfused if the hemoglobin concentration dropped below 7 g/dL and were maintained between 7 and 9 g/dL. In the liberal transfusion group, patients received transfusion for hemoglobin levels less than 10 g/dL, and their hemoglobin values were maintained between 10 and 12 g/dL. Consistent with other studies, the average hemoglobin value and red cells units transfused were significantly lower in the restrictive trigger group. There was no statistical difference in 30-day mortality between the 2 groups, although there was a trend toward lower mortality in the restrictive transfusion group (18.7% vs 23.3%). The restrictive transfusion group did have lower rates of myocardial infarction (0.07% vs 2.9%, $P = .02$) and pulmonary edema (5.3% vs 10.7%, $P<.01$) than the liberal strategy group. Those patients with underlying ischemic heart disease showed no difference in the 30-day mortality rate between the 2 transfusion groups. Although this study took place in the critical care setting, it provides useful information even for perioperative patients.

A meta-analysis evaluated all 10 randomized clinical trials pertaining to red cell transfusion triggers.[27,28] Several important conclusions were drawn from data that were pooled from the various studies. Firstly, a restrictive transfusion trigger had a lower likelihood of red blood cell transfusion by 42% (relative risk [RR], 0.58; 95% confidence interval [CI], 0.51–0.77), saving an average of 0.93 units of red cells per transfused patient. Secondly, there were 24% fewer cardiac events in the restrictive trigger groups, although the statistical significance was borderline (RR, 0.76; 95% CI, 0.57–1.00). Thirdly, patients in the restrictive trigger groups had, on average, 5.6% lower hematocrit levels than the liberal trigger groups. Fourthly, there was no statistically significant difference in the length of hospital stay between the restrictive and liberal trigger groups. Finally, there was no increase in mortality seen in the restrictive trigger groups when compared with those with liberal transfusion triggers. Actually, restrictive transfusion triggers were associated with a one-fifth lower mortality (RR, 0.80; 95% CI, 0.63–1.02), although this was not statistically significant (P = .07). It should be noted that 83% of the data on mortality was taken from the TRICC trial. This meta-analysis, however, found insufficient evidence pertaining to restrictive transfusion triggers in the setting of cardiovascular disease, hematologic disorders, and renal failure. The authors of the review concluded that additional randomized clinical trials need to be done in various clinical settings, especially in those with underlying cardiovascular disease.

There is a multicenter, randomized clinical trial called functional outcomes in cardiovascular patients undergoing surgical hip fracture repair (FOCUS) currently underway that is evaluating red cell transfusion strategy in hip fracture patients with cardiovascular disease or cardiovascular disease risk factors in up to 2000 patients.[29] The results should be available in late 2009.

TREATMENT OF ANEMIA
Reversible Causes

In the case of iron deficiency anemia, the underlying cause, such as blood loss, should be identified and treated. Therefore, a thorough gastrointestinal evaluation is often indicated. The supplementation of iron, however, should also be initiated. Iron is most easily given in the oral form, the least expensive of which is ferrous sulfate. Ferrous sulfate provides 65 mg of elemental iron per 325 mg tablet. It is recommended that adults receive 150 to 200 mg of elemental iron per day in deficiency states. Oral iron is more readily absorbed in an acidic gastric environment and, therefore, often given with ascorbic acid and while avoiding antacids. Reticulocytosis is generally seen in 7 to 10 days, and the hemoglobin level should increase by 1 g/dL every 2 to 3 weeks. If patients have failed oral iron therapy or if iron loss exceeds capacity for oral iron absorption, intravenous iron therapy may be necessary. Common clinical scenarios in which this occurs include patients with inflammatory bowel disease, intestinal malabsorption from celiac disease, patients intolerant to oral iron therapy, or patients undergoing cancer chemotherapy. Of the intravenous iron preparations, ferric gluconate and iron sucrose are generally believed to have the best safety profile. Studies and systematic reviews, however, suggest that low–molecular-weight iron dextran may have a comparable toxicity profile to iron sucrose.[30–33]

Anemia resulting from vitamin B12 or folate deficiency is also easily treated with supplementation. Folate deficiency should be treated with folic acid, 1 mg/d for up to 4 months, or until the patient's anemia is corrected. Vitamin B12 deficiency is usually treated with intramuscular cobalamin injections. The dosage of cobalamin may vary depending on the severity of the anemia and symptoms, from 1000 µg daily for 7 days, to 1000 µg every 1 to 4 weeks. Studies have also shown that oral cobalamin supplementation of 1000 to 2000 µg/d for 4 months, may be at least as effective as parenteral cobalamin, but this requires greater patient compliance.[34,35] Reticulocytosis may be expected in 3 to 5 days, and hemoglobin levels should rise within 10 days.

Patients with anemia of chronic disease, chronic renal insufficiency, zidovudine-treated HIV-infected patients, and other hematologic diseases may benefit from use of erythropoietin before surgery. In many patients, erythropoietin raises the hemoglobin concentration enough to reduce the need for allogeneic blood transfusion after surgery.[36,37] The target hemoglobin concentration should be no greater than 12 g/dL to avoid potential risks associated with erythropoietin (ie, thromboembolism,[38,39] serious cardiovascular events,[40,41] and mortality[39]), and all patients should receive thromboembolism prophylaxis. The authors recommend against using erythropoietin in patients with cancer because there are some studies that demonstrate increased risk for tumor progression or recurrence.[42–44]

Red Cell Transfusion Guidelines

The old adage of transfusing red cells such that the hemoglobin is greater than 10 g/dL and the hematocrit is more than 30% before surgery no longer applies. The evidence to date suggests that a more conservative threshold for transfusion can be used in most patients. Updated guidelines from the American Society of Anesthesiology recommend transfusion if hemoglobin level is less than 6 g/dL, and that transfusion is rarely necessary when the level is more than 10 g/dL.[45] When hemoglobin concentrations fall between 6 and 10 g/dL, the guidelines state that transfusion decisions should be based on indication of organ ischemia, risk for or ongoing bleeding, intravascular volume status, and susceptibility to complications of inadequate oxygenation.

A special mention should be made about preoperative transfusions in patients with sickle cell disease, because the perioperative complication rate in this patient population can be as high as 67%.[46] Surgical stress and trauma can increase the rate of anemia and sickle cell formation, and red cell transfusions are often used to preserve oxygen-carrying capacity and to dilute the sickle cells. A randomized clinical trial evaluated transfusion regimens in patients undergoing 602 surgical procedures.[47] Patients were randomly assigned to either an aggressive transfusion strategy, which maintained a preoperative hemoglobin level of 10 g/dL and a hemoglobin S level of 30% or less, or a conservative strategy, in which transfusions were given to maintain a hemoglobin concentration of 10 g/dL regardless of the hemoglobin S level. There was no difference in the rate of serious complications between the 2 groups, but transfusion-related complications were twice as likely in the aggressive strategy group (odds ratio, 2.15; 95% CI, 1.23–3.77). A Cochrane Database review concluded that although a conservative transfusion strategy seems as effective in preoperative patients as an aggressive regimen, further studies are needed to determine the best possible course of therapy and whether preoperative transfusion is required in all surgical settings.[48]

In the authors' opinion, a transfusion threshold of 7 g/dL can be used safely in most perioperative patients, provided that they have no underlying ischemic heart disease and are asymptomatic. The optimal threshold is unknown in patients with cardiovascular disease, for there is no randomized evidence available. The authors recommend carefully evaluating each patient's symptoms and signs and not basing the transfusion decision solely on a hemoglobin concentration. Those patients who are symptomatic from their anemia should be transfused as needed. The optimal rate of red cell administration should be guided by the clinical situation. Active exsanguination may require transfusion rates as high as 5 to 10 units of red cells within 10 to 15 minutes, whereas those patients at risk for volume overload should be transfused at 1 mL/kg/h. Most patients may be transfused at 1 unit of red cells every 1 to 2 hours, and a hemoglobin level rise of 1 g/dL should be expected per unit of red cells transfused.[49] After each red cell unit is transfused, a repeat hemoglobin level should be obtained, and the patient should be reevaluated.

SUMMARY

Anemia produces a unique set of challenges in the preoperative patient. An efficient evaluation of anemia relies on a detailed history and physical examination and a systematic approach to the diagnostic testing. The presence of anemia and the use of perioperative blood transfusions have potential ramifications on the surgical outcome. Although evidence suggests that a lower transfusion threshold may be appropriate in most preoperative patients, the decision to transfuse must be individualized to the patient and the clinical setting.

REFERENCES

1. Whitaker BI, Green J, King MR, et al. The 2007 national blood collection and utilization survey report. Washington, DC: Department of Health and Human Services; 2007.
2. Cook SS, Epps J. Transfusion practice in central Virginia. Transfusion 1991;31: 355–60.
3. Eisenstaedt RS. Modifying physicians' transfusion practice. Transfus Med Rev 1997;11:27–37.
4. Friedman EA, Burns TL, Shork MA. A study of national trends in transfusion practice. Springfield (VA): National Technical Information Service; 1980.
5. Wells AW, Mounter PJ, Chapman CE, et al. Where does blood go? Prospective observational study of red cell transfusion in north England. BMJ 2002;325:803–4.
6. Carson JL, Duff A, Poses RM, et al. Effect of anaemia and cardiovascular disease on surgical mortality and morbidity. Lancet 1996;348:1055–60.
7. Carson JL, Noveck H, Berlin JA, et al. Mortality and morbidity in patients with very low postoperative Hb levels who decline blood transfusion. Transfusion 2002;42: 812–8.
8. Leung JM, Weiskopf RB, Feiner J, et al. Electrocardiographic ST-segment changes during acute, severe isovolemic hemodilution in humans [In Process Citation]. Anesthesiology 2000;93:1004–10.
9. Toy P, Feiner J, Viele MK, et al. Fatigue during acute isovolemic anemia in healthy, resting humans. Transfusion 2000;40:457–60.
10. Weiskopf RB, Kramer JH, Viele M, et al. Acute severe isovolemic anemia impairs cognitive function and memory in humans. Anesthesiology 2000;92:1646–52.
11. Weiskopf RB, Viele MK, Feiner J, et al. Human cardiovascular and metabolic response to acute, severe isovolemic anemia. JAMA 1998;279:217–21.
12. Spahn DR, Zollinger A, Schlumpf RB, et al. Hemodilution tolerance in elderly patients without known cardiac disease. Anesth Analg 1996;82:681–6.
13. Spahn DR, Schmid ER, Seifert B, et al. Hemodilution tolerance in patients with coronary artery disease who are receiving chronic β-adrenergic blocker therapy. Anesth Analg 1996;82:687–94.
14. Madjdpour C, Spahn DR, Weiskopf RB. Anemia and perioperative red blood cell transfusion: a matter of tolerance. Crit Care Med 2006;34:S102–8.
15. Wu WC, Schifftner TL, Henderson WG, et al. Preoperative hematocrit levels and postoperative outcomes in older patients undergoing noncardiac surgery. JAMA 2007;297:2481–8.
16. Shander A, Goodnough LT. Do preoperative anemia and polycythemia affect clinical outcome in patients undergoing major surgery? Nat Clin Pract Cardiovasc Med 2008;5:20–1.
17. Marik PE, Corwin HL. Efficacy of red blood cell transfusion in the critically ill: a systematic review of the literature. Crit Care Med 2008;36:2667–74.

18. Carson JL, Reynolds RC, Klein HG. Bad bad blood? Crit Care Med 2008;36: 2707–8.
19. Blair SD, Janvrin SB, McCollum CN, et al. Effect of early blood transfusion on gastrointestinal haemorrhage. Br J Surg 1986;73:783–5.
20. Bracey AW, Radovancevic R, Riggs SA, et al. Lowering the hemoglobin threshold for transfusion in coronary artery bypass procedures: effect on patient outcome. Transfusion 1999;39:1070–7.
21. Carson JL, Terrin ML, Barton FB, et al. A pilot randomized trial comparing symptomatic vs. hemoglobin-level-driven red blood cell transfusions following hip fracture. Transfusion 1998;38:522–9.
22. Fortune JB, Feustel PJ, Saifi J, et al. Influence of hematocrit on cardiopulmonary function after acute hemorrhage. J Trauma 1987;27:243–9.
23. Hebert PC, Wells G, Blajchman MA, et al. A multicenter, randomized, controlled clinical trial of transfusion requirements in critical care. Transfusion Requirements in Critical Care Investigators, Canadian Critical Care Trials Group. N Engl J Med 1999;340:409–17 [see comments].
24. Johnson RG, Thurer RL, Kruskall MS, et al. Comparison of two transfusion strategies after elective operations for myocardial revascularization. J Thorac Cardiovasc Surg 1992;104:307–14.
25. Lotke PA, Barth P, Garino JP, et al. Predonated autologous blood transfusions after total knee arthroplasty: immediate versus delayed administration. J Arthroplasty 1999;14:647–50.
26. Topley E, Fischer MR. The illness of trauma. Br J Clin Pract 1956;1:770–6.
27. Carson JL, Hill S, Carless P, et al. Transfusion triggers: a systematic review of the literature. Transfus Med Rev 2002;16:187–99.
28. Hill SR, Carless PA, Henry DA, et al. Transfusion thresholds and other strategies for guiding allogeneic red blood cell transfusion. Cochrane Database Syst Rev 2002;(2):CD002042.
29. Carson JL, Terrin ML, Magaziner J, et al. Transfusion trigger trial for functional outcomes in cardiovascular patients undergoing surgical hip fracture repair (FOCUS). Transfusion 2006;46:2192–206.
30. Auerbach M, Goodnough LT, Picard D, et al. The role of intravenous iron in anemia management and transfusion avoidance. Transfusion 2008;48:988–1000.
31. Critchley J, Dundar Y. Adverse events associated with intravenous iron infusion (low-molecular-weight iron dextran and iron sucrose): a systematic review. Transfus Altern Transfus Med 2007;9:8–36.
32. Moniem KA, Bhandari S. Tolerability and efficacy of parenteral iron therapy in hemodialysis patients, a comparison of preparations. Transfus Altern Transfus Med 2007;9:37–42.
33. Sav T, Tokgoz B, Sipahioglu MH, et al. Is there a difference between the allergic potencies of the iron sucrose and low molecular weight iron dextran? Ren Fail 2007;29:423–6.
34. Eussen SJ, de Groot LC, Clarke R, et al. Oral cyanocobalamin supplementation in older people with vitamin B12 deficiency: a dose-finding trial. Arch Intern Med 2005;165:1167–72.
35. Kuzminski AM, Del Giacco EJ, Allen RH, et al. Effective treatment of cobalamin deficiency with oral cobalamin. Blood 1998;92:1191–8.
36. Faris PM, Ritter MA, Abels RI. The effects of recombinant human erythropoietin on perioperative transfusion requirements in patients having a major orthopaedic operation. The American Erythropoietin Study Group. J Bone Joint Surg Am 1996;78:62–72.

37. Laupacis A, Feagan B, Wong C. Effectiveness of perioperative recombinant human erythropoietin in elective hip replacement. COPES Study Group. Lancet 1993;342:378.

38. Bennett CL, Silver SM, Djulbegovic B, et al. Venous thromboembolism and mortality associated with recombinant erythropoietin and darbepoetin administration for the treatment of cancer-associated anemia. JAMA 2008;299:914–24.

39. Phrommintikul A, Haas SJ, Elsik M, et al. Mortality and target haemoglobin concentrations in anaemic patients with chronic kidney disease treated with erythropoietin: a meta-analysis. Lancet 2007;369:381–8.

40. Drueke TB, Locatelli F, Clyne N, et al. Normalization of hemoglobin level in patients with chronic kidney disease and anemia. N Engl J Med 2006;355: 2071–84.

41. Singh AK, Szczech L, Tang KL, et al. Correction of anemia with epoetin alfa in chronic kidney disease. N Engl J Med 2006;355:2085–98.

42. Henke M, Laszig R, Rube C, et al. Erythropoietin to treat head and neck cancer patients with anaemia undergoing radiotherapy: randomised, double-blind, placebo-controlled trial. Lancet 2003;362:1255–60.

43. Henke M, Mattern D, Pepe M, et al. Do erythropoietin receptors on cancer cells explain unexpected clinical findings? J Clin Oncol 2006;24:4708–13.

44. Longmore GD. Do cancer cells express functional erythropoietin receptors? N Engl J Med 2007;356:2447.

45. Practice guidelines for perioperative blood transfusion and adjuvant therapies: an updated report by the American Society of Anesthesiologists Task Force on perioperative blood transfusion and adjuvant therapies. Anesthesiology 2006; 105:198–208.

46. Vichinsky EP, Neumayr LD, Haberkern C, et al. The perioperative complication rate of orthopedic surgery in sickle cell disease: report of the National Sickle Cell Surgery Study Group. Am J Hematol 1999;62:129–38.

47. Vichinsky EP, Haberkern CM, Neumayr L, et al. A comparison of conservative and aggressive transfusion regimens in the perioperative management of sickle cell disease. The Preoperative Transfusion in Sickle Cell Disease Study Group. N Engl J Med 1995;333:206–13 [see comments].

48. Hirst CW, Williamson L. Preoperative blood transfusions for sickle cell disease. Cochrane Database Syst Rev 2001;3:CD003149.

49. Wiesen AR, Hospenthal DR, Byrd JC, et al. Equilibration of hemoglobin concentration after transfusion in medical inpatients not actively bleeding. Ann Intern Med 1994;121:278–80.

Perioperative Anticoagulant Management

Paul J. Grant, MD[a], Daniel J. Brotman, MD[b], Amir K. Jaffer, MD[c],*

KEYWORDS

- Perioperative care • Anticoagulation
- Venous thromboembolism • Risk factors
- Warfarin • Heparin

The oral anticoagulant warfarin is a common medication that requires special consideration in the perioperative period. Although some procedures do not require warfarin interruption, the majority will necessitate its temporary cessation due to the risk of bleeding. Determining whether patients will benefit from the temporary use of a heparin product while warfarin is discontinued perioperatively (so-called "bridging" therapy) needs to take into consideration the risk of bleeding balanced with the risk of thromboembolism. Perioperative care also requires minimizing the risk of venous thromboembolism (VTE). Understanding the patient-specific and procedure-specific risks for VTE is paramount to employ optimal risk reduction strategies. This review uses a case-based approach to present the topics of perioperative warfarin management and postoperative VTE prevention.

THE PERIOPERATIVE MANAGEMENT OF WARFARIN
Clinical Vignette 1: Does Warfarin Need to be Discontinued?

A 78-year-old man with a history of atrial fibrillation, ischemic stroke, and hypertension is scheduled to have cataract surgery. He is taking warfarin with an international normalized ratio (INR) goal of 2.0 to 3.0. How should his warfarin be managed in preparation for his upcoming surgery?

This case illustrates the first question that should be asked for any patient taking warfarin who is planning to undergo surgery: Does the planned procedure require cessation of warfarin? Although most surgical interventions call for holding this

[a] Division of General Medicine, Department of Internal Medicine, University of Michigan Medical School, 3119 Taubman Center, Box 5376, 1500 East Medical Center Drive, Ann Arbor, MI 48109-5376, USA
[b] Hospitalist Program, Department of Medicine, Johns Hopkins University, 600 North Wolfe Street/Park 307, Baltimore, MD 21287, USA
[c] Division of Hospital Medicine, Department of Medicine, University of Miami Miller School of Medicine, 1120 NW 14th Street, 933 CRB (C216), Miami, FL 33136, USA
* Corresponding author.
E-mail address: ajaffer@med.miami.edu (A.K. Jaffer).

Med Clin N Am 93 (2009) 1105–1121
doi:10.1016/j.mcna.2009.05.002
0025-7125/09/$ – see front matter © 2009 Elsevier Inc. All rights reserved.

medication, it is important to recognize procedures that can safely be performed while on warfarin. Procedures that do not pose any significant increased risk of bleeding while on warfarin include:

- Cataract extractions and trabeculectomies[1,2]
- Many gastrointestinal procedures such as upper endoscopy and colonoscopy with or without biopsy, endoscopic retrograde cholangiopancreatography (ERCP) without sphincterotomy, biliary stent insertion without sphincterotomy, endosonography without fine needle aspiration, and push enteroscopy[3]
- Dental procedures such as restorations, endodontics, prosthetics, uncomplicated extractions, and dental hygiene treatment[4]
- Dermatologic procedures including Mohs micrographic surgery and simple excisions[5]
- Joint and soft tissue aspirations and injections[6]
- Minor podiatric procedures such as nail avulsions and phenol matrixectomies[7]

The patient in this clinical vignette may continue his warfarin perioperatively as cataract surgery is considered a "bloodless" procedure that does not require discontinuation of anticoagulation therapy.

Clinical Vignette 2: Rapid Reversal of Anticoagulation

A 44-year-old woman presents to the emergency department with severe right upper quadrant abdominal pain. Acute cholecystitis is diagnosed and the surgical team plans to take her to the operating room as soon as possible. However, the patient is on warfarin therapy for a deep vein thrombosis (DVT) diagnosed 3 months ago. Her INR is 2.8. What is the best way to reverse her anticoagulation in preparation for surgery?

Reversal of anticoagulation is often required when emergent or urgent procedures are necessary. Reversal of anticoagulation is typically achieved with the administration of fresh frozen plasma (FFP) or vitamin K. FFP has an immediate onset of action but its effects are short-lived. FFP exposure does not cause resistance to anticoagulation with warfarin postoperatively. Clinical trials have been unable to demonstrate an accurate dose-prediction model for INR reversal using FFP, thus dosing is largely empiric.[8] The INR should be monitored after initial FFP administration and every few hours subsequently to determine if additional treatment is needed to achieve the INR goal. As with any blood product, FFP treatment carries the risk of transfusion-related adverse events. The patient in this vignette should receive FFP as she is to undergo surgery as soon as possible.

For less urgent situations, such as surgery to be performed within 24 to 96 hours, vitamin K is the treatment of choice. Intravenous vitamin K will provide more rapid INR reversal than other routes of administration. A retrospective study found that 1 mg of intravenous vitamin K reversed anticoagulation to an INR <1.4 in a median time of 27 hours.[9] The most notable adverse events to intravenous vitamin K were dyspnea and chest tightness during infusion, which occurred in approximately 2% of patients. At this dosage of vitamin K, there was no resistance to postoperative anticoagulation. Vitamin K given orally is the most common method of administration and does not pose the same potential side effects as intravenous delivery. Dosages of 1.0 to 2.5 mg of oral vitamin K will correct supratherapeutic INRs (>4.5) to a therapeutic range within 24 to 48 hours.[10,11] One could extrapolate from these data that using similar doses of vitamin K will lower therapeutic INR values (ie, 2.0–3.0) to levels considered safe for surgery (typically an INR <1.5).[12] For certain procedures, however, such as neurosurgery, it may be desirable to have a near-normal INR (ie, <1.2).

Oral vitamin K is only available in 5-mg tablets in the United States. These tablets are scored allowing for easy administration of 2.5 mg. Lower doses can be administered by having the patient drink the intravenous preparation. Although subcutaneous delivery of vitamin K used to be commonplace, it has been shown that absorption by this route is not predictable and thus no longer recommended.[13,14]

WHO SHOULD RECEIVE BRIDGING THERAPY?

If anticoagulation reversal is required before surgery, there will always be some risk of thromboembolism. This risk is dependent on the following factors: the underlying indication for warfarin therapy, the patient's risk factors for thromboembolism, the duration of anticoagulation cessation, and whether the anticoagulation is completely or only partially reversed. Although the first 2 variables are not modifiable, perioperative bridging therapy with heparin allows us to influence the amount of time the patient is not anticoagulated. Patients at high risk for thromboembolism are likely to benefit from bridging therapy, whereas low-risk patients are unlikely to benefit and may be exposed to unnecessary risk. Although there are currently no randomized controlled trials on perioperative bridging to help guide recommendations, the first randomized clinical trial sponsored by the National Institutes of Health (NIH) for patients with atrial fibrillation on warfarin needing surgery is about to start and will enroll approximately 2500 patients. Patients will be randomized to bridging therapy with dalteparin or placebo. Until this study is completed, observational studies and guidelines must guide management of these patients.[15,16] The following clinical vignettes address perioperative warfarin management for the 3 most common indications for this medication: atrial fibrillation, mechanical heart valves, and venous thromboembolism.

Clinical Vignette 3: The Patient with Atrial Fibrillation

An 82 year-old woman with a history of atrial fibrillation, hypertension, congestive heart failure, and stroke is scheduled to undergo a nephrectomy. She has no previous history of VTE and is on chronic warfarin therapy. What is the best way to manage this patient's anticoagulation perioperatively?

Atrial fibrillation is a common condition associated with an increased long-term risk of stroke. The rate of ischemic stroke averages 5% per year.[17] This risk increases with age as the annual risk of stroke attributable to atrial fibrillation is 1.5% in those aged 50 to 59 years and 23.5% in those aged 80 to 89 years.[17]

The CHADS-2 risk classification is a validated tool designed to estimate the annual stroke risk in patients with atrial fibrillation by assigning points to risk factors.[18] This scheme assigns 1 point each for Congestive heart failure, Hypertension, Age ≥75 years, and Diabetes mellitus; and 2 points for a history of Stroke or transient ischemic attack (TIA). White and colleagues used an administrative database to suggest that the CHADS-2 score could be applied to predict the perioperative risk of stroke in patients with atrial fibrillation.[19] For example, patients with a CHADS-2 score of 5 or 6 are considered high risk for stroke and therefore may benefit from perioperative bridging. Other scenarios that pose a high risk for stroke and thus warrant perioperative bridging include rheumatic atrial fibrillation,[20] atrial fibrillation with a history of cardioembolic stroke,[21] and atrial fibrillation with a mechanical heart valve.[22]

The patient in this clinical vignette has atrial fibrillation and many other stroke risk factors including advanced age, hypertension, congestive heart failure, and previous stroke. Her CHADS-2 score is 5 indicating a high annual risk for stroke. This patient would be a good candidate for perioperative bridging therapy.

Clinical Vignette 4: The Patient with a Mechanical Heart Valve

A 54-year-old man with a history of hyperlipidemia and obesity is on chronic warfarin therapy for his aortic mechanical valve (bileaflet; St. Jude valve). He is scheduled to undergo major surgery that will require interruption of his warfarin. Does this patient require perioperative bridging therapy?

Without anticoagulation therapy, the risk for arterial thromboembolism (which includes stroke, systemic embolism, and valvular thrombosis) is estimated to be 4% per year[23] with a lifetime risk as high as 34% in patients with mechanical heart valves.[22] Factors that affect this risk include the type of valve and the valve position. Older models of mechanical valves, such as the ball-in-cage and tilting disk types, pose a higher risk of thromboembolism compared with the modern bileaflet type (ie, St. Jude), which offers the least resistance to blood flow and are thus lower risk.[23] Furthermore, mechanical valves in the mitral position double the risk for thromboembolism over those in the aortic position.[23]

The 2008 American College of Chest Physicians (ACCP) clinical practice guidelines for the perioperative management of antithrombotic therapy assessed perioperative bridging anticoagulation in 14 prospective cohort studies in patients with a mechanical heart valve.[15] The overall risk for perioperative arterial thromboembolism was 0.83% with no reported cases of mechanical valve thrombosis. The investigators caution that interpretation of these results is limited as there are no published trials that have a comparator group of patients who do not receive perioperative bridging anticoagulation when warfarin is discontinued.[15]

Other risk factors need to be considered in determining if bridging therapy is appropriate in patients with mechanical heart valves. The presence of atrial fibrillation or valve replacement surgery within the preceding few months both significantly increase the risk of thromboembolism.[22] Similar to patients with atrial fibrillation, the history of stroke or stroke risk factors (such as age, congestive heart failure, hypertension, and diabetes) will also increase the risk of thromboembolism.[15]

The patient in clinical vignette 4 has a newer model mechanical valve in the aortic position and no other significant risk factors for thromboembolism or stroke. For this patient, perioperative bridging therapy would not be recommended given his low risk for thromboembolism. In addition to the 2008 ACCP guidelines,[15] the latest American College of Cardiology/American Heart Association guidelines for the management of patients with valvular heart disease also supports this recommendation.[16]

Clinical Vignette 5: The Patient with a History of Venous Thromboembolism

A 58-year-old woman is scheduled to undergo a right-sided mastectomy for the recent diagnosis of breast cancer. She is currently on warfarin therapy for a pulmonary embolism (PE) that was diagnosed 2 months ago. The patient has no other medical issues and denies any other history of venous thromboembolic events. How should this patient's warfarin be managed perioperatively?

In contrast to patients with atrial fibrillation and mechanical heart valves, who are at risk for arterial thromboembolism and stroke, patients with prior VTE are at risk for recurrent VTE (ie, DVT and PE). Risk stratification to determine if perioperative bridging is recommended largely depends on how recently the previous VTE event occurred. The risk is highest in the first 4 weeks with an estimated recurrence of 0.3% to 1.3% per day without anticoagulation.[24] This risk drops to 0.03% to 0.2% per day over the next 4 to 12 weeks, and to less than 0.05% per day after 12 weeks.[24] Given these numbers, elective surgery should be postponed for a minimum of 1 month from the VTE event to provide continuous anticoagulation during this time.

Perioperative heparin bridging is recommended for patients with a history of VTE within the preceding 3 months[15,24] and can be considered for VTE events within the past 3 to 6 months.[24] A single VTE event that occurred more than 6 to 12 months ago is unlikely to justify bridging therapy. Patients with a prior VTE event and a known thrombophilia (such as deficiency of protein C, protein S, or antithrombin; antiphospholipid antibody syndrome; and homozygous factor V Leiden mutation) are also candidates for heparin bridging. Even without a diagnosed defect, if a patient has a clinically apparent thrombophilia based on recurrent or unprovoked VTE events, perioperative bridging should be employed.[15,24]

In contrast to the prevention of arterial thromboembolic events and strokes, which have never been convincingly shown to be preventable with parenteral perioperative anticoagulation, the literature is clear that perioperative VTE events can be reduced with the subcutaneous administration of low-dose heparin (unfractionated heparin or low molecular weight heparin [LMWH]).[25] By using low-dose heparin, effective anticoagulation for VTE risk reduction can be initiated 12 to 24 hours postoperatively. This is sooner than the 24 to 72 hours generally required before full-dose anticoagulation can be started.

The patient in clinical vignette 5 should undergo bridging treatment with heparin as her PE occurred less than 3 months ago. This patient has active cancer, which is also likely to increase her risk of VTE thus reinforcing the decision for perioperative bridging. Prophylactic-dose heparin products can be used in the immediate postoperative period, followed by full-dose anticoagulation when safe from a surgical perspective.

Box 1 summarizes heparin bridging recommendations for specific patient populations based on perioperative thromboembolic risk.

HOW TO BRIDGE WITH HEPARIN PERIOPERATIVELY

For patients who require discontinuation of warfarin before surgery, the 2 main options for perioperative bridging include unfractionated heparin (UFH) or LMWH. Although no randomized controlled trials on perioperative bridging exist, published studies assessing bridging with LMWH far outnumber those for UFH.[15] The use of therapeutic-dose intravenous UFH for perioperative bridging has significantly declined over the years due to the benefits of LMWH. Compared with UFH, LMWH has improved bioavailability, a more predictable dose response, a longer plasma half-life, and less interaction with platelets, endothelial cells, macrophages, and plasma proteins.[26] In addition, the risk of heparin-induced thrombocytopenia, a significant risk for thrombosis, is considerably lower with LMWH (~1%) compared with UFH (~3%).[27]

Another advantage of LMWH is its ability to be administered in the outpatient setting and without laboratory monitoring, translating into significant cost savings. One study demonstrated a lower mean total health care cost of more than $13,000 by using LMWH for perioperative bridging instead of UFH.[28] Although it is recommended *not* to routinely monitor Factor Xa levels in patients receiving LMWH,[15] in selected patient groups it may be appropriate to guide treatment. These include patients with severe renal insufficiency (ie, creatinine clearance <30 mL/min), those who are significantly over or under weight, and those who are pregnant.[29]

Despite the noted benefits of LMWH, some clinical circumstances may favor UFH for bridging. For example, in patients with severely reduced renal function (ie, creatinine clearance <10 mL/min or on dialysis), a potential for medication noncompliance, a language barrier, or an unsuitable home environment to support therapy, it may be

---

Box 1

Evaluating perioperative risk for thromboembolism: who should be bridged?

High risk for thromboembolism—bridging advised

- Known thrombophilia as documented by a thromboembolic event and 1 of the following: protein C deficiency, protein S deficiency, antithrombin III deficiency, homozygous factor V Leiden mutation, or antiphospholipid antibody syndrome
- Thrombophilia suggested by recurrent (2 or more) arterial or idiopathic venous thromboembolic events (not including primary atherosclerotic events, such as stroke or myocardial infarction due to intrinsic cerebrovascular or coronary disease)
- Venous or arterial thromboembolism within the preceding 3 months
- Rheumatic atrial fibrillation
- Acute intracardiac thrombus visualized by echocardiogram
- Atrial fibrillation plus mechanical heart valve in any position
- Older model mechanical valve (single disk or ball-in-cage) in mitral position
- Recently placed mechanical valve (<3 months)
- Atrial fibrillation with history of cardioembolism

Intermediate risk for thromboembolism—bridging decision on a case by case basis

- Newer model mechanical valve (ie, St. Jude) in mitral position
- Older model mechanical valve in aortic position
- Atrial fibrillation without a history of cardiac embolism but with multiple risks for cardiac embolism (ie, low ejection fraction (<40%), hypertension, older than 75 years, diabetes, history of stroke or TIA)
- Venous thromboembolism more than 3 to 6 months ago

Low risk for thromboembolism—bridging not advised

- One remote venous thromboembolism (>6 months ago)
- Intrinsic cerebrovascular disease (such as carotid atherosclerosis) without recurrent strokes or TIAs
- Atrial fibrillation without multiple risks for cardiac embolism
- Newer model mechanical valve in aortic position (ie, St. Jude)

Abbreviation: TIA, transient ischemic attack.

From Jaffer AK, Brotman DJ, Chukwumerije N. When patients on warfarin need surgery. Cleve Clin J Med 2003;70:973–84. Reprinted with permission. Copyright © 2000 Cleveland Clinic. All rights reserved.

---

judicious to choose UFH for bridging. When using UFH for perioperative bridging, the patient should be hospitalized approximately 36 hours after the last dose of warfarin (typically 2–3 days before surgery). The intravenous infusion should be discontinued 4 to 6 hours before surgery.[15] For surgery that carries a high risk of bleeding, consideration can be given to checking the activated partial thromboplastin time (aPTT) before incision. If bridging with LMWH, the last dose should be administered approximately 24 hours before surgery.[30] If using full-dose LMWH twice daily, the full dose can be given 24 hours before surgery, but with once daily dosing, it may be prudent to reduce the dose or to wait a full 36 hours before surgery.[15] **Fig. 1** illustrates a suggested perioperative bridging protocol using LMWH.

Preoperatively

Ensure patient does not have any contraindications to LMWH bridging such as:
- allergy to LMWH
- history of HIT
- severe thrombocytopenia
- extremes of weight (severely underweight of overweight)
- creatinine clearance < 15 ml/min (weight-based dosing if 15-30 ml/min)
- poor patient reliability
- inability to administer injections

Provide bridging instructions:
- stop warfarin 5 days before surgery (if INR 2-3)
- stop warfarin 6 days before surgery (if INR 3-4.5)
- start LMWH* 36 hours after last warfarin dose
- administer last dose of LMWH 24 hours prior to procedure†
- check INR on morning of surgery to ensure <1.5 and in some cases <1.2

Postoperatively

- restart LMWH* approximately 24 hours post procedure or consider thromboprophylaxis dosing of LMWH on post-op day 1 if patient is at high risk for bleeding (discuss with surgeon)
- restart warfarin at patient's usual dose on the evening of the surgical day
- check INR daily until patient is discharged and periodically thereafter until INR is therapeutic
- check CBC on post-op days 3 and 7 to monitor platelets
- discontinue LMWH when INR is therapeutic for two consecutive days

Fig. 1. Perioperative bridging strategy using LMWH. *Enoxaparin 1 mg/kg every 12 hours or 1.5 mg/kg every 24 hours or dalteparin 120 U/kg every 12 hours or 200 U/kg every 24 hours, or tinzaparin 175 U/kg every 24 hours. †Take full dose if using twice daily LMWH dosing, take two thirds dose if using once daily LMWH. CBC, complete blood count; HIT, heparin-induced thrombocytopenia; INR, international normalized ratio; LMWH, low molecular weight heparin.

Bridging therapy with LMWH has been controversial for patients with mechanical heart valves.[31] This controversy largely stemmed from the maternal and fetal deaths of 2 out of 8 pregnant women who took part in an enoxaparin thromboprophylaxis trial in South Africa. The enoxaparin package insert then stated that the medication "… has not been adequately studied for thromboprophylaxis in patients with mechanical prosthetic heart valves …" (Enoxaparin sodium package insert, June 7, 2007). However, based on the cumulative published bridging data, which includes a few poorly done studies using UFH,[32–34] many experts, including those who drafted the latest ACCP guidelines on the perioperative management of antithrombotic therapy,[15] endorse the use of LMWH for perioperative bridging in patients with mechanical heart valves.

POSTOPERATIVE PREVENTION OF VENOUS THROMBOEMBOLISM

The importance of preventing VTE in surgical patient is undisputed. VTE is the second most common postoperative medical complication and third most common cause of excess mortality in the postoperative patient.[35] Moreover, PE is recognized as the most common preventable cause of hospital death.[36] Without prophylaxis, the risk of developing venographically apparent DVT among surgical patients is striking, with estimates of 15% to 40% in general surgery patients,[37] 40% to 60% in lower extremity orthopedic patients,[25] and greater than 60% in trauma patients.[38] Data from randomized controlled trials and meta-analyses have demonstrated little or no increased rates of clinically important bleeding with prophylactic (low-dose) unfractionated heparin (LDUH), LMWH, or warfarin.[25] Given the high incidence of VTE, its significant morbidity and mortality, and the effective prevention strategies available, VTE prophylaxis must be a priority in the postoperative setting.[39] Unfortunately, studies continue to demonstrate that compliance rates for effective VTE prophylaxis remain poor. A recent multinational study involving more than 68,000 patients revealed that only 58.5% of surgical patients received appropriate VTE prophylaxis.[40]

Although thromboprophylactic therapies are effective, they are not perfect. It is estimated that pharmacologic prophylaxis will reduce the risk of VTE by more than 50% in surgical patients.[41] Despite this impressive risk reduction, breakthrough VTE is still a common problem given the high baseline rates of thrombosis. Therefore, clinicians caring for the perioperative patient should ensure that: (1) all patients undergo VTE risk assessment to help guide appropriate prophylaxis following surgery, and (2) a high index of suspicion for VTE is maintained, even when a patient is receiving appropriate prophylaxis.

VENOUS THROMBOEMBOLISM RISK ASSESSMENT

In addition to perioperative status, there are numerous other risk factors that predispose patients to VTE (**Box 2**). In general, the more risk factors present, the higher the risk of VTE.[42] In surgical patients, the overall risk of VTE depends not only on the patient's baseline comorbidities and risk factors but also on procedure related factors such as type of surgery, type of anesthesia, and duration of anesthesia.[25,43] The latest ACCP guidelines on prevention of VTE[25] recommend that hospitals develop a formal VTE prevention protocol for all medical and surgical inpatients. These guidelines favor the use of group-specific risk stratification (ie, patients undergoing major orthopedic surgery) over individualizing risk assessment given the lack of validated data to determine individual risk. In addition, individualized risk assessment can be cumbersome, which may lead to suboptimal compliance. **Table 1** summarizes the recommended VTE prophylaxis strategy for each of the main surgical groups.

OPTIONS FOR VENOUS THROMBOEMBOLISM PROPHYLAXIS

VTE prophylaxis options can be broadly classified into 2 categories: mechanical and pharmacologic. Mechanical prophylactic choices include graded compression stockings (GCS), intermittent pneumatic compression (IPC) devices, venous foot pumps (VFPs), and even inferior vena cava (IVC) filters. Pharmacologic options include parenteral anticoagulants (LDUH, LMWH, and fondaparinux) and oral anticoagulants such as warfarin. Newer agents such as direct thrombin inhibitors and anti-Xa inhibitors also exist but are currently not approved for thromboprophylaxis.

NONINVASIVE MECHANICAL PROPHYLAXIS

Mechanical options for VTE prevention are appealing as they pose no risk of bleeding. Thus, they provide an appropriate choice for postoperative surgical patients with a substantial risk of bleeding such as those with recent hemorrhage or neurosurgery patients. Furthermore, mechanical options such as IPC devices and GCS have shown

Box 2
Risk factors for VTE
Advanced age
Acute medical illness
Recent surgery
Trauma (major trauma or lower extremity injury)
Malignancy
History of DVT or PE
Immobility (confined to bed or chair) or lower extremity paresis
Obesity (BMI >30)
Smoking
Ischemic stroke
Inflammatory bowel disease
Congestive heart failure
Nephrotic syndrome
Myeloproliferative disorder
Venous insufficiency or varicose veins
Active collagen vascular disease
Thrombophilia (inherited or acquired)
Family history of thrombophilia or frequent unprovoked DVT or PE
Central venous catheterization
Pregnancy (including the post-partum period)
Estrogen use (oral contraception, HRT, SERM therapy)
Atherosclerosis
Abbreviations: BMI, body mass index; DVT, deep venous thrombosis; HRT, hormone replacement therapy; PE, pulmonary embolism; SERM, selective estrogen receptor modulator.

efficacy in VTE prevention in patients after general and orthopedic surgery in systematic reviews.[44,45] Dual prophylaxis strategies with mechanical devices in addition to pharmacologic prophylaxis may improve efficacy over pharmacologic prophylaxis alone in selected patient populations.[25] Although mechanical prophylaxis seems to be helpful, our experience suggests that compliance is often poor, and ambulation may be discouraged when IPC devices are employed. Furthermore, these devices have not been studied with the same rigor as pharmacologic agents for VTE prophylaxis. Given these issues, the latest ACCP guidelines advocate pharmacologic prophylaxis for most postoperative patients in the absence of active bleeding or contraindications to pharmacologic agents.[25]

PHARMACOLOGIC PROPHYLAXIS
Aspirin

Aspirin has been evaluated for VTE prevention in trials involving various types of surgical patients. In the Pulmonary Embolism Prevention (PEP) trial, 13,356 hip fracture patients were randomized to receive either aspirin or placebo, with additional

Table 1	
Recommended VTE prophylaxis strategies for the surgical patient	
Type of Surgery	**VTE Prophylaxis Options**
Minor general, gynecologic, urologic, and vascular procedures without VTE risk factors[a] Laparoscopic and arthroscopic procedures without VTE risk factors[a]	No routine pharmacologic prophylaxis recommended Early and frequent ambulation
Major gynecologic procedures without risk factors[a] Coronary artery bypass surgery	LMWH or LDUH, or IPC
Laparoscopic procedures with risk factors[a]	LDUH or LMWH or fondaparinux Consider mechanical VTE prophylaxis in combination with any of the above
Neurosurgery	LMWH or LDUH, or IPC Consider mechanical VTE prophylaxis in combination with any of the above for higher risk patients
Major gynecologic, vascular, thoracic, urologic, bariatric, and general surgical procedures with risk factors[a]	LDUH or LMWH or fondaparinux Consider mechanical VTE prophylaxis in combination with any of the above for gynecologic, urologic, bariatric, and general surgical procedures
Lower extremity orthopedic surgery: Total hip arthroplasty Total knee arthroplasty Hip fracture surgery	LMWH or fondaparinux or warfarin

Typical dosing: LMWH, enoxaparin 40 mg sc daily, dalteparin 5000 IU sc daily; fondaparinux 2.5 mg sc daily, warfarin to INR goal of 2–3.

Abbreviations: INR, international normalized ratio; IPC, intermittent pneumatic compression; LDUH, low-dose unfractionated heparin; LMWH, low molecular weight heparin; VTE, venous thromboembolism.

[a] The risk factors are presented in **Box 2**.

Data from Geerts WH, Bergqvist D, Pineo GF, et al. Prevention of venous thromboembolism. American College of Chest Physicians evidence-based clinical practice guidelines (8th edition). Chest 2008;133:381S–453S.

forms of thromboprophylaxis at the discretion of the treating physician.[46] In this study, aspirin exposure significantly reduced the incidence of DVT and PE. However, other studies have shown that aspirin, if used alone, has less efficacy for VTE prevention than LMWH.[47] The ACCP provides a strong recommendation *against* the use of aspirin for VTE prophylaxis in surgical patients.[25]

Low-Dose Unfractionated Heparin

LDUH has been studied extensively in randomized controlled trials (RCTs) in general surgery patients. Most trials evaluated LDUH 5000 U 1 to 2 hours before surgery and then 5000 U subcutaneously twice a day or three times a day until patients were ambulating or discharged from the hospital. In a meta-analysis of 46 RCTs, LDUH significantly decreased the rate of DVT, PE, and overall mortality.[48] This meta-analysis also suggested that LDUH three times a day was more efficacious than LDUH twice a day without increasing the risk of bleeding, but this was based on an indirect comparison.

Low Molecular Weight Heparin

LMWH has been studied extensively and compared with placebo and LDUH in general surgery patients. Multiple meta-analyses have been published evaluating LDUH versus LMWH, and there seems to be little difference in relative efficacy. However, one meta-analysis concluded that there was a decreased rate of clinical VTE with LWMH following surgery.[41] This meta-analysis demonstrated that LMWH doses of less than 3400 IU daily have comparable efficacy with LDUH with less bleeding, whereas doses greater than 3400 IU daily yielded slightly improved efficacy but with somewhat higher bleeding rates.[25,41] For reference, LMWH doses greater than 3400 IU daily include enoxaparin 40 mg subcutaneously daily and dalteparin 5000 IU subcutaneously daily.

Warfarin

VTE prophylaxis with warfarin is generally reserved for patients undergoing lower extremity orthopedic surgery due to the need for extended therapy after hospital discharge. A meta-analysis[49] demonstrated that warfarin was superior to placebo for the prevention of VTE in orthopedic surgery patients. Warfarin was also more effective than IPC devices for preventing proximal DVT. However, this meta-analysis also revealed that warfarin was less effective than LMWH in preventing DVT without any difference in major bleeding or wound hematoma.[49] Despite some concerns about postoperative orthopedic patients being unprotected for the first several days after initiation of warfarin thromboprophylaxis,[50] the ACCP gives a strong recommendation for warfarin use as a viable option in this population.[25]

Synthetic Pentasaccharide

Fondaparinux is a synthetic pentasaccharide that mediates the interaction of heparin with antithrombin and inhibits factor Xa. This drug has essentially 100% bioavailability and has a half-life of 17 hours permitting once daily administration. Another advantage of this agent, unlike UFH and LMWH, is that it is not believed to cause heparin-induced thrombocytopenia (HIT).[51] Fondaparinux is excreted in the urine and is contraindicated in patients with a creatinine clearance less than 30 mL/min.

A meta-analysis of randomized double-blind trials assessing VTE risk reduction in patients undergoing lower extremity orthopedic surgery demonstrated a significant benefit of fondaparinux over the LMWH enoxaparin.[52] However, a higher incidence of major bleeding was noted with fondaparinux. Fondaparinux has also demonstrated efficacy in general surgery patients. The PEGASUS trial compared fondaparinux with the LMWH dalteparin in 2927 patients undergoing major abdominal surgery.[53] Although no difference was observed in the overall rates of VTE or bleeding, in patients who underwent abdominal cancer surgery (approximately 70% of the overall sample), the incidence of VTE was significantly lower in the fondaparinux group. These studies suggest that fondaparinux has somewhat greater anticoagulant activity than LMWH at the doses studied.

SPECIAL CONSIDERATIONS FOR PERIOPERATIVE VTE PROPHYLAXIS
Clinical Vignette 6: The Low-risk Surgical Patient

A 36-year-old man developed an inguinal hernia while working as a furniture mover. The patient is a nonsmoker, has a BMI of 22, and denies any previous medical history. He is scheduled to have his hernia repaired by laparoscopic technique. What is the recommended method of VTE prophylaxis for this patient?

Although most patients will require pharmacologic VTE prophylaxis in the perioperative setting, some patients are at low enough risk for VTE such that drug therapy is not recommended. This is a young patient (<40 years) without any VTE risk factors (see **Box 2**) who is scheduled to undergo minor surgery. In low-risk patients such as the man described here, the ACCP guidelines recommend against the use of specific prophylaxis other than early and frequent ambulation.[25]

Clinical Vignette 7: The Patient at High Risk for Postoperative Venous Thromboembolism

A 78-year-old woman with a history of obesity and venous insufficiency presents for an elective total hip replacement due to severe osteoarthritis. She currently feels well and has no complaints. What is the recommended strategy for VTE prophylaxis in this high-risk patient?

Patients undergoing lower extremity orthopedic surgery are among the highest risk group of patients for development of postoperative VTE. There are 3 pharmacologic options for VTE prophylaxis in this patient, all of which receive the strongest recommendation from the most recent ACCP guidelines: LMWH, fondaparinux, and warfarin.[25] These agents are also recommended for patients undergoing elective total knee replacement surgery. Although published data are lacking, the optimal timing of prophylaxis is likely as follows: LMWH should be started either 12 hours preoperatively, or 12 to 24 hours postoperatively, fondaparinux should be started 6 to 8 hours postoperatively, and warfarin should be initiated on the evening of the surgical day.[25] The duration of prophylaxis has been addressed in many trials including systematic reviews.[54,55] The data are clear that patients who undergo total hip replacement benefit from extended VTE prophylaxis for 4 to 5 weeks postoperatively using any of the agents listed earlier. Venous thrombosis following knee replacement tends to occur sooner than following hip replacement, so the efficacy of prolonged prophylaxis is less clear. At least 10 to 14 days of pharmacotherapy should be used following knee replacement surgery.

Clinical Vignette 8: The Surgical Patient with Abdominal or Pelvic Cancer

A 60-year-old man was recently diagnosed with colon cancer and is scheduled to undergo a hemi-colectomy. It is unclear if the cancer has spread to regional lymph nodes. The patient has a history of hypertension and diabetes mellitus. What is the best VTE prophylaxis strategy for this patient?

Given the diagnosis of cancer, this patient's risk for postoperative VTE is high. Options for VTE prevention include LMWH, LDUH three times a day, or fondaparinux (all with equally high recommendations) with the consideration of adding a mechanical method such as GCS or IPC device (a weaker recommendation).[25] A double-blind multicenter trial assessed the optimal duration of VTE prophylaxis in patients undergoing surgery for abdominal or pelvic cancer.[56] All patients received enoxaparin for 6 to 10 days postoperatively, but those randomized for an additional 21 days of enoxaparin prophylaxis noted a significantly reduced incidence of VTE. Thus, extended prophylaxis with LMWH is recommended for patients undergoing surgery for abdominal or pelvic cancer.[25]

Clinical Vignette 9: The Patient with an Indwelling Epidural Catheter

A 64 year-old man with a history of severe osteoarthritis has undergone total knee replacement surgery. For optimal pain control, the anesthesiologist has left the epidural catheter in place. What precautions need to be taken while using pharmacologic VTE prophylaxis in this patient?

The timing of prophylactic anticoagulation is further complicated when neuraxial anesthesia is employed. The delivery of anesthetic to the neuraxis requires insertion of a needle or catheter into the epidural space. In this scenario, the concomitant use of prophylactic anticoagulation may increase the risk of paraspinal hematomas. The ACCP and the American Society of Regional Anesthesiology (ASRA) agree that pharmacologic VTE prophylaxis can still be used in parallel with neuraxial anesthesia, as long as precautions are taken to reduce the risk of bleeding.[25,57] Specific recommendations for LMWH include waiting 10 to 12 hours after a prophylactic dose of LMWH before inserting the epidural catheter, waiting 10 to 12 hours after the last dose before removing the catheter, and waiting at least 2 hours after removal of the catheter to restart LMWH. These precautions, including those recommended for LDUH, warfarin, and fondaparinux, are outlined in **Table 2**.

Clinical Vignette 10: Inferior Vena Cava Filters

A 46-year-old woman presents to the emergency department after a being involved in a devastating motor vehicle accident. She has numerous bone fractures involving her lower extremities and pelvis, significant blood loss, and a ruptured spleen. She is being rushed to the operating room for an urgent splenectomy. What methods of VTE prophylaxis are appropriate for this patient?

This patient has a clear contraindication to pharmacologic VTE prophylaxis. However, her risk for VTE is high given the multiple fractures, the need for surgery, and anticipated prolonged hospital stay with immobility. Although there are some data to suggest that the prophylactic use of retrievable IVC filters may benefit trauma patients with a contraindication to drug prophylaxis,[58] meta-analyses of prospective studies have found no difference in the rates of PE among trauma patients with or without IVC filters.[59,60] Given the current data, the ACCP recommends against the use of IVC filters as thromboprophylaxis in trauma patients.[25] They further state that IVC filter insertion is only indicated for patients with a proven proximal DVT who have either an absolute contraindication for full-dose anticoagulation, or require major

Table 2			
VTE prophylaxis management for patients receiving neuraxial anesthesia/analgesia			
	Before Neuraxial Technique	Before Catheter Removal	After Catheter Removal
LDUH	No contraindication	No contraindication	No contraindication
LMWH			
- Single daily dosing	Wait 10–12 h after last dose	Wait 10–12 h after last dose	Wait 2 h before resuming
- Twice daily dosing	Wait 10–12 h after last dose	Not recommended for use while catheter in place	Wait 2 h before resuming
Warfarin	INR <1.5	INR ≤1.5	Resume therapy to INR goal
Fondaparinux	Currently not recommended in conjunction with neuraxial anesthesia/analgesia		

Abbreviations: LDUH, low-dose unfractionated heparin; LMWH, low molecular weight heparin; VTE, venous thromboembolism.

Data from Horlocker TT, Wedel DJ, Benzon H, et al. Regional anesthesia in the anticoagulated patient: defining the risks (the Second ASRA Consensus Conference on Neuraxial Anesthesia and Anticoagulation). Reg Anesth Pain Med 2003;28:172–97.

surgery in the near future. The best option for VTE prophylaxis for this patient is to employ optimal mechanical measures such as IPC devices. Although limited, there are prospective randomized data reporting benefit when using these devices in trauma patients.[61] It should be emphasized that pharmacologic prophylaxis using LMWH should be instituted as soon as it is considered safe.[25]

SUMMARY

The perioperative management of warfarin is a common issue that requires careful attention by the perioperative consultant. If warfarin interruption is required, a thorough assessment balancing the perioperative risks of thromboembolism versus bleeding will determine if heparin bridging therapy is indicated. Being familiar with an appropriate bridging protocol for LMWH and UFH is important to minimize perioperative risk. In addition, reducing the risk of VTE is a top priority in perioperative medicine, and requires understanding the patient-specific and procedure-specific VTE risk factors. The consultant should also be comfortable with the various mechanical and pharmacologic prophylactic options available, including knowledge of the timing and duration of prophylactic anticoagulation to maximize VTE risk reduction and to limit the risk of bleeding.

REFERENCES

1. Dunn AS, Turpie AG. Perioperative management of patients receiving oral anticoagulants: a systematic review. Arch Intern Med 2003;163(8):901–8.
2. Konstantatos A. Anticoagulation and cataract surgery: a review of the current literature. Anaesth Intensive Care 2001;29(1):11–8.
3. Eisen GM, Baron TH, Dominitz JA, et al. Guideline on the management of anticoagulation and antiplatelet therapy for endoscopic procedures. Gastrointest Endosc 2002;55(7):775–9.
4. Wahl MJ. Dental surgery in anticoagulated patients. Arch Intern Med 1998; 158(15):1610–6.
5. Billingsley EM. Intraoperative and postoperative bleeding problems in patients taking warfarin, aspirin, and nonsteroidal antiinflammatory agents. A prospective study. Dermatol Surg 1997;23(5):381–3 [discussion: 384–5].
6. Thumboo J, O'Duffy JD. A prospective study of the safety of joint and soft tissue aspirations and injections in patients taking warfarin sodium. Arthritis Rheum 1998;41(4):736–9.
7. Lanzat M, Danna AT, Jacobson DS. New protocols for perioperative management of podiatric patients taking oral anticoagulants. J Foot Ankle Surg 1994;33(1): 16–20.
8. Frazee LA, Bourquet CC, Gutierrez W, et al. Retrospective evaluation of a method to predict fresh-frozen plasma dosage in anticoagulated patients. Am J Ther 2008;15(2):111–8.
9. Shields RC, McBane RD, Kuiper JD, et al. Efficacy and safety of intravenous phytonadione (vitamin K1) in patients on long-term oral anticoagulant therapy. Mayo Clin Proc 2001;76(3):260–6.
10. Crowther MA, Donovan D, Harrison L, et al. Low-dose oral vitamin K reliably reverses over-anticoagulation due to warfarin. Thromb Haemost 1998;79(6): 1116–8.
11. Weibert RT, Le DT, Kayser SR, et al. Correction of excessive anticoagulation with low-dose oral vitamin K1. Ann Intern Med 1997;126(12):959–62.

12. White RH, McKittrick T, Hutchinson R, et al. Temporary discontinuation of warfarin therapy: changes in the international normalized ratio. Ann Intern Med 1995; 122(1):40–2.

13. Crowther MA, Douketis JD, Schnurr, et al. Oral vitamin K lowers the international normalized ratio more rapidly than subcutaneous vitamin K in the treatment of warfarin-associated coagulopathy. A randomized, controlled trial. Ann Intern Med 2002;137(4):251–4.

14. Dezee KJ, Shimeall WT, Douglas KM, et al. Treatment of excessive anticoagulation with phytonadione (vitamin K): a meta-analysis. Arch Intern Med 2006;166(4): 391–7.

15. Douketis JD, Berger PB, Dunn AS, et al. The perioperative management of antithrombotic therapy: American College of Chest Physicians Evidence-Based Clinical Practice Guidelines (8th Edition). Chest 2008;133:299S–339S.

16. Bonow RO, Carabello BA, Chatterjee K, et al. ACC/AHA 2006 guidelines for the management of patients with valvular heart disease: a report of the American College of Cardiology/American Heart Association Task Force on Practice Guidelines (Writing Committee to Develop Guidelines for the Management of Patients With Valvular Heart Disease). American College of Cardiology Web Site. Available at: http://www.acc.org/clinical/guidelines/valvular/index.pdf. Accessed December 20, 2008.

17. Wolf PA, Abbott RD, Kannel WB. Atrial fibrillation as an independent risk factor for stroke: the Framingham Study. Stroke 1991;22:983–8.

18. Gage BF, Waterman AD, Shannon W, et al. Validation of clinical classification schemes for predicting stroke: results from the National Registry of Atrial Fibrillation. JAMA 2001;285:2864–70.

19. White RH, Kaatz S, Douketis J, et al. Comparison of the 30-day incidence of ischemic stroke and bleeding after major surgery in patients with or without atrial fibrillation (AF). J Thromb Haemost 2007;5(Suppl 1):O-M-035.

20. Cerebral Embolism Task Force. Cardiogenic brain embolism. Arch Neurol 1986; 43(1):71–84.

21. Atrial Fibrillation Investigators Risk factors for stroke and efficacy of antithrombotic therapy in atrial fibrillation. Analysis of pooled data from five randomized controlled trials [erratum appears in Arch Intern Med 1994;154(19):2254]. Arch Intern Med 1994;154(13):1449–57.

22. Bettadapur MS, Griffin BP, Asher CR. Caring for patients with prosthetic heart valves. Cleve Clin J Med 2002;69(1):75–87.

23. Cannegieter SC, Rosendaal FR, Briet E. Thromboembolic and bleeding complications in patients with mechanical heart valve prostheses. Circulation 1994; 89(2):635–41.

24. Jaffer AK, Brotman DJ, Chukwumerije N. When patients on warfarin need surgery. Cleve Clin J Med 2003;70(11):973–84.

25. Geerts WH, Bergqvist D, Pineo GF, et al. Prevention of venous thromboembolism: American College of Chest Physicians Evidence-Based Clinical Practice Guidelines (8th Edition). Chest 2008;133:381S–453S.

26. Hirsh J, Dalen J, Anderson DR, et al. Oral anticoagulants: mechanism of action, clinical effectiveness, and optimal therapeutic range. Chest 2001;119(1 Suppl):8S–21S.

27. Warkentin TE, Levine MN, Hirsh J, et al. Heparin-induced thrombocytopenia in patients treated with low-molecular-weight heparin or unfractionated heparin. N Engl J Med 1995;332(20):1330–5.

28. Spyropoulos AC, Frost FJ, Hurley JS, et al. Costs and clinical outcomes associated with low-molecular-weight heparin vs unfractionated heparin for

perioperative bridging in patients receiving long-term oral anticoagulant therapy. Chest 2004;125:1642–50.

29. Hirsh J, Raschke R. Heparin and low-molecular-weight heparin: the Seventh ACCP Conference on Antithrombotic and Thrombolytic Therapy. Chest 2004; 126(Suppl):188S–203S.
30. O'Donnell MJ, Kearon C, Johnson J, et al. Preoperative anticoagulant activity after bridging low-molecular-weight heparin for temporary interruption of warfarin. Ann Intern Med 2007;146(3):184–7.
31. Anticoagulation in Prosthetic Valves and Pregnancy Consensus Report Panel and Scientific Round Table Discussion. Anticoagulation and enoxaparin use in patients with prosthetic heart valves and/or pregnancy. Volume 3. Clinical cardiology consensus reports. Atlanta (GA): American Health Consultants; 2002 . p. 1–20.
32. Tinker JH, Tarhan S. Discontinuing anticoagulant therapy in surgical patients with cardiac valve prostheses. Observations in 180 operations. JAMA 1978;239:738–9.
33. Katholi RE, Nolan SP, McGuire LB. Living with prosthetic heart valves. Subsequent noncardiac operations and the risk of thromboembolism or hemorrhage. Am Heart J 1976;92:162–7.
34. Katholi RE, Nolan SP, McGuire LB. The management of anticoagulation during noncardiac operations in patients with prosthetic heart valves. A prospective study. Am Heart J 1978;96:163–5.
35. Zhan C, Miller MR. Excess length of stay, charges, and mortality attributable to medical injuries during hospitalization. JAMA 2003;290:1868–74.
36. Shojania KG, Duncan BW, McDonald KM, et al. Making health care safer: a critical analysis of patient safety practices; evidence report/technology assessment, No. 43 (prepared by the University of California at San Francisco-Stanford Evidence-based Practice Center under contract no. 290-97-0013). AHRQ Publication No. 01-E058, Rockville, MD. Agency for Healthcare Research and Quality. Available at: www.ahrq.gov/clinic/ptsafety/. Accessed November 9, 2008.
37. Clagett GP, Reisch JS. Prevention of venous thromboembolism in general surgical patients: results of meta-analysis. Ann Surg 1988;208:227–40.
38. Kudsk KA, Fabian TC, Baum S, et al. Silent deep vein thrombosis in immobilized multiple trauma patients. Am J Surg 1989;158:515–9.
39. Geerts WH, Pineo GF, Heit JA, et al. Prevention of venous thromboembolism: the seventh ACCP conference on antithrombotic and thrombolytic therapy. Chest 2004;126(Suppl 3):338S–400S.
40. Cohen AT, Tapson VF, Bergmann JF, et al. ENDORSE investigators. Venous thromboembolism risk and prophylaxis in the acute hospital care setting (ENDORSE study): a multinational cross-sectional study [erratum appears in Lancet 2008;371(9628):1914]. Lancet 2008;371(9610):387–94.
41. Mismetti P, Laporte S, Darmon JY, et al. Meta-analysis of low molecular weight heparin in the prevention of venous thromboembolism in general surgery. Br J Surg 2001;88(7):913–30.
42. Anderson FA Jr, Spencer FA. Risk factors for venous thromboembolism. Circulation 2003;107(23 Suppl 1):I9–16.
43. Jaffer AK, Barsoum WK, Krebs V, et al. Duration of anesthesia and venous thromboembolism after hip and knee arthroplasty. Mayo Clin Proc 2005;80(6):732–8.
44. Amaragiri SV, Lees TA. Elastic compression stockings for prevention of deep vein thrombosis. Cochrane Database Syst Rev 2000;3:CD001484.
45. Freedman KB, Brookenthal KR, Fitzgerald RH Jr, et al. A meta-analysis of thromboembolic prophylaxis following elective total hip arthroplasty. J Bone Joint Surg Am 2000;82(7):929–38.

46. Prevention of pulmonary embolism and deep vein thrombosis with low dose aspirin: Pulmonary Embolism Prevention (PEP) trial. Lancet 2000;355:1295–302.

47. Gent M, Hirsh J, Ginsberg JS, et al. Low-molecular-weight heparinoid orgaran is more effective than aspirin in the prevention of venous thromboembolism after surgery for hip fracture. Circulation 1996;93(1):80–4.

48. Collins R, Scrimgeour A, Yusuf S, et al. Reduction in fatal pulmonary embolism and venous thrombosis by perioperative administration of subcutaneous heparin. Overview of results of randomized trials in general, orthopedic, and urologic surgery. N Engl J Med 1988;318(18):1162–73.

49. Mismetti P, Laporte S, Zufferey P, et al. Prevention of venous thromboembolism in orthopedic surgery with vitamin K antagonists: a meta-analysis. J Thromb Haemost 2004;2(7):1058–70.

50. Brotman DJ, Jaffer AK, Hurbanek JG, et al. Warfarin prophylaxis and venous thromboembolism in the first 5 days following hip and knee arthroplasty. Thromb Haemost 2004;92(5):1012–7.

51. Hirsh J, Bauer KA, Donati MB, et al. Parenteral anticoagulants: American College of Chest Physicians Evidence-Based Clinical Practice Guidelines (8th Edition). Chest 2008;133(6):141S–59S.

52. Turpie AG, Bauer KA, Eriksson BI, et al. Fondaparinux vs enoxaparin for the prevention of venous thromboembolism in major orthopedic surgery: a meta-analysis of 4 randomized double-blind studies. Arch Intern Med 2002;162(16):1833–40.

53. Agnelli G, Bergqvist D, Cohen AT, et al. Randomized clinical trial of postoperative fondaparinux versus perioperative dalteparin for prevention of venous thromboembolism in high-risk abdominal surgery. Br J Surg 2005;92(10):1212–20.

54. Hull RD, Pineo GF, Stein PD, et al. Extended out-of hospital low-molecular-weight heparin prophylaxis against deep venous thrombosis in patients after elective hip arthroplasty: a systematic review. Ann Intern Med 2001;135:858–69.

55. O'Donnell M, Linkins LA, Kearon C, et al. Reduction of out-of-hospital symptomatic venous thromboembolism by extended thromboprophylaxis with low-molecular-weight heparin following elective hip arthroplasty: a systematic review. Arch Intern Med 2003;163:1362–6.

56. Bergqvist D, Agnelli G, Cohen AT, et al, for the ENOXACAN II investigators. Duration of prophylaxis against venous thromboembolism with enoxaparin after surgery for cancer. N Engl J Med 2002;346:975–80.

57. Horlocker TT, Wedel DJ, Benzon H, et al. Regional anesthesia in the anticoagulated patient: defining the risks (the second ASRA consensus conference on neuraxial anesthesia and anticoagulation). Reg Anesth Pain Med 2003;28:172–97.

58. Offner PJ, Hawkes A, Madayag R, et al. The role of temporary inferior vena cava filters in critically ill surgical patients. Arch Surg 2003;138(6):591–4.

59. Velmahos GC, Kern J, Chan LS, et al. Prevention of venous thromboembolism after injury: an evidence-based report; part II. Analysis of risk factors and evaluation of the role of vena caval filters. J Trauma 2000;49:140–4.

60. McMurty AL, Owings JT, Anderson JT, et al. Increased use of prophylactic vena cava filters in trauma patients failed to decrease overall incidence of pulmonary embolism. J Am Coll Surg 1999;189:314–20.

61. Fisher CG, Blachut PA, Salvian AJ, et al. Effectiveness of pneumatic leg compression devices for the prevention of thromboembolic disease in orthopaedic trauma patients: a prospective, randomized study of compression alone versus no prophylaxis. J Orthop Trauma 1995;9:1–7.

Preoperative Preparation of the Surgical Patient with Neurologic Disease

Adam Schiavi, MD, PhD[a], Alexander Papangelou, MD[a],
Marek Mirski, MD, PhD[b,c,d,e],*

KEYWORDS

- Preoperative • Neurologic disease • Management
- Perioperative • Surgery

The amount of neurologic disease in the general population is a difficult number to assess accurately. This is, in part, because of the wide-sweeping scope of neurologic disease. The International Classification of Diseases has the highest number of conditions attributable to neurologic disease, many of which are uncommon. An epidemiologic study in 2000 from the United Kingdom by MacDonald and colleagues[1] showed an incidence of neurologic disease of 0.6% in an 18-month period in 1995 to 1996, with stroke and seizure disorders topping the list, but including more uncommon disorders as well. The lifetime prevalence of neurologic disease (per 1000) from that time was 6%. More recently, a US epidemiologic study from 2007 examined rates of more common neurologic disorders, such as stroke and migraine, but did not include more generalized data.[2] For the purposes of this article, however, it is sufficient to say that neurologic disease is neither uncommon nor inconsequential, and indeed serious and chronic neurologic conditions are likely to appear in patients for whom surgery has been deemed necessary.

[a] Division of Neuroanesthesia and Neurosciences Critical Care Medicine, Department of Anesthesiology and Critical Care Medicine, Johns Hopkins Medical Institutions, 600 North Wolfe Street/Meyer 8-140, Baltimore, MD 21287, USA
[b] Department of Anesthesiology and Critical Care Medicine, Johns Hopkins Medical Institutions, 600 North Wolfe Street/Meyer 8-140, Baltimore, MD 21287, USA
[c] Department of Neurology and Neurosurgery, Johns Hopkins Medical Institutions, 600 North Wolfe Street/Meyer 8-140, Baltimore, MD 21287, USA
[d] Neurosciences Critical Care Division, Johns Hopkins Medical Institutions, Baltimore, MD 21287, USA
[e] Division of Neuroanesthesiology, Johns Hopkins Medical Institutions, 600 North Wolfe Street/Meyer 8-140, Baltimore, MD 21287, USA
* Corresponding author. Department of Anesthesiology and Critical Care Medicine, Johns Hopkins Medical Institutions, 600 North Wolfe Street/Meyer 8-140, Baltimore, MD 21287.
E-mail address: mmirski@jhmi.edu (M. Mirski).

Med Clin N Am 93 (2009) 1123–1130
doi:10.1016/j.mcna.2009.05.005
0025-7125/09/$ – see front matter © 2009 Elsevier Inc. All rights reserved.

medical.theclinics.com

The target audience of this article is anyone who will be evaluating patients for what is likely to be elective surgery, because truly lifesaving surgery would generally proceed regardless of coexisting medical issues. An internist or family practitioner will frequently be consulted by a surgeon to do a preoperative evaluation. Higher-risk patients will frequently be evaluated in an anesthesiology preoperative clinic. Additionally, these higher-risk patients frequently have a cardiologist or pulmonologist who are asked to help with the assessment. Although there may be significant overlap with the more common perioperative medical problems, patients with severe or chronic neurologic disease may also have unique perioperative risk as a result of their neurologic issues. Occasionally, a neurologist may be asked to evaluate these patients as well. Those who typically do preoperative evaluations (internists, family practitioners, anesthesiologists) will benefit from this article if their patient has not specifically been evaluated by a neurologist. The neurologist asked to do a preoperative assessment for the neurologic patient may benefit as well from more general considerations of perioperative risk assessment.

GENERAL CONSIDERATIONS IN PREOPERATIVE PREPARATION

It is important that the purpose of the preoperative evaluation and preparation of any patient is not simply to "clear" a patient for surgery. This terminology is misleading and implies absence of significant risk if clearance for surgery has been given. First and foremost it is important for all practitioners to realize that risk always coexists with any surgical procedure. The purpose of the preoperative assessment is to identify modifiable risk factors and to optimize medically specific issues before surgery. In addition, the preoperative assessment is meant to uncover comorbidities that may not be easily discoverable during the brief, routine preoperative anesthetic review on the day of surgery, and to make such information readily available well before the time of surgery.

Typically, if any patient develops a new neurologic problem or an exacerbation of an existing one, elective surgery should be rescheduled until the issue can be managed properly. Referral should be made to a neurologist and communication with the surgeon and anesthesiologist to that effect should be made.

PREOPERATIVE HISTORY AND PHYSICAL EXAMINATION

A full history and physical examination should be considered standard in any preoperative evaluation, typically focusing on the cardiovascular and pulmonary systems and the airway. For the neurologic patient, particular attention should be paid to the neurologic examination. Although a neurologist may perform a comprehensive evaluation, the non-neurologist must also be willing to perform a fairly detailed neurologic examination when appropriate. Along with a routine neurologic history and examination of the cranial nerves and gross motor and sensory systems, careful documentation of any deficits must specifically be recorded for comparative purposes with the postoperative neurologic state. Current medications and a social history concerning smoking, alcohol, and illicit drug use must be obtained in the history. Discussions about management of current non-neurologic medications are discussed elsewhere in this issue.

Specific to the preexisting neurologic disease, preoperative studies may include an electroencephalogram, electrophysiological muscle or sensory studies, and neurologic imaging such as cerebral angiography or CT or MRI of the brain and spinal cord. It is important to review and to document pertinent findings from these tests and to discuss with the patient's neurologist if further evaluation is necessary. It may be prudent to repeat some tests to identify any interval changes before surgery.

If there are perioperative complications, it would again be important to have a recent preoperative baseline assessment.

It is always essential for the anesthesiologist to have detailed information about cardiac and pulmonary testing to optimize the perioperative care. Such data take on more significance if neurologic disease alters these physiologic systems. Muscular dystrophy, for example, frequently manifests itself in young people who may not otherwise have a reason to have cardiac testing. These myopathies frequently have primary cardiac manifestations which may compromise cardiac function. Similarly, in myasthenia gravis, baseline pulmonary function testing is often vital information to gauge a patient's fitness for extubation and need for intensive care monitoring postoperatively.

Of special importance are neurologic patients suffering from cerebral vascular disease, as they comprise a large fraction of neurologic patients and are prone to ischemic risks during surgery. Management of blood pressure during surgery is of great consequence in patients who suffer from carotid or vertebral artery stenosis, a known cerebral aneurysm, or recent stroke or transient ischemic attack. A vascular imaging study such as a magnetic resonance angiogram, CT angiogram, or contrast-injected cerebral angiogram have become critical for surgeons and anesthesiologists to estimate the risks for surgery and optimal perioperative blood pressure control. Understanding the results of neuroimaging tests is also a key in assessing the risks for surgery and anesthesia in patients with central nervous system tumors, as the localization of such mass lesions is critical in defining potential hemodynamic liability and postoperative deficits.

SPECIFIC CONSIDERATIONS AS THEY RELATE TO CERTAIN NEUROLOGIC CONDITIONS
Disturbances of Consciousness

Processes such as delirium are beyond the scope of this article. However, counseling should be provided to chronic encephalopathy (eg, dementia) patients and/or their families that the recovery period after a major surgery can be prolonged. Patients with an already susceptible brain (eg, dementia, history of stroke or brain trauma) are more predisposed to injury and postoperative cognitive dysfunction. There is a nonmodifiable risk that these patients may never return to their neurologic and cognitive baseline after more substantial surgeries and those requiring cardiac bypass.[3,4] Therefore, the risks and benefits of proceeding with such surgery should be carefully explained and weighed. The uses of certain medications such as neuroleptics are commonly prescribed to patients with agitated alterations of behavior, and should be documented. Discontinuation of this class of drugs may have consequences of acute dystonic reactions, whereas continuation of neuroleptics may also be risky—leading to the risk for neuroleptic malignant syndrome with general anesthesia. There are case reports of neuroleptic malignant syndrome developing after the withdrawal of neuroleptics for cardiac surgery.[5] This same concept applies to patients with cerebral palsy.[6]

Cerebrovascular Disorders

This term encompasses a large patient population, which includes those with a history of stroke, intracerebral hemorrhage, and/or intracranial atherosclerosis and/or vasculopathy (eg, vasculitis). These patients often have a substantial history of risk factors such as hypertension, diabetes, dyslipidemia, and cardiac arrhythmias. Any workup of these patients must include thorough cardiac testing including ECG, echocardiogram and possibly cardiac stress testing. These patients often have vascular disease with significant end organ damage. Complete blood count and complete metabolic panel should be drawn up to evaluate for such injury. The greatest risk factor for perioperative stroke is a history of prior stroke.[7,8] Specific information needs to be given to the anesthesiologist in cases of substantial cerebrovascular disease. The baseline neurologic deficits must be clearly defined and intracranial vascular anatomy should be elucidated when known. Any preoperative imaging should be made available. Substantial intracranial arterial stenosis, in particular of the posterior circulation, may be especially perfusion dependent. This can occasionally be shown clinically by the presence of recurrent, sometimes stereotypic transient ischemic attacks. In these situations, blood pressure management intraoperatively for maintenance of adequate cerebral perfusion pressure is paramount.

Understanding the patient's baseline blood pressure range is key for maintaining cerebral perfusion under general anesthesia. There is evidence in the cardiac anesthesia literature that dropping the mean arterial pressure by at least 10 mm Hg from the preoperative baseline increases the risk for stroke by approximately four fold[9] despite a confluence of ischemic stroke risks for diminished perfusion and the risk for microembolic stroke following cardioplegic washout during the unclamping period. However, the concept of keeping the blood pressure as close as possible to baseline in this patient population is important and should be considered the safest practice.

Stroke prophylactic agents such as aspirin and warfarin should be maintained in the perioperative period, if at all possible. There is a growing body of evidence that this is safe in the majority of surgical procedures.[10–12] Coordination between the primary care physician , neurologist, and surgeon is necessary to maintain maximal prophylaxis during the high risk perioperative period.

Spine Disease

It is helpful to characterize spine disease as either chronic or acute. Chronic spine disease commonly refers to nerve root disorders or spinal cord compression typically caused by degenerative disk disease, spondylosis, scoliosis, and tumors. Acute disorders include disk herniation, epidural abscess, and traumatic injury. In patients with spine disease, knowledge of the type, location, and duration are critical in the preparation for surgery. Preoperative assessment should focus on neurologic deficits and possible ventilatory compromise from phrenic nerve involvement or control of the airway as a result of cervical disease and restricted neck flexion and extension (or immobilization by collars, halo vests, etc). Severe spine deformities necessitate pulmonary function testing to evaluate the extent of restrictive lung disease present. Scoliosis and ankylosing spondylitis are but two common examples of conditions which reduce functional residual capacity and vital capacity, and pulmonary function testing provides risk analysis information regarding the potential for extended ventilatory support postoperatively. This information is also helpful to properly manage such ventilator settings and to evaluate for fitness of extubation following surgery. Traction or cervical immobilization can limit neck movement requiring preparation for special techniques to secure the airway. A patient with cervical myelopathy similarly may need to have advance preparation to safely secure the airway because manipulation of the cervical spine may lead to further injury. If a patient has had an acute spinal cord injury and has any deficits as a result, it is important to elucidate a thorough history including what the injury was, when the injury occurred, and what specific neurologic deficits have resulted. Knowledge of the injury will allow the perioperative team to safely move and position the patient. Autonomic instability is common and can be difficult to manage intraoperatively. Proper preparation of medications is needed therefore this information must be communicated to the anesthesia team.

Chronic Pain Syndromes

Pain can be categorized as somatic (eg, back pain), visceral (eg, pancreatic tumor), or neuropathic (eg, nerve injury). Narcotics can be used to treat pain in any of these categories. The dose of narcotics is frequently escalated over time as the patient becomes more tolerant to their effects. More recently, adjuvant pain medications are playing an increasing role in the management of chronic pain. It is essential to get accurate assessment of outpatient narcotic use to deduce the development of narcotic tolerance, which is helpful in assessing perioperative requirements. To manage pain preoperatively, and to avoid any symptoms of withdrawal, patients should be told to continue their current dose of narcotic medications and be specifically instructed to take them the morning of surgery. Adjuvant analgesic medications should be specifically screened for side effects. Some anticonvulsant medications now are commonly used for neuropathic pain syndromes—gabapentin, carbamazepine, and so on. The latter frequently induces a syndrome of inappropriate antidiuretic hormone secretion, thus a preoperative electrolyte panel would be important. Preoperative planning may also include the use of neuroaxial techniques which can substantially reduce the need for additional narcotic medications perioperatively. Special attention should be given to patients with complex regional pain syndrome. Information about current therapy and an accurate description of the affected area should be provided so that proper intraoperative planning can be made.

Headache

Headache disorders are a heterogeneous group of diseases, broadly categorized as primary or secondary. Primary headache disorders include migraines, cluster, pseudotumor cerebri, hemicrania continuum, and exertional headaches. Secondary headaches are because of more ominous processes such as intracranial masses, giant cell arteritis, and hydrocephalus. Prophylactic medications should be continued, if possible, for primary headache disorders. An assessment of baseline intracranial pressure (ICP) should be provided for patients with pseudotumor cerebri, as cerebral perfusion pressure needs to be maintained at acceptable levels during general anesthesia. Similarly, a general assessment of ICP must be made for patients with intracranial mass lesions. All patients, including ambulatory patients with only a mild headache or even no symptoms at the time of their preoperative visit who have an intracranial mass, should be assessed by imaging studies to ensure good documentation of the size of the lesion and degree of mass effect and edema. Baseline deficits should be independently established, as patients often may not appreciate subtle but important findings such as cognitive disturbances, cranial nerve deficits, visual changes, or subtle weakness and sensory loss. Antiepileptic drugs should be continued when applicable, and a history of recent steroid use for secondary headache disorders should be communicated.

Seizure Disorders

Epilepsy is a broad term encompassing the various seizure disorders. They may be partial, focal, or generalized. Patients with epilepsy are known to have an increased risk for perioperative seizure secondary to the choice of anesthetic or physiologic derangement.[13,14] In evaluating the patient with epilepsy, it is important to obtain a complete history, including the type of seizure disorder and its characteristics so that the perioperative team can recognize if and when the patient has a seizure. Additionally, any underlying causes such as anatomic and/or structural or metabolic abnormalities must be elucidated and corrected if possible, especially if there are metabolic derangements that may increase the risk for perioperative seizure, such as uremia, hypoglycemia, and drug toxicity or withdrawal. Most seizure patients are treated with antiepileptic drugs (AED). The AED regimen should be reviewed and drug levels should be obtained before surgery. The medications should be continued during the perioperative period. Clinical signs of toxicity, such as ataxia, dizziness, and confusion should be investigated and corrected. Most AEDs at toxic or even therapeutic levels may cause liver dysfunction and possibly bone marrow suppression. Liver function tests, a complete blood count, and a metabolic panel should be performed before surgery.

Muscular Dystrophies

Patients with Duchenne and Becker muscular dystrophy suffer from a progressive loss of muscle mass. They are susceptible to multiple perioperative complications, including to the respiratory, cardiac, and musculoskeletal systems. The possible presence of cardiac or pulmonary dysfunction needs to be evaluated and communicated. Consideration should be made for pulmonary function testing and echocardiography even in the asymptomatic patient, as limited physical activity reduces the opportunity to otherwise discern the hemodynamic and ventilatory capabilities under surgical stress. The activity level may still provide some clue as to the presence of cardiopulmonary dysfunction. The presence of compensated heart failure should modify the anesthetic plan and preparation. When heart failure is uncompensated, surgery should be delayed. Acute rhabdomyolysis can result from the use of certain inhalational anesthetic agents, as Duchenne's muscular dystrophy is a risk for malignant hyperthermia. Because of the risk association between muscular dystrophy and malignant hyperkalemia after paralysis with succinylcholine, the use of this depolarizing neuromuscular relaxant has fallen out of favor in the field of pediatric anesthesia.

Multiple Sclerosis

Multiple Sclerosis (MS) may be divided into 4 subtypes: relapsing/remitting (80% of cases), primary progressive, secondary progressive, and progressive relapsing. Patients with MS typically have multiple, unassociated, demyelinating lesions of the brain and spinal cord that are separated by space and time. At outset, such lesions are often associated with symptoms that are either transient and reversible or leave mild neurologic deficits. As the disease advances over time, a secondary progressive stage ensues where more permanent deficits accumulate. With further advancement, usually over many years, the lesions and deficits tend to result in progressively worsening motor weakness and paresthesias. The time course of the disease is important to elucidate any medications used for spasticity such as dantrolene, or baclofen. If a patient is having an exacerbation of MS, surgery should be delayed if possible until the resolution of the acute symptoms. The stress of surgery and anesthesia alone may lead to an exacerbation, so patients should be counseled in this regard so as to make an informed decision to pursue elective surgery and for prophylaxis to prevent an exacerbation.[15] In advanced stages, patients may have the same problem list to the anesthesiologist and surgeon as a patient with a moderate to severe stroke: cognitive dysfunction, cranial nerve deficits, poor airway mechanics—all imposing an increased risk for perioperative complications.

Myasthenia Gravis and Lambert-Eaton Myasthenic Syndrome

Myasthenia gravis (MG) is a postsynaptic neuromuscular junction disorder involving what is believed to be autoimmune destruction of the acetylcholine receptor.[16] The disease course is typically intermittent with complete or partial remission. Muscle weakness worsens with continual use; therefore there is typically ocular muscle involvement and respiratory weakness, as well as weakness of the postural muscles of the neck and back. Bulbar involvement can lead to dysarthria, dysphagia, and aspiration. In preparing the myasthenic patient for surgery, it is important to assess the severity and recent history of disease, current treatments, and any other concomitant illnesses. Preoperative pulmonary function testing can be very helpful to the perioperative team to determine the ability for a patient to be extubated after surgery. Anticholinesterase drugs such as pyridostigmine (Mestinon) are often used to treat MG. It is important to discriminate recent worsening neurologic symptoms between an MG exacerbation (myasthenic crisis) from pyridostigmine (cholinesterase) toxicity. The former is often precipitated by a mild infection or stress (pregnancy is common in female MG patients). An edrophonium test or careful assessment of the patient's symptoms following an additional dose of cholinesterase inhibitor may be used to differentiate between the two entities. A thorough history of infectious symptoms, coupled with a simple laboratory evaluation (especially urine analysis) as well as a preoperative pregnancy test in females of child-bearing age, is warranted. If a patient is having worsening symptoms, elective surgery should be postponed until more aggressive treatment such as immunotherapy or plasmapherisis can be performed. However, a thymectomy may be indicated in a patient with continuing muscle weakness as a treatment.[17]

Guillain-Barré Syndrome/Chronic Inflammatory Demyelinating Polyradiculopathy

The demyelinating polyradiculopathies have a broad medical phenotype. Often, patients with Guillain-Barré Syndrome (GBS) make a full or near complete recovery; however, other syndromes can be neurologically devastating, especially over time. With chronic inflammatory demyelinating polyradiculopathy, there tends to be a relapsing, remitting course, with benefits achieved using immunotherapy and periodic intravenous immunoglobulin therapy. Again, it is important for the anesthesiologist to know the current immunotherapeutic regimen and the baseline neurologic examination. Stress dose steroids may need to be administered by the anesthesiologist when appropriate. These patients often have preexisting peripheral nerve damage, and may be predisposed to further compression during surgery.

In addition, conditions such as GBS may lead to significant dysautonomia. The presence of a dysautonomia should be made clear to the anesthesiologist so that preparations for hemodynamic fluctuation can be made. Blood pressure augmenting agents such as fludrocortisone and midodrine should be continued in the perioperative period, since hypotension tends to be more problematic and injurious intraoperatively.

SUMMARY

This article emphasizes some key points in the preoperative evaluation of patients with neurologic disease. Patients with neurologic disease are commonly encountered, and their illness is often complicated by significant comorbid disease. It is important to think of the patient as a whole rather than the sum of his or her systems. While it is tempting to consider the traditional preoperative evaluation from a "cardiac clearance" point of view, we must resist this urge, and evaluate which risk factors we can modify and hopefully mitigate to optimize the perioperative period.

REFERENCES

1. MacDonald BK, Cockerell OC, Sander JW, et al. The incidence and lifetime prevalence of neurological disorders in a prospective community-based study in the UK. Brain 2000;123:665–76.
2. Hirtz D, Thurman DJ, Gwinn-Hardy K, et al. How common are the "common" neurologic disorders? Neurology 2007;68:326–37.
3. Gao L, Taha R, Gauvin D, et al. Postoperative cognitive dysfunction after cardiac surgery. Chest 2005;128(5):3664–70.
4. Benedict RH. Cognitive function after open-heart surgery: are postoperative neuropsychological deficits caused by cardiopulmonary bypass? Neuropsychol Rev 1994;4(3):223–55.
5. Stotz M, Thummler D, Schurch M, et al. Fulminant neuroleptic malignant syndrome after perioperative withdrawal of anti-Parkinsonian medication. Br J Anaesth 2004;93:868–71.
6. Tsuchiya N, Morimura E, Hanafusa T, et al. Postoperative neuroleptic malignant syndrome that occurred repeatedly in a patient with cerebral palsy. Paediatr Anaesth 2007;17(3):281–4.
7. Limburg M, Wijdicks EFM, Li H. Ischemic stroke after surgical procedures: clinical features, neuroimaging, and risk factors. Neurology 1998;50:895–901.
8. Lekprasert V, Akavipat P, Sirinan C, et al. Perioperative stroke and coma in Thai Anesthesia Incidents Study (THAI Study). J Med Assoc Thai 2005;88:S113–7.
9. Gottesman RF, Sherman PM, Grega MA, et al. Watershed strokes after cardiac sugery. Stroke 2006;37:2306–11.
10. Maulaz AB, Bezerra DC, Michel P, et al. Effect of discontinuing aspirin therapy on the risk of brain ischemic stroke. Arch Neurol 2005;62:1217–20.
11. Genewein U, Haeberli A, Straub PW, et al. Rebound after cessation of oral anticoagulant therapy: the biochemical evidence. Br J Haematol 1996;92:479–85.
12. Larson BJ, Zumberg MS, Kitchens CS. A feasibility study of continuing dose-reduced warfarin for invasive procedures in patients with high thromboembolic risk. Chest 2005;127:922–7.
13. Iijima T, Nakamura Z, Iwao Y, et al. The epileptogenic properties of the volatile anesthetics sevoflurane and isoflurane in patients with epilepsy. Anesth Analg 2000;91:989–95.
14. Voss LJ, Sleigh JW, Barnard JP, et al. The howling cortex: seizures and general anesthetic drugs. Anesth Analg 2008;107(5):1689–703.
15. Dickerman RD, Schneider SJ, Stevens QE, et al. Prophylaxis to avert exacerbation/relapse of multiple sclerosis in affected patients undergoing surgery. Surgical observations and recommendations. J Neurosurg Sci 2004;48:135–7.
16. Abel M, Eisenkraft JB. Anesthetic implications of myasthenia gravis. Mt Sinai J Med 2002;69:31–7.
17. Vincent A, Newsom-Davis J, Newton P, et al. Acetylcholine receptor antibody and clinical response to thymectomy in myasthenia gravis. Neurology 1983;33:1276–82.

Emergency and Urgent Surgery

Kevin M. Schuster, MD[a],*, Kimberly A. Davis, MD, FACS[a],
Stanley H. Rosenbaum, MD[b]

KEYWORDS

- Surgery • Emergencies • Diagnosis • Treatment
- Preoperative • Management

In patients who require emergency surgical intervention, the management of significant medical comorbidities requires rapid coordination between the surgeon, the anesthesiologist, and the primary medical team. In urgent nonelective surgeries, the medical consultant has a more significant role. Coordination of care in this population is equally important, as urgency of care for the surgical disease needs to be balanced with necessary preoperative diagnostic testing and medical optimization. Every major surgical discipline performs procedures on an emergency or urgent basis that are either life- or limb-saving. This review concentrates on life-threatening surgical emergencies managed by general surgeons and the noncardiac subspecialties of general surgery.

PROVIDERS OF EMERGENCY SURGICAL CARE

Any discussion of urgent and emergency surgery would not be complete without a review of the current crisis in emergency care, as highlighted by the Institute of Medicine's committee on the future of emergency care in the US health system entitled "Hospital Based Emergency Care at the Breaking Point."[1] Central among the issues discussed included overcrowding and boarding of nonfunded and underfunded patients in the nation's shrinking number of emergency departments, as well as the problem of minimal surge capacity. Also considered was the issue of unavailability of surgical specialists to cover emergency calls, due to issues of uncompensated care and perceived higher malpractice risk for off-hours emergency care. Emergency rooms across California have reported difficulty maintaining subspecialist coverage, with plastic surgery, otolaryngology, dentistry, psychiatry, and neurosurgery the most problematic.[2] This situation is not limited to the state of California but is

[a] Department of Surgery, Section of Trauma, Surgical Critical Care, and Surgical Emergencies, Yale University, School of Medicine, 330 Cedar Street, BB 310, New Haven, CT 06520, USA
[b] Department of Anesthesiology, Yale University School of Medicine, Yale-New Haven Hospital, 789 Howard Avenue, PO Box 208051, New Haven, CT 06520-8051, USA
* Corresponding author.
E-mail address: kevin.schuster@yale.edu (K.M. Schuster).

Med Clin N Am 93 (2009) 1131–1148
doi:10.1016/j.mcna.2009.05.011
0025-7125/09/$ – see front matter © 2009 Elsevier Inc. All rights reserved.

medical.theclinics.com

universal, and has generated an ever-increasing volume of transferred patients requiring emergency surgical care.[3] Increased transfer requirements may delay necessary surgery and result in patients presenting for surgery with compromised physiology, thereby complicating preoperative assessment and management.

The trauma surgical community, long-standing providers of emergency care to critically ill and injured patients, has begun a critical evaluation of emergency surgery, reevaluating their scope of practice in an effort to address the problems of limited access to care. Changes in the field of trauma, with increased attention to nonoperative management of a variety of injuries, have resulted in a decreased number of operative trauma cases.[4] This situation, combined with the expanding concern regarding lifestyle issues among residents, has resulted in decreased resident interest in trauma as a career due to a paucity of operative cases available for a fully trained general surgeon.[5] To offset some of these factors the major trauma organizations, including the American Association for the Surgery of Trauma and the American College of Surgeons Committee on Trauma, are developing the new discipline of Acute Care Surgery. Although the final practice and training paradigms have yet to be fully delineated, this specialty will be designed to provide care for a broad variety of patients, focusing not only on trauma but also on emergency general surgery and surgical critical care.[6] Currently, a fellowship is offered after completion of a general surgical residency; training includes special emphasis on vascular, thoracic, endoscopic, and hepatobiliary procedures performed on an emergency basis. The ultimate scope of practice may depend more on its acceptance by subspecialties and their willingness to train these physicians. In combination with Residency Review Committee (RRC)-approved surgical critical care fellowships, the acute care surgery fellowships will ensure that these surgeons are well prepared to provide perioperative medical management in conjunction with the anesthesiologist. This potential solution to the crisis of access to emergency surgery is attractive on many levels, as it will serve to recruit trainees into the field while providing care for those patients who might otherwise go without.

PREPARATION OF THE PATIENT FOR EMERGENCY SURGERY

Patients who require emergency or urgent operations present with severe metabolic derangements that require rapid intervention. These derangements commonly range from mild perfusion deficits to severe shock. Such shock may be hypovolemic as in the case of a trauma patient, septic as in the case of intestinal ischemia or hollow viscus perforation, or multifactorial such as in a patient with intestinal ischemia who develops myocardial ischemia and dysfunction. The recommendations made by the authors of the Surviving Sepsis Campaign guideline include early goal-directed resuscitation (EGDR).[7] Many patients with emergency general surgical conditions present with septic physiology and should be resuscitated in a goal-oriented fashion. The timing of emergency operative intervention then becomes an important issue. EGDR can be successfully continued intraoperatively by anesthesia staff.[8] However, the completeness of preoperative resuscitation may be an important determinant in the outcome and the appropriate timing of an immediately necessary operation is often difficult to establish.

Many patients presenting with intra-abdominal catastrophes have sepsis and septic shock. In addition to aggressive resuscitation with fluids and correction of vasomotor tone with pressors, these patients require source control as soon as their physiologic stability allows intervention. The most minimal procedure that achieves source control is generally appropriate.[7] Source control may be achievable at the beside in the intensive care unit (ICU), for example endoscopic biliary decompression in ascending cholangitis, or ultrasound-guided abdominal abscess or empyema drainage. In addition to source control, early institution of broad-spectrum antibiotics should if possible follow acquisition of cultures but should not be delayed solely for the purpose of obtaining culture material. Delay in initiation of effective antimicrobial therapy has a time-dependent effect on mortality for patients presenting with hypotension due to an infection.[9]

Although patients with intra-abdominal emergencies often present with fever, some with severe sepsis may be hypothermic. In the setting of elective colorectal surgery, hypothermia has been associated with an increased incidence of wound infection and longer hospital stay.[10] Hypothermia also leads to increased mortality in patients who are admitted to the intensive care unit postoperatively.[11] Hypothermia is consistently associated with acidosis and coagulopathy as part of the lethal triad often discussed in the context of trauma and damage control surgery.[12] Patients undergoing general anesthesia are at high risk for developing core hypothermia due to peripheral vasodilation and a loss of ability to maintain a gradient between their core temperature and the ambient environment.[13] Because of the negative effects of hypothermia on coagulation and wound infection, it should be aggressively corrected preoperatively, as it will only be exacerbated by general anesthesia. Correcting hypothermia is difficult in these patients as the most common methods such as gastric or bladder irrigation or forced air warming are either limited or impossible intraoperatively. Preoperative warming using fluid warmers and ongoing intraoperative warming therefore become key to regaining and maintaining normothermia. Having the patient's body surface warmed for the induction of general anesthesia is critical to compensate for the loss of vasomotor tone that occurs with the induction of general anesthetics.[14] To this end, patients should be covered with warm blankets and forced warm air methods used.[15] Intravenous fluids and to an even greater extent blood and blood products should be warmed for the prevention of further heat loss.[16] Blood and blood products should not be withheld for the prevention of hypothermia; however, limiting their use as much as is feasible may also improve outcome in the emergency surgical patient requiring intensive care.[17,18] Like resuscitation, the advantages of preoperative normothermia must be balanced with the risk of delaying a necessary operation.

The stress of critical illness often induces hyperglycemia.[19] The level of hyperglycemia that is detrimental and the degree of control that is important remains controversial.[20] In 2001, Van den Berghe and colleagues published the first of two studies documenting a mortality benefit to tight glycemic control (blood glucose 80–110 mg/dL).[21,22] The benefit was observed in cohorts of cardiac and noncardiac surgical patients. Postoperative morbidity was also reduced, including decreases in ventilator days, renal dysfunction, bloodstream infection, transfusion requirements, and polyneuropathy.[21] Intraoperative hyperglycemia has also been shown to have independent detrimental effects in cardiac surgical patients.[23] Defining an appropriate management strategy has recently been complicated by several prospective randomized studies of tight glycemic control demonstrating unacceptably high rates of hypoglycemia.[24] Although there are few data on preoperative control of hyperglycemia in the emergency surgical patient, based on the currently available literature in other similar settings it would seem prudent to maintain blood glucose less than 150 mg/dL in accordance with the surviving sepsis campaign guidelines.[7]

Obtaining an adequate medical history is always advantageous in the care of these patients. However, this is often difficult when the patients are compromised by their acute disease. They may also be elderly, poor historians, or residents of extended care facilities. Knowledge of a patient's baseline mental status is important as it allows the clinician to determine deviations from baseline in the postoperative period as an early indicator of potential complications. Knowledge of the patient's preoperative functional status is helpful in predicting ultimate recovery from the disease process, as well as the time frame for recovery. The effects of medication should be considered as these may block physiologic responses; for example, b-blockers mask tachycardia and are taken commonly in patients with hypertension or known coronary artery disease.[25] Warfarin, aspirin, and clopidogrel are also common medications among the elderly that negatively impact surgical bleeding and postoperative renal function.

Before proceeding with emergency surgical intervention, it is important to determine whether the patient has advanced directives. Patients presenting with surgical emergencies or urgencies are often elderly with multiple comorbidities or a terminal condition. These patients may have a preference for pain relief over extension of life.[26] The decision to pursue surgical therapy in a terminally ill patient will often involve the patient and family, the surgeon, the physician treating the terminal disease, and the emergency physician. This decision involves the autonomy of two individuals, the patient or their representative and the surgeon. Communication between the surgeon and the patient's physician is essential to establish a clear understanding of the risk of perioperative morbidity and mortality as well as the impact of the acute condition on the patient's chronic or terminal disease. An open discussion between the patient and surgeon, with family and other physicians involved, is then important to establish the patient's wishes. The surgeon's autonomy is also important as adherence to the ethical principles of nonmaleficence and beneficence may guide the surgeon to elect not to perform an operation that he or she feels would not improve the patient's condition or alter the patient's outcome. Rarely, a conflict may arise between physicians or between physicians and family, a situation best avoided by open communication among all the individuals involved.

Once operative intervention has been agreed on, the status of any do-not-resuscitate (DNR) orders must be addressed. As recently as 1994 few institutions had policies governing DNR orders in the perioperative setting.[27] The American College of Surgeons (ACS) and the American Society of Anesthesiologists (ASA) have developed statements regarding DNR orders.[28,29] Fundamental to these two sets of guidelines is the principle that DNR orders should neither be suspended implicitly nor followed explicitly. Patients exposed to anesthesia are at increased risk from transient insults that are reversible by resuscitation.[30] Following DNR orders explicitly may result in potentially preventable death. However, the suspension of DNR orders denies patients autonomy of care and exposes them to procedures they would not otherwise accept. The ASA guidelines suggest that either goal-directed or procedure-directed care be applied.[29] Goal-directed care allows flexibility for the providers as the patient will define their goals of care and the clinicians will provide procedures consistent with those goals. This strategy places more autonomy with the providers. An alternative is procedure-directed care whereby the patient is provided with a checklist of procedures that he or she will allow in the perioperative period. Similarly, the ACS guidelines recommend customizing the advanced directive to remain consistent with the patient's goals during the perioperative period.[30] This should be clearly documented in the medical record and communicated to the entire operative team. In the setting of a patient who is noncommunicative and documentation is unclear, some US statutes have required continuing life-sustaining treatments.[31]

SPECIFIC LIFE-THREATENING SURGICAL EMERGENCIES
Trauma

Addressing the broad range of surgical problems encountered in a trauma patient is beyond the scope of this review. Most of the perioperative physiology after trauma can be summarized as hypoperfusion secondary to hemorrhagic shock, requiring resuscitation of the intravascular and extravascular spaces, with attention to the prevention of hypothermia, acidosis, and coagulopathy. However, elderly trauma patients represent a unique and increasing subset of the trauma population, and it is in this group of patients that medical comorbidities will be most prevalent. The segment of the population over the age of 65 years will more than double by 2030 and represents the most rapidly growing part of the population.[32] Although trauma is the leading cause of death in the first 4 decades of life, it remains among the top 10 causes of death in all age groups.[33] Risk of death from moderate injury increases progressively beyond the age of 40 years, whereas minor trauma has an increased mortality in persons older than 65 years.[34] Rates of injury-related death are actually highest in those older than 70 years. In individuals 65 years and older, falls are the most common cause of injury-related death, followed by motor vehicle crashes. Deaths are but the extreme example of the problem. For every death from a fall there are more than 30 falls that result in nonfatal significant injury.[35] These patients will commonly require operative intervention to manage the orthopedic or other injuries they have sustained. Rapid preoperative assessment, risk stratification, and optimization will be required for these often complex patients in cases for which operative intervention can be delayed. Orthopedists currently will often consult their medical or surgical intensivist colleagues for assistance with the timing of necessary operative intervention and optimization of the patient's condition preoperatively. In the 1980s the concept of "early total care" was introduced. This concept implied that immediate (<24 hours) surgical repair of all orthopedic injuries improved patient outcome.[36,37] Subsequent studies have cast doubt on these findings for patients with multiple traumatic injuries.[38,39] Orthopedists have more recently adopted damage control techniques in unstable or borderline patients as outlined later. Orthopedic damage control, with initial minimal operation such as external fixation, has been successfully used to delay definitive open reduction and internal fixation, with good clinical results.[40,41]

Damage Control Surgery

The idea that all goals of surgical care should be met with one definitive and complete operation was challenged by trauma surgeons in the 1980s and early 1990s. The concept that patient survival could be improved by controlling major hemorrhage and contamination, followed by ICU-based resuscitation and a later return to the operating room to complete repairs, was not completely new. Pringle, Halstead, and Schroeder each reported on the control of liver hemorrhage by packing, followed by later reexploration.[42–44] This became the standard of care throughout World War II, at which time surgical techniques were believed to have advanced to the point whereby it was felt all injuries could be repaired at the time of initial surgery. A resurgence of liver packing and later reexploration occurred as several groups reported on improved survival with this technique.[45–47] The techniques of damage control were expanded to include nonhepatic trauma in an effort to prevent the lethal triad of hypothermia, coagulopathy, and acidosis.[48,49] In addition to packing for hemorrhage control, in damage control gastrointestinal injuries are rapidly controlled without restoring intestinal continuity, major vascular injuries are shunted, biliary and urinary injuries are drained, and the abdomen is closed in a temporary fashion. It was in 1993 that Rotondo and colleagues borrowed the term Damage Control from the US Navy, a term describing a naval vessel's ability to absorb damage and maintain mission integrity.[50,51] Rotondo and colleagues demonstrated improved survival in severe penetrating trauma by applying a staged approach and delaying definitive repairs.[50] The approach of carrying out minimal rapid procedures to control major hemorrhage has been expanded to include thoracic injuries, extremity vascular injuries, and, as described above, orthopedic injuries.[52] Support for the application of damage control techniques to nontraumatic abdominal disease has been variable.[53] Patients suffering from sepsis due to an intra-abdominal source will often display the characteristics of hypothermia, coagulopathy, and acidosis, which may make them amenable to damage control techniques. For patients in whom closure would result in elevated intra-abdominal pressure, there is a role for maintaining an open abdomen.[54] Simply leaving the abdomen open, however, should not be confused with true temporizing or damage control techniques. In patients suffering from an intra-abdominal sepsis, who will tolerate definitive operative management and abdominal closure, maintaining an open abdomen for planned reexploration offers no benefit and may be harmful.[55–57]

Abdominal Compartment Syndrome

Patients after hemorrhagic shock or with sources of sepsis are often resuscitated with large volumes of intravenous fluid to specific therapeutic end points.[7,58] The institution of goal-directed therapy with aggressive volume resuscitation often results in intra-abdominal hypertension (IAH) and, occasionally, abdominal compartment syndrome (ACS) secondary to the development of systemic inflammatory response syndrome and visceral edema. A spectrum of disease, IAH is simply increased intra-abdominal pressure without physiologic manifestations, whereas ACS describes the hemodynamic, pulmonary, and renal complications associated with pressures greater than 25 mmHg. Intra-abdominal hypertension and ACS was identified in 50% and 8% of a mixed cohort of intensive care patients, respectively.[59] Although surgical patients are at slightly higher risk, any patient requiring fluid resuscitation can develop ACS.[60] Current standard therapy for ACS is surgical decompression, although other nonsurgical therapies may also be applied.[61,62] Surgical decompression usually results in prompt improvement in hemodynamic instability and organ dysfunction.[63] Abdominal compartment syndrome therefore is an acute surgical emergency requiring prompt intervention. Abdominal decompression, although potentially lifesaving, creates the difficult problem of the open abdomen. The ability to attain primary closure of the abdomen has been reported to range from 20% to 80% of patients following decompression after trauma.[64,65] The timing of closure is also important as one group reported a 12% complication rate if the abdomen was closed within 8 days versus a 52% complication rate after 8 days.[65] The most common complications included wound infection, abscess, and fistula. Patients whose abdomen cannot be closed primarily usually have skin grafts placed over the abdominal viscera until they can undergo abdominal wall reconstruction at 6 to 12 months. This time delay is necessary for conversion from dense inflammatory adhesions between intra-abdominal viscera and the overlying skin graft to more easily dissected chronic adhesions.

Incarcerated Hernia

An abdominal hernia generally involves a failure of containment of abdominal structures within the abdominal cavity. These usually involve the anterior abdominal wall but may involve the diaphragm, the posterior abdominal wall and retroperitoneum, or the pelvic floor. Patients with acute incarceration typically present with an acutely occurring painful abdominal wall mass or a mass at the site of a previously known reducible hernia, with or without bowel obstruction. Internal hernias may also occur when there is a defect in an intra-abdominal structure through which another intra-abdominal structure may pass. Symptomatic incarcerated hernias are a surgical emergency, as delays in intervention result in strangulation and associated bowel ischemia. Diagnosis is generally based on physical examination findings for external hernias, although abdominal radiographs or CT scanning may identify bowel obstruction. Signs of strangulation include tenderness or erythema at the hernia site, fever, tachycardia, and leukocytosis. Kulah and colleagues quoted morbidity and mortality rates for urgent surgical repair of incarcerated hernias as 20% and 3%, respectively.[66] These rates are significantly higher than for elective repair.[67] Factors related to complications included advanced age, preexisting disease, and delayed presentation.[66] In another review of incarcerated external hernias in patients older than 65 years who required urgent repair, 82% were inguinal, 7% were ventral/incisional, and 10% were umbilical. One third of patients experienced perioperative complications and associated mortality was 5%, which increased to 20% when bowel resection was required due to bowel ischemia.[68] Risk factors for bowel resection for inguinal hernias include older age, female gender, and femoral hernias.[69] Because these patients often present with bowel obstruction or strangulation, their physiologic status is more a reflection of the effects of the incarceration. These patients should be treated based on the status of their intestinal complication, and optimized in concert with timely operative intervention.

Although the standard surgical dogma dictates the elective repair of all inguinal hernias, this has recently been challenged. Two prospective randomized studies have demonstrated that a policy of watchful waiting in patients with asymptomatic or minimally symptomatic inguinal hernias results in outcomes equivalent to operative repair.[70,71] If adoption of this approach becomes widespread, this may lead to the presentation of more acutely incarcerated hernias, although this remains unclear. Based on the known risk factors for obstruction and strangulation in groin hernias (older age, femoral location, and short duration of hernia), it seems prudent to offer these patients elective repair.[72]

Methods of repair will vary based on surgeon preference. Laparoscopic and open approaches are currently acceptable for elective hernia repair, and laparoscopic repair has been reported for incarcerated hernias.[73,74] Laparoscopic repair, however, requires general anesthesia with pneumoperitoneum, a consideration in the management of patients with significant comorbidities. A laparoscopic approach should only be taken by a surgeon proficient in elective laparoscopic hernia repair.[75] Mesh repair in uncontaminated surgical fields has been shown to result in a decreased recurrence rate, although prosthetics cannot be safely used in patients with bowel ischemia or injury.[76,77]

Bowel Obstruction

Bowel obstruction describes a wide variety of disease processes, some of which require urgent surgical management and others which may at least initially be managed nonoperatively. In 1994 more than 300,000 patients underwent adhesiolysis, most of which were for bowel obstruction.[78] Considering that as many as 80% of cases of bowel obstruction are managed nonoperatively, this represents a small fraction of the patients admitted with bowel obstruction. Bowel obstruction is generally classified based on whether it involves the small or large bowel, whether it is a mechanical or functional obstruction, and, in the case of mechanical obstruction, if it is partial or complete. Classification of the obstruction based on these 3 criteria helps formulate important management decisions.

Small bowel obstruction usually presents with abdominal pain, often colicky, nausea, vomiting, and lack of flatus. If ischemia is present the pain may have the classic quality of being out of proportion to tenderness on physical examination. Small bowel obstruction is most commonly caused by adhesions (up to 75% of cases), but may also be caused by hernia, malignancy, inflammatory bowel disease, ischemia, intussusception, infections, radiation, graft-versus-host disease (GVHD), intramural hemorrhage, stones (gallstones, enteroliths), Meckel's diverticulum, and other generalized inflammatory disorders such as lupus.[79] Important historical questions include prior abdominal surgery, inflammatory bowel disease, cancer, radiation, pelvic inflammatory disease, endometriosis, or other intestinal disease. Examination is important to assess the degree of abdominal distension, tympany, tenderness, bowel sounds, and location and quality of scars, as patients are often poor historians in terms of prior surgery. The presence of hernia should be carefully excluded. The degree of distension may give a clue as to the location of the obstruction, as distension increases with more distal obstructions. Hernia and distension are often difficult to assess in obese patients. Rectal or stomal digital examination is mandatory in patients who have not had recent surgery in these areas to identify stool or malignancies as the causative factors.

The diagnostic algorithm should focus on the classification of the obstruction as well as on determining the likelihood of ischemia. A complete blood count (CBC) to assess for leukocytosis and lactic acid assists in the identification of ischemia, although these are neither sensitive nor specific for mesenteric ischemia.[79] Azotemia and electrolyte abnormalities are common and in the case of ileus may contribute to the pathophysiology. The blood counts should be obtained to help assess the degree of volume depletion present in these patients and to assist in fluid resuscitation and electrolyte repletion. Women of child-bearing age should have at least a qualitative β-human chorionic gonadotropin (β-hCG) measurement. Radiographic evaluation begins with supine and upright views of the abdomen. These films should be evaluated for bowel dilatation, colonic and rectal air, and air fluid levels. Often the transition point, that is, the location of obstruction, can be determined based on these radiographs alone, although the sensitivity of plain films is low (40%–80%).[80,81] CT scanning has become a standard imaging modality for bowel obstruction as it has a sensitivity of 94% to 100% and specificity of 90% to 95%.[82] Current CT technology with multiplanar reformats provides greater diagnostic confidence in terms of location and cause of obstruction.[79] CT may determine whether the obstruction is complete or partial, and the presence of a closed loop obstruction or intestinal ischemia. Signs of ischemia on CT scan include thickened bowel wall, pneumatosis intestinalis, absence of wall or vascular enhancement, portal venous gas, ascites, and inflammatory changes in the fat. The results of CT imaging often change the management of bowel obstruction,[83] and should therefore be used in cases where diagnosis is in question, or obstruction fails to resolve rapidly with nonoperative management. Small bowel follow-up studies have been reported to result in more frequent and rapid resolution of bowel obstruction, but this was not confirmed in a recent meta-analysis.[84]

Initial management of the patient should focus on fluid resuscitation and the concept that the patient is being prepared for surgery. Medical management should focus on the patient's underlying comorbidities. Fluid resuscitation should be guided based on hemodynamic response and urine output. Monitoring of urine output is critical, and if there is any question of adequate urine output a Foley catheter should be placed. For patients with emesis, a nasogastric tube for decompression can provide symptomatic relief. Antiemetics can be administered judiciously, but for patients at risk for aspiration, nasogastric decompression is more prudent. Prophylaxis for deep venous thrombosis should be administered as these patients will often be bed-bound or destined for surgery. There are no data available regarding antibiotic administration except for immediate preoperative prophylaxis or in the setting of a known infectious cause.

Standard therapy for mechanical small bowel obstruction is prompt surgery. This is especially true for patients with clinical signs of bowel ischemia including fever, leukocytosis, peritonitis, acidosis, patients with radiographic signs of a closed loop obstruction or bowel ischemia, or patients with a complete obstruction. Patients with a partial obstruction, those in the immediate postoperative period, and those with obstruction from primary bowel inflammation such as inflammatory bowel disease or GVHD can generally be managed nonoperatively, as small bowel obstruction has been reported to resolve in up to 81% of cases without operation.[85,86] Bowel obstruction that fails to resolve with nonoperative management after 48 hours will generally not resolve with more prolonged periods of observation.[85] Although no study has demonstrated worsened mortality with delay in operation for patients without intestinal ischemia, it may be more likely to result in morbidity and the need for bowel resection.[87] Although laparoscopic or open approaches are feasible, laparoscopy has been reported to be a successful operative modality in 60% of patients requiring operative intervention,[88] with a conversion rate to an open procedure of 20% to 65%.[89,90]

Large bowel obstruction is most commonly due to neoplasm. Other causes include inflammation/infection, volvulus, stricture, intussusception, and fecal impaction. Colonic obstruction typically presents with abdominal pain, abdominal distension, and obstipation.[91] Complications such as ischemia and perforation are, as in small bowel obstruction, heralded by fever, leukocytosis, tachycardia, and peritonitis on physical examination. Diagnosis by plain radiographs has a sensitivity of 84% and specificity of 72%, whereas CT scanning provides valuable diagnostic information in terms of cause and location.[92,93] Initial management is centered on resuscitation and correction of electrolyte abnormalities. Unlike with small bowel obstruction, emesis is uncommon and the need for nasogastric decompression is also less common. Definitive management is usually surgical, although for malignant obstructions colonic stents may be useful in cases of poor surgical risk or widely metastatic disease. Volvulus may be reduced endoscopically, which is usually successful in cases of sigmoid volvulus but less so in cecal volvulus.[94] Surgical resection is mandatory in cases of recurrence and should be considered after successful reduction due to high recurrence rates. Patients with obstruction due to acute diverticulitis or other acute infectious causes should be treated with antibiotics, percutaneous drainage of abscesses, and careful monitoring of colonic diameter and serial abdominal examinations for signs of peritonitis.

Acute colonic pseudo-obstruction, Ogilvie syndrome, is a pancolonic dilatation without mechanical obstruction. The pathogenesis of this disorder is believed to involve autonomic dysregulation and occurs most commonly in association with another acute illness. Management generally involves fluid resuscitation and bowel rest with rectal decompression and nasogastric decompression. Narcotic and anticholinergic medications should be minimized. Although absolute cecal diameter is often implicated as determining the risk of perforation, the major risk factor is duration of overdistension in patients with a cecal diameter greater than 10 cm.[95] Therefore, in addition to the interventions mentioned earlier, therapy with an acetylcholinesterase inhibitor or colonoscopic decompression should be undertaken if there is no clinical improvement within 24 hours. In a randomized controlled crossover trial design, neostigmine resulted in a 94% success rate in improving abdominal distension and a low rate of recurrence, with 11% developing recurrent colonic distension.[96] Success rates for colonoscopic decompression vary from 61% to 95%.[97] Surgery is indicated for failure of less invasive modalities and generally includes resection with or without reanastomosis if contamination is present at operation. Open and percutaneous cecostomy have been described but significant complications of these procedures have also been noted.[91]

Gastrointestinal Bleeding

Bleeding from the gastrointestinal tract is generally separated into upper and lower sources with the point of separation being the ligament of Treitz. Upper gastrointestinal bleeding (UGIB) is most commonly caused by peptic ulcers, gastritis, and esophageal or gastric varicies.[98] Elements of the history that become important are any history of UGIB, recent hematemesis, hematochezia, melena, or "coffee-ground" emesis, use of nonsteroidal anti-inflammatory drugs (NSAIDs) or aspirin, chronic abdominal pain, use of oral anticoagulants or antiplatelet medications, smoking, alcoholism, liver disease, or any history of aortic or other abdominal vascular surgery. Patients with severe bleeding may present with melena (75%), hematemesis (50%), or hematochezia (14%).[99–101] They require rapid assessment of volume status and correction of hemorrhage with crystalloids, blood and blood products, and appropriate surgical or nonsurgical intervention. A rectal examination is mandatory to assess the character of any rectal blood. Abdominal examination is important to identify an intra-abdominal catastrophe. Nasogastric aspirates by tube insertion will help to confirm the diagnosis of UGIB although a negative aspirate does not rule out an UGI source. Definitive diagnosis requires upper endoscopy within 24 hours.[102] Successful control of hemorrhage is common, but depends on endoscopic findings.[103,104] Patients without evidence of UGIB should be evaluated for a lower GI source, again by lower endoscopy. Bleeding scans and visceral arteriography should be reserved for patients with an unclear source of hemorrhage. Surgery is indicated in either scenario for ongoing hemodynamic instability not responsive to resuscitation, and for all patients requiring more than 6 units of red cell transfusion, in the face of normal coagulation parameters.

Resuscitation should be aggressively administered in all patients with hemodynamic compromise. Transfusion goals are lower than a normal hemoglobin and hematocrit, even in patients with underlying coronary artery disease.[17] Any coagulopathy should be corrected, as should thrombocytopenia if the platelet count is less than 100,000/mm^3. If UGIB is suspected, proton pump inhibitors are generally administered with an intravenous bolus followed by an infusion, although this has not been shown to reduce mortality.[105] If the patient has a history or stigmata of liver disease, an octreotide infusion should also be considered.

Gastrointestinal Perforation

Perforation may be due to obstruction, ischemia, direct injury from a foreign body or endoscope, direct injury from an object penetrating the abdominal wall, malignancy, or a local infectious or inflammatory process, and most result in secondary peritonitis. The peritonitis may be chemical in nature or infectious as the intraluminal acidity and bacterial burden vary along the length of the intestine.[106] With the possible exception of patients with a penetrating injury or an obvious endoscopic perforation, presentation is usually with acute-onset abdominal pain. Although it is important to include the time course and the nature of the abdominal pain as well as associated and antecedent symptoms in the history, attention should be specifically directed to identify the use of steroids or NSAIDs, and prior surgeries. Physical examination should identify hernias, scars, tenderness, masses, and signs of peritonitis. Basic preoperative laboratory evaluation may assist in the diagnosis. Serum lactate may be helpful in the diagnosis of visceral ischemia, and a liver profile and serum lipase may be helpful in excluding biliary tract and pancreatic causes of pain. Patients with frank peritonitis on examination should be referred for urgent surgical exploration without further imaging. Patients without obvious peritonitis on physical examination will require further radiologic evaluation. Plain radiographs have low sensitivity.[107] The finding of pneumoperitoneum on these easily obtained radiographs, however, may obviate further workup and rapid surgical intervention. The accuracy of helical CT of the abdomen with water-soluble enteric contrast as reported in the literature is generally greater than 90% for most disease processes and can be rapidly performed in most institutions.[108–110] Management of these patients requires aggressive resuscitation with crystalloids and blood component therapy as necessary, broad-spectrum intravenous antibiotics, and emergency operation for source control. A short delay may be necessary to optimize hemodynamics before operative intervention, to minimize worsening of hypotension at the induction of anesthesia.

Mesenteric Ischemia

Acute mesenteric ischemia is difficult to diagnose, as these patients often present with generalized abdominal pain and other nonspecific symptoms, and has an associated mortality rate of 59% to 93%.[79,111] Acute ischemia may be embolic with occlusion of a portion of the superior mesenteric artery, thrombotic, or nonocclusive and the result of generalized poor perfusion. Patients with embolic disease typically present with more acute onset of pain with little antecedent history and often have an underlying cardiac dysrhythmia or structural abnormality. Thrombosis is a much more ominous diagnosis, with a mortality rate of 90%.[112] Venous thrombosis is much less common but presents in a similar fashion, has a significant mortality rate, and is often associated with a hypercoaguable state.[113] Nonocclusive mesenteric ischemia may occur in patients with atherosclerotic lesions of the mesenteric vessels in states of relative hypoperfusion such as in cardiogenic or distributive shock. The differential diagnosis is extremely broad and includes almost any process that causes abdominal pain. The diagnostic test of choice has become multidetector row CT angiography, which when bowel wall and angiographic findings were combined, resulted in a 96% sensitivity and 94% specificity.[114] Laboratory values are nonspecific.

The ischemia results in a significant fluid deficit due to capillary leak and is exacerbated by a generalized systemic inflammatory response. Because the goal of therapy is rapid restoration of perfusion, aggressive fluid administration, particularly in the case of nonocclusive mesenteric ischemia, is usually required. Because bacterial translocation secondary to mucosal slough is likely, broad-spectrum antibiotics covering bowel flora are prudent, although there is little literature to support this approach. Emergency surgical therapy is almost always indicated for confirmation of the diagnosis, resection of nonviable bowel, and restoration of arterial flow through the mesenteric circulation. For thrombotic disease, endovascular therapy has been reported for the treatment of acute mesenteric ischemia without peritoneal signs and involves the use of catheter-directed thrombolytics. Schoots and colleagues reviewed the literature on this treatment modality and identified 48 patients treated with this technique, of whom 43 survived with successful resolution of the occlusion with only 13 requiring laparotomy.[115] Mesenteric venous thrombosis in the absence of bowel ischemia may be managed by anticoagulation alone, with a concurrent workup to identify the cause of the patient's hypercoagulability.

Necrotizing Soft Tissue Infections

Skin and soft tissue infections are among the most common encountered in the emergency room. Differentiating between a life-threatening necrotizing soft tissue infection (NSTI) and a more superficial severe cellulitis can often be a considerable diagnostic challenge, especially in the early stages of disease. The findings often considered pathognomonic, crepitus and blistering, are commonly absent.[116] Soft tissue gas is also uncommon on plain radiographs and CT scans.[116] Most commonly these patients do present with systemic illness including signs of systemic inflammatory response syndrome or septic shock. The pain is often out of proportion to the degree of erythema and induration often extends beyond the borders of the erythema.[117] The erythema is often rapidly spreading despite seemingly appropriate intravenous antibiotics. Routine laboratory evaluation should also include blood cultures. Tissue cultures at the time of operation should be obtained if the patient is systemically ill. C-reactive protein levels may also be helpful in distinguishing necrotizing infections from more benign cellulitis. In addition to the C-reactive protein, white blood cell count, hemoglobin, sodium, creatinine, and glucose levels can be combined in the Laboratory Risk Indicator for Necrotizing Fasciitis Score (LRINEC), a scoring system that may have the ability to distinguish necrotizing from nonnecrotizing soft tissue infections.[118] Although gas may be absent on CT scan or MRI, these tests may be helpful for identifying the depth of inflammation, the extent of tissue edema, and involvement of the fascia or muscle. The ultimate diagnosis, however, is generally based on clinical examination or findings at the time of surgical debridement.

Initial management of these patients should follow the guidelines as described for any other septic process. Broad-spectrum antibiotics that cover the typical organisms of Group A streptococcus, *Clostridium perfringens*, *Staphylococcus aureus*, and *Vibrio vulnificus* should be rapidly administered. Recommended antibiotics include combined therapy with ampicillin-sulbactam, clinidamycin, and ciprofloxacin.[119] As these guidelines were written before the abundance of recent literature demonstrating the high prevalence of community-acquired methicillin-resistant *S. aureus* (CA-MRSA), all patients with a necrotizing infection should have initial antibiotic therapy that also covers CA-MRSA. Although broad-spectrum antibiotic therapy is necessary, early wide surgical debridement of infected and necrotic tissue is the cornerstone of therapy. If the diagnosis is not clear, surgical incision with direct inspection of the tissue for viability may be necessary. These patients will most commonly require multiple repeat operative debridements as the full extent of tissue necrosis may not be appreciable at the initial operation.

SUMMARY

Several common themes run through this article. Most importantly, patients presenting with general surgical emergencies are hypovolemic, and require early aggressive resuscitative efforts. Although these efforts may safely be accomplished preoperatively in a select subset of patients, it is often the combined efforts of surgeons, anesthesiologists, and internists that optimize these critically ill patients in the intraoperative and postoperative period. Early surgical consultation and intervention can be lifesaving. The aggressiveness of the surgical intervention is patient- and disease-specific, and requires frequent and open communication between all health care providers, the patient, and his or her family.

REFERENCES

1. Institute of Medicine, Committee on the Future of Emergency Care in the U.S. Health System. Hospital Based Emergency Care at the Breaking Point. Washington, DC: National Academy Press; 2006.
2. Rudkin SE, Oman J, Langdorf MI, et al. The state of ED on-call coverage in California. Am J Emerg Med 2004;22:575–81.
3. Menchine MD, Baraff LJ. On-call specialists and higher level of care transfers in California emergency departments. Acad Emerg Med 2008;15:329–36.
4. Jurkovich GJ. Acute care surgery: the trauma surgeon's perspective. Surgery 2007;141:293–6.
5. Richardson JD, Miller FB. Will future surgeons be interested in trauma care? Results of a resident survey. J Trauma 1992;32:229–33.
6. Britt LD. Acute care surgery: a proposed training curriculum. Surgery 2007;141: 304–6.
7. Dellinger RP, Levy MM, Carlet JM, et al. Surviving sepsis campaign: international guidelines for management of severe sepsis and septic shock: 2008. Crit Care Med 2008;36:296–327.
8. Gan TJ, Soppitt A, Maroof M, et al. Goal-directed intraoperative fluid administration reduces length of hospital stay after major surgery. Anesthesiology 2002;97: 820–6.
9. Kumar A, Roberts D, Wood K, et al. Duration of hypotension before initiation of effective antimicrobial therapy is the critical determinant of survival in human septic shock. Crit Care Med 2006;34:1589–96.
10. Kurz A, Sessler DI, Lenhardt R. Perioperative normothermia to reduce the incidence of surgical-wound infection and shorten hospitalization. N Engl J Med 1996;334:1209–15.
11. Slotman GJ, Jed EH, Burchard KW. Adverse effects of hypothermia in postoperative patients. Am J Surg 1985;149:495–501.
12. Lee JC, Peitzman AB. Damage-control laparotomy. Curr Opin Crit Care 2006;12: 346–50.
13. Plattner O, Xiong J, Sessler D, et al. Rapid core-to-peripheral tissue heat transfer during cutaneous cooling. Anesth Analg 1996;82:925–30.
14. Vanni SM, Braz JR, Modolo NS, et al. Preoperative combined with intraoperative skin-surface warming avoids hypothermia caused by general anesthesia and surgery. J Clin Anesth 2003;15(2):119–25.
15. Putzu M, Casati A, Berti M, et al. Clinical complications, monitoring and management of perioperative mild hypothermia: anesthesiological features. Acta Biomed 2007;78:163–9.
16. Smith CE, Gerdes E, Sweda S, et al. Warming intravenous fluids reduces perioperative hypothermia in women undergoing ambulatory gynecological surgery. Anesth Analg 1998;87:37–41.
17. Hebert PC, Wells G, Blajchman MA, et al. A multicenter randomized, controlled clinical trial of transfusion requirements in critical care. N Engl J Med 1999;340:409–17.
18. Sarani B, Dunkman J, Dean L. Transfusion of fresh frozen plasma in critically ill surgical patients is associated with an increased risk of infection. Crit Care Med 2008;36:1114–8.
19. McCowen KC, Malhotra A, Bistrain BR. Stress-induced hyperglycemia. Crit Care Clin 2001;17:107–24.
20. Marik PE, Varon J. Intensive insulin therapy in the ICU: is it now time to jump off the bandwagon. Resuscitation 2007;74:191–3.

21. van den Berghe G, Wouters P, Weekers F, et al. Intensive insulin therapy in critically ill patients. N Engl J Med 2001;345:1359–67.

22. Van den Bergh G, Wilmer A, Hermans G, et al. Intensive insulin therapy in medical intensive care patients. N Engl J Med 2006;354:449–61.

23. Gandhi GY, Nuttall GA, Abel MD, et al. Intraoperative hyperglycemia and perioperative outcomes in cardiac surgery patients. Mayo Clin Proc 2005;80:862–6.

24. Vanhorebeek I, Langouche L, Van den Berghe G. Tight blood glucose control with insulin in the ICU facts and controversies. Chest 2007;132:268–78.

25. Fishkind D, Paris BE, Aronow WS. Use of digoxin, diuretics, beta blockers, angiotensin-converting enzyme inhibitors, and calcium channel blockers in older patients in an academic hospital-based geriatrics practice. J Am Geriatr Soc 1997;45:809–12.

26. Somogyi-Zalud E, Zhong Z, Hamel MB, et al. The use of life-sustaining treatments in hospitalized persons aged 80 and older. J Am Geriatr Soc 2002;50:930–4.

27. Margolis JO, McGrath BJ, Kussin PS, et al. Perioperative do not resuscitate (DNR) orders: a survey of major institutions. Anesthesiology 1994;81:A1311.

28. Committee on Ethics, American College of Surgeons. Statement on advance directives by patients: "Do Not Resuscitate" in the operating room. Bull Am Coll Surg 1994;79:29.

29. American Society of Anesthesiologists. Ethical guidelines for the anesthesia care of patients with do-not-resuscitate orders or other directives that limit care; 1999 Directory of Members. Park Ridge (IL): American Society of Anesthesiologists; 1999. p. 470–1.

30. Cohen CB, Cohen PJ. Do-not-resuscitate orders in the operating room. N Engl J Med 1991;325:1879–82.

31. Ewanchuk M, Brindley PG. Ethics review: perioperative do-not-resuscitate orders – doing 'nothing' when 'something' can be done. Crit Care 2006;10(4):219.

32. Available at: http://www.census.gov/ipc/www/usinterimproj/. Accessed July 1, 2008.

33. CDC Injury Research Agenda. Atlanta (GA): Department of Health and Human Services, Centers for Disease Control and Prevention; 2002.

34. Morris JA Jr, MacKenzie EJ, Damiano AM, et al. Mortality in trauma patients: the interaction between host factors and severity. J Trauma 1990;30:1476–82.

35. Binder S. Injuries among older adults: the challenge of optimizing safety and minimizing unintended consequences. Inj Prev 2002;8(Suppl 4):IV2–4.

36. Johnson KD, Cadambi A, Seibert GB. Incidence of adult respiratory distress syndrome in patients with multiple musculoskeletal injuries: effect of early operative stabilization of fractures. J Trauma 1985;25:375–84.

37. Bone LB, Johnson KD, Weigelt J, et al. Early versus delayed stabilization of fractures. A prospective randomized study. J Bone Joint Surg Am 1989;71:336–40.

38. Reynolds MA, Richardson JD, Spain DA. Is timing of fracture fixation important for the patient with multiple trauma? Ann Surg 1995;222:470–81.

39. Pape HC, Auf'm'Kolk M, Paffrath T. Primary intramedullary fixation in polytrauma patients with associated lung contusion – a cause of posttraumatic ARDS? J Trauma 1993;34:540–8.

40. Scalea TM, Boswell SA, Scott JE, et al. External fixation as a bridge to intramedullary nailing for patients with multiple injuries and with femur fractures: damage control orthopedics. J Trauma 2000;48:613–23.

41. Nowotarski PJ, Turen CH, Brumback RJ, et al. Conversion of external fixation to intramedullary nailing for fractures of the shaft of the femur in multiply injured patients. J bone Joint Surg Am 2000;82:781–8.

42. Pringle JH. Notes on the arrest of hepatic hemorrhage due to trauma. Ann Surg 1908;48:541–9.
43. Halsted WS. The employment of fine silk in preference to catgut and the advantages of transfixing tissues and vessels in controlling hemorrhage. Also an account of the introduction of gloves, gutta-percha tissue and silver foil. JAMA 1913;60:1119.
44. Schroeder WE. The process of liver hemostasis: reports of cases. Surg Gynecol Obstet 1906;2:52.
45. Calne R, Macmaster P, Pentlow B. The treatment of major liver trauma by primary packing with transfer of the patient for definitive treatment. British Journal of Surgery 1978;66:338–9.
46. Feliciano DV, Mattox KL, Jordan GL Jr. Intra-abdominal packing for control of hepatic hemorrhage: a reappraisal. J Trauma 1981;21:285–90.
47. Svoboda JA, Peter ET, Dang CV, et al. Severe liver trauma in the face of coagulopathy: a case for temporary packing and early reexploration. Am J Surg 1982; 144:717–21.
48. Stone HH, Strom PR, Mullins RJ. Management of the major coagulopathy with onset during laparotomy. Ann Surg 1983;197:532–5.
49. Talbert S, Trooskin SZ, Scalea T, et al. Packing and re-exploration for patients with non-hepatic injuries. J Trauma 1992;33:121–5.
50. Rotondo MF, Schwab CW, McGonigal MD, et al. Damage control: an approach for improved survival in exsanguinating penetrating abdominal injury. J Trauma 1993;35:375–83.
51. Department of Defense. Surface ship survivability. Washington, DC: Naval War Publication; 1996. p. 3–20.31.
52. Loveland JA, Boffard KD. Damage control in the abdomen and beyond. Br J Surg 2004;91:1095–101.
53. Jansen JO, Loudon MA. Damage control surgery in a non-trauma setting. Br J Surg 2007;94:789–90.
54. Moore AFK, Hargrest R, Martin M, et al. Intra-abdominal hypertension and the abdominal compartment syndrome. Br J Surg 2004;91:1102–10.
55. Hau T, Ohmann C, Wolmershauser A, et al. Planned relaparotomy vs relaparotomy on demand in the treatment of intra-abdominal infections. Arch Surg 1995; 130:1193–7.
56. Christou NV, Barie PS, Dellinger EP, et al. Surgical Infection Society intra-abdominal infections study. Prospective evaluation of management techniques and outcome. Arch Surg 1993;128:193–8.
57. van Ruler O, Mahler CW, Boer KR, et al. Comparison of on-demand vs planned relaparotomy strategy in patients with sever peritonitis: a randomized trial. JAMA 2007;298:865–72.
58. Rivers E, Nguyen B, Havstad S, et al. Early goal-directed therapy in the treatment of severe sepsis and septic shock. N Engl J Med 2001;345: 1368–77.
59. Malbrain ML, Chiumello D, Wilmer A, et al. Prevalence of intra-abdominal hypertension in critically ill patients: a multicenter epidemiological study. Intensive Care Med 2004;30:822–9.
60. Malbrain ML, Chiumello D, Pelosi P, et al. Incidence and prognosis of intraabdominal hypertension in a mixed population of critically ill patients: a multiple-center epidemiological study. Crit Care Med 2005;33:315–22.
61. Maerz L, Kaplan LJ. Abdominal compartment syndrome. Crit Care Med 2008; 36:S212–5.

62. De Waele JJ, Hoste EA, Malbrain ML. Decompressive laparotomy for abdominal compartment syndrome – a critical analysis. Crit Care 2006;10(2):R51.

63. An G, West MA. Abdominal compartment syndrome: a concise clinical review. Crit Care Med 2008;36:1304–10.

64. Fabian TC. Damage control in trauma: laparotomy wound management acute to chronic. Surg Clin North Am 2007;87:73–93.

65. Miller RS, Morris JA Jr, Diaz JJ, et al. Complications after 344 damage-control open celiotomies. J Trauma 2005;59:1365–74.

66. Kulah B, Kulacoglu IH, Oruc T, et al. Presentation and outcome of incarcerated external hernias in adults. Am J Surg 2001;181:101–4.

67. Primatesta P, Goldacre MJ. Inguinal hernia repair: incidence of elective and emergency surgery readmission and mortality. Int J Epidemiol 1996;25:835–9.

68. Kulah B, Duzgun AP, Moran M, et al. Emergency hernia repairs in elderly patients. Am J Surg 2001;182:455–9.

69. Kurt N, Oncel M, Ozkan Z, et al. Risk and outcome of bowel resection in patients with incarcerated groin hernias: retrospective study. World J Surg 2003;27:741–3.

70. O'Dwyer PJ, Norrie J, Alani A, et al. Observation or operation for patients with asymptomatic inguinal hernia. Ann Surg 2006;244:167–73.

71. Fitzgibbons RJ, Giobbie-Hurder A, Gibbs J, et al. Watchful waiting vs repair of inguinal hernia in minimally symptomatic men a randomized clinical trial. JAMA 2006;295:285–92.

72. Rai S, Chandra SS, Smile SR. A study of the risk of strangulation and obstruction in groin hernias. Aust N Z J Surg 1998;68:650–4.

73. Shah RH, Sharma A, Khullar R, et al. Laparoscopic repair of incarcerated ventral abdominal wall hernias. Hernia 2008;12:457–63.

74. Ferzli G, Shapiro K, Chaudry G, et al. Laparoscopic extraperitoneal approach to acutely incarcerated inguinal hernia. Surg Endosc 2004;18:228–31.

75. Claridge JA, Croce MA. Abdominal wall. In: Britt LD, Trunkey DD, Feliciano DV, editors. Acute care surgery principles and practice. New York: Springer; 2007. p. 435–49.

76. Luijendijk RW, Hop WC, van der Tol MP, et al. A comparison of suture repair with mesh repair for incisional hernia. N Engl J Med 2000;343:392–8.

77. Gray SH, Vick CC, Graham LA, et al. Variation in mesh placement for ventral hernia repair: an opportunity for process improvement? Am J Surg 2008;196:201–6.

78. Ray NF, Denton WG, Thamer M, et al. Abdominal adhesiolysis: inpatient care and expenditures in the United States in 1994. J Am Coll Surg 1998;186:1–9.

79. Herbert GS, Steele SR. Acute and chronic mesenteric ischemia. Surg Clin North Am 2007;87:1115–34.

80. Frager D, Medwid SW, Baer JW, et al. CT of small-bowel obstruction: value in establishing the diagnosis and determining the degree and cause. AJR Am J Roentgenol 1994;162:37–41.

81. Caoili EM, Paulson EK. CT of small-bowel obstruction: another perspective using multiplanar reformations. AJR Am J Roentgenol 2000;183:899–906.

82. Sinha R, Verma R. Multidetector row computed tomography in bowel obstruction. Part 1. Small bowel obstruction. Clin Radiol 2005;60:1058–67.

83. Taourel PG, Fabre JM, Pradel JA, et al. Value of CT in the diagnosis and management of patients with suspected acute small-bowel obstruction. AJR Am J Roentgenol 1995;165:1187–92.

84. Abbas SM, Bisset IP, Parry BR. Meta-analysis of oral water-soluble contrast agent in the management of adhesive small bowel obstruction. Br J Surg 2007;94:404–11.

85. Brolin RE, Kransa MJ, Mast BA. Use of tubes and radiographs in the management of small bowel obstruction. Ann Surg 1987;206:126–33.
86. Cox MR, Gunn IF, Eastman MC, et al. The safety and duration of non-operative treatment for adhesive small bowel obstruction. Aust N Z J Surg 1993;63: 367–71.
87. Margenthaler JA, Longo WE, Virgo KS, et al. Risk factors for adverse outcomes following surgery for small bowel obstruction. Ann Surg 2006;243:456–64.
88. Fischer CP, Doherty D. Laparoscopic approach to small bowel obstruction. Semin Laparosc Surg 2002;9:40–5.
89. Borzellino G, Tasselli S, Zerman G, et al. Laparoscopic approach to postoperative adhesive obstruction. Surg Endosc 2004;18:686–90.
90. Léon EL, Metzger A, Tsiotos GG, et al. Laparoscopic management of small bowel obstruction: indications and outcome. J Gastrointest Surg 1998;2: 132–40.
91. Lopez-Kostner F, Hool GR, Lavery IC. Management and causes of acute large-bowel obstruction. Surg Clin North Am 1997;77:1265–90.
92. Chapman AH, McNamara M, Porter G. The acute contrast enema in suspected large bowel obstruction: value and technique. Clin Radiol 1992;46:273–8.
93. Sinha R, Verma R. Multidetector row computed tomography in bowel obstruction. Part 2. Large bowel obstruction. Clin Radiol 2005;60:1068–75.
94. Mangiante EC, Croce MA, Fabian TC, et al. Sigmoid volvulus: a four-decade experience. Am Surg 1989;55:41–4.
95. Johnson CD, Rice RP, Kelvin FM, et al. The radiological evaluation of gross cecal distension: emphasis on cecal ileus. AJR Am J Roentgenol 1985;145:1211–7.
96. Ponec RJ, Saunders MD, Kimmey MB. Neostigmine for the treatment of acute colonic pseudo-obstruction. N Engl J Med 1999;341:137–41.
97. Saunders MD. Acute colonic pseudo-obstruction. Best Pract Res Clin Gastroenterol 2007;21:671–87.
98. Silverstein FE, Gilbert DA, Tedesco FJ, et al. The national ASGE survey on upper gastrointestinal bleeding: 1. Study design and baseline data. Gastrointest Endosc 1981;27:73–9.
99. Peter DJ, Doughtery JM. Evaluation of the patient with gastrointestinal bleeding: an evidence based approach. Emerg Med Clin North Am 1999;17:239–61.
100. Wilcox CM, Alexander LN, Cotsonis G. A prospective characterization of upper gastro-intestinal hemorrhage presenting with hematochezia. Am J Gastroenterol 1997;92:231–5.
101. Borgman MA, Spinella PC, Perkins JG, et al. The ratio of blood products transfused affects mortality in patients receiving massive transfusions at a combat support hospital. J Trauma 2007;63:805–13.
102. Lin HJ, Wang K, Perng CL, et al. Early or delayed endoscopy for patients with peptic ulcer bleeding. A prospective randomized study. J Clin Gastroenterol 1996;22:267–71.
103. Adler DG, Leighton JA, Davila RE. ASGE guideline: the role of endoscopy in acute non-variceal upper-GI hemorrhage. Gastrointest Endosc 2004;60:497–504.
104. Rollhauser C, Fleischer DE. Nonvariceal upper gastrointestinal bleeding. Endoscopy 2002;34:111–8.
105. Leontiadis GI, Sharma VK, Howden CW. Systemic review and meta-analysis: proton-pump inhibitor treatment for ulcer bleeding reduces transfusion requirements and hospital stay-results from the Cochran Collaboration. Aliment Pharmacol Ther 2005;22:169–74.
106. Guarner F. Enteric flora in health and disease. Digestion 2006;73:5–12.

107. MacKersie AB, Lane MJ, Gerhardt RT, et al. Nontraumatic acute abdominal pain: unenhanced helical CT compared with three-view acute abdominal series. Radiology 2005;239:114–22.

108. Urban BA, Fishman EK. Tailored helical CT evaluation of acute abdomen. Radiographics 2000;20:725–49.

109. Ahn SH, Mayo-Smith WW, Murphy BL, et al. Acute nontraumatic abdominal pain in adult patients: abdominal radiography compared with CT evaluation. Radiology 2002;225:159–64.

110. Yoshito T, Yamada S, Aoki J, et al. Effect of contrast-enhanced computed tomography on diagnosis and management of acute abdomen in adults. Clin Radiol 2002;57:507–13.

111. Brandt LJ, Boley SJ. AGA technical review on intestinal ischemia. American Gastrointestinal Association. Gastroenterology 2000;118:954–68.

112. Schoots IG, Koffeman GI, Legemate DA, et al. Systematic review of survival after acute mesenteric ischaemia according to disease aetiology. Br J Surg 2004;91:17–27.

113. Rhee RY, Gloviczki P, Mendonca CT, et al. Mesenteric venous thrombosis: still a lethal disease in the 1990s. J Vasc Surg 1994;20:688–97.

114. Kirkpatrick ID, Kroeker MA, Greenberg HM. Biphasic CT with mesenteric CT angiography in the evaluation of acute mesenteric ischemia: initial experience. Radiology 2003;229:91–8.

115. Schoots IG, Levi MM, Reekers JA, et al. Thrombolytic therapy for acute superior mesenteric artery occlusion. J Vasc Interv Radiol 2005;16:317–29.

116. Elliott DC, Kufera JA, Myers RA. Necrotizing soft tissue infections. Risk factors for mortality and strategies for management. Ann Surg 1996;224:672–83.

117. Abrahamian FM, Talan DA, Moran GJ. Management of skin and soft-tissue infections in the emergency department. Infect Dis Clin North Am 2008;22:89–116.

118. Wong CH, Khin LW, Heng KS, et al. The LRINEC (Laboratory Risk Indicator for Necrotizing Fasciitis) score: a tool for distinguishing necrotizing fasciitis from other soft tissue infections. Crit Care Med 2004;32:1535–41.

119. Stevens DL, Bisno AL, Chambers HF, et al. Practice guidelines for the diagnosis and management of skin and soft-tissue infections. Clin Infect Dis 2005;41:1373–406.

Index

Note: Page numbers of article titles are in **boldface** type.

Med Clin N Am 93 (2009) 1149–1160
doi:10.1016/S0025-7125(09)00096-0
0025-7125/09/$ – see front matter © 2009 Elsevier Inc. All rights reserved.

Moving?

Make sure your subscription moves with you!

To notify us of your new address, find your **Clinics Account Number** (located on your mailing label above your name), and contact customer service at:

Email: journalscustomerservice-usa@elsevier.com

800-654-2452 (subscribers in the U.S. & Canada)
314-447-8871 (subscribers outside of the U.S. & Canada)

Fax number: 314-447-8029

Elsevier Health Sciences Division
Subscription Customer Service
3251 Riverport Lane
Maryland Heights, MO 63043

*To ensure uninterrupted delivery of your subscription,
please notify us at least 4 weeks in advance of move.